AF801186

Advances in Pediatric Extremity Fracture Management

Federico Canavese

Advances in Pediatric Extremity Fracture Management

A Curated Literature Overview

Springer

Federico Canavese
Department of Orthopaedics
IRCCS Istituto Giannina Gaslini
Genoa, Italy

ISBN 978-3-032-33305-6 ISBN 978-3-032-33306-3 (eBook)
https://doi.org/10.1007/978-3-032-33306-3

© The Editor(s) (if applicable) and The Author(s), under exclusive license to Springer Nature Switzerland AG 2026

This work is subject to copyright. All rights are solely and exclusively licensed by the Publisher, whether the whole or part of the material is concerned, specifically the rights of translation, reprinting, reuse of illustrations, recitation, broadcasting, reproduction on microfilms or in any other physical way, and transmission or information storage and retrieval, electronic adaptation, computer software, or by similar or dissimilar methodology now known or hereafter developed.
The use of general descriptive names, registered names, trademarks, service marks, etc. in this publication does not imply, even in the absence of a specific statement, that such names are exempt from the relevant protective laws and regulations and therefore free for general use.
The publisher, the authors and the editors are safe to assume that the advice and information in this book are believed to be true and accurate at the date of publication. Neither the publisher nor the authors or the editors give a warranty, expressed or implied, with respect to the material contained herein or for any errors or omissions that may have been made. The publisher remains neutral with regard to jurisdictional claims in published maps and institutional affiliations.

This Springer imprint is published by the registered company Springer Nature Switzerland AG
The registered company address is: Gewerbestrasse 11, 6330 Cham, Switzerland

If disposing of this product, please recycle the paper.

Auto-summaries can be generated by either an abstractive or extractive auto-summarization:

- An extraction-based summarizer identifies the most important sentences of a text and uses the original sentences to create the summary.
- An abstraction-based summarizer creates new text based on deep learning. New phrases are created to summarize the content.

The auto-summaries you will find in this book have been generated via an abstractive summarization approach.

Each chapter was carefully edited by Dr. Federico Canavese. The author selected the papers which were then auto-summarized. The author have edited the auto-summaries to support the understanding of the original content. You will find the author's reviews and guidance on the auto-summaries in their chapter introductions.

In curated literature overview books, authors are defined as those who curate the content for the book by selecting the papers to be auto-summarized and by organizing the output into a meaningful order. Next to the thoughtful curation of the papers, the author should guide the readers through the auto-summaries and make transparent why they selected the papers.

The ultimate goal is to provide a current literature review of Springer Nature publications on a given topic in order to support readers in overcoming information overload and to help them dive into a topic faster; to identify interdisciplinary overlaps; and to present papers which might not have been on the readers' radar.

Please note, that the selected papers are not used to train a LLM while the auto-summaries are created.

Preface

The management of paediatric extremity fractures is a rapidly evolving area of orthopaedic practice. As any clinician will know, these fractures are both common and complex in children. This is due to their relationship with a developing skeleton and the high levels of activity typical of childhood. Advances in imaging, biomaterials, surgical techniques and care pathways over the past two decades have transformed how specialists diagnose, analyse, and treat these injuries. The objective of this book, *Advances in Pediatric Extremity Fracture Management: A Curated Literature Overview*, is to bring clarity, synthesis, and clinical insight to this rapidly expanding body of knowledge. As Editor, I had a very specific vision for this volume: to create a comprehensive yet concise resource that aligns the best available evidence with daily clinical practice. Instead of creating a traditional textbook, we summarised, interpreted, and organised literature from Springer Nature to highlight progress, controversies, and emerging trends in the management of extremity fractures in skeletally immature patients.

In recent years, clinicians have been faced with a significant increase in the volume of scientific publications. This wealth of information is invaluable, but it also poses a challenge: how to go through it effectively, identify what truly matters, and translate this into clinical and surgical practice.

To help readers navigate the material efficiently, this book is organised into thematic sections that follow anatomical and conceptual logic. Each chapter begins with a summary of information retrieved from the literature, followed by articles containing this information and an extensive bibliography on the subject. The aim was not merely to report findings, but also to interpret and present them clearly.

Paediatric extremity fracture management will continue to evolve. I hope that *Advances in Pediatric Extremity Fracture Management: A Curated Literature Overview* will serve as a trusted resource on this journey, a companion that summarises what we know today and inspires ongoing curiosity, collaboration, and improvement.

I hope this text will resonate with paediatric and adult orthopaedic surgeons, as well as residents, fellows, and all other professionals dedicated to improving musculoskeletal care for children.

Enjoy the read!

Genova, Italy　　　　Federico Canavese

Contents

Guide to the Bibliographic Sections

The bibliography section of each chapter includes a list of the articles summarized in that chapter, along with additional articles cited within the bibliographies of those summarized works. These specifically represent the sources from which data or content has been drawn while preparing the research highlights. Accordingly, not all references from the original article's bibliography are included—only those that have been directly referred to or used.

About the Author

Federico Canavese is Full Professor of Orthopaedics and Traumatology at the University of Genoa and Head of the Pediatric Orthopedic Department at the IRCCS Istituto Giannina Gaslini in Genoa, Italy.

Born in Turin, Italy, he completed his orthopaedic residency in Montpellier, France, under Professor Alain Diméglio. He then undertook a 3-year paediatric orthopaedic fellowship at the Shriners Hospital for Children in Portland, USA, and the Hospital for Sick Children in Toronto, Canada. Following this, he joined the University Hospital of Geneva in Switzerland, where he worked with Professor André Kaelin.

Professor Canavese earned a Ph.D. in Animal Pathology from the Universities of Bologna and Udine, Italy, focusing on thoracic and pulmonary growth and the effects of spinal arthrodesis on neural structures. He later served as Head of the Pediatric Orthopedic Department and Full Professor of Pediatric Orthopedic Surgery at the Universities of Clermont-Ferrand and Lille in France. He also completed a 1-year clinical professorship at Guangzhou Women and Children's Hospital in China.

His clinical interests include paediatric spinal disorders, cerebral palsy, and paediatric traumatology. Fluent in Italian, French, English, and conversational Spanish, he regularly participates in humanitarian missions caring for children in developing countries.

Professor Canavese is the author of more than 270 peer-reviewed publications, over 80 book chapters, and 8 books, and serves on several editorial boards in orthopaedic surgery journals.

Clavice Fracture

1

Introduction by the Author

Clavicle fractures are a common injury in children of all ages. They occur at a rate of 29–100 per 100,000 children and adolescents per year, and they affect males more often. Overall, 69% of clavicle fractures occur in the middle shaft.

The standard method of diagnosis is to take anteroposterior radiographs of the clavicle to identify the location and displacement of the fracture. Recent evidence has shown that ultrasound can diagnose clavicle fractures without exposing children to ionizing radiation. However, although ultrasonography is a valuable diagnostic tool, it may not always be definitive. Additionally, deep learning models have been developed to date infant fractures. This has the potential to impact the diagnosis and management of suspected abuse cases.

Currently, conservative treatment is the gold standard for treating displaced and non-displaced clavicle fractures in children.

However, there is an ongoing debate about whether surgical treatment is necessary for adolescents with displaced and shortened clavicle fractures. Several papers have investigated the role of surgical fixation in older patients, especially adolescents with midshaft clavicle fractures of more than 2 cm, who generally have high functional demands.

The risk of clavicle deformity and shortening is a concern with nonoperative treatment, especially in adolescents, who have limited bone remodeling capacity. Although conservative treatment is the standard for treating clavicle fractures in children and adolescents, elastic stable intramedullary nailing and plate fixation also provide satisfactory clinical outcomes for older patients with displaced midshaft fractures. However, evidence about their superiority to conservative management of such injuries is lacking. Original research and

© The Author(s), under exclusive license to Springer Nature Switzerland AG 2026

F. Canavese, *Advances in Pediatric Extremity Fracture Management*,
https://doi.org/10.1007/978-3-032-33306-3_1

review papers, including meta-analyses, have failed to identify any advantages in terms of healing rates, complications, or functional outcomes when comparing conservative treatment with different forms of surgical treatment, such as open reduction and surgical fixation with plates and screws or elastic stable intramedullary nailing. In particular, patients treated conservatively have a higher risk of nonunion and malunion, while patients treated surgically have a higher risk of refracture. Despite these differences, however, functional outcomes are comparable.

1.1 Machine Generated Summaries

Disclaimer: The summaries in this chapter were generated from Springer Nature publications using abstractive AI auto-summarization: An abstraction-based summarizer creates new text based on deep learning. New phrases are created to summarize the content. As the constituted sentences are machine selected, they may not fully reflect the body of the work, so we strongly advise that the original content is read and cited. The auto-generated summaries were curated by the author(s) to meet Springer Nature publication standards.

Deep Learning of Birth-Related Infant Clavicle Fractures: A Potential Virtual Consultant for Fracture Dating [72]

This is a machine-generated summary of:

Tsai, Andy; Grant, P. Ellen; Warfield, Simon K.; Ou, Yangming; Kleinman, Paul K. Deep learning of birth-related infant clavicle fractures: a potential virtual consultant for fracture dating [72]
Published in: Pediatric Radiology (2022)
Link to original: https://doi.org/10.1007/s00247-022-05380-0
Copyright of the summarized publication:
The Author(s), under exclusive licence to Springer-Verlag GmbH Germany, part of Springer Nature 2022
All rights reserved.

If you want to cite the papers, please refer to the original.

For technical reasons we could not place the page where the original quote is coming from.

Research Highlights

Dating fractures in cases of suspected infant abuse is crucial for establishing a timeline of traumatic events. Traditional methods rely on radiographic features and expert radiologist interpretation, which can be imprecise. Now, a new study by Andy Tsai and colleagues explores the use of deep learning to objectively date infant clavicle fractures, addressing limitations of previous methodologies.

The study utilized a deep learning model adapted from face-age estimation techniques to date birth-related clavicle fractures. Researchers conducted a retrospective analysis using dedicated clavicle radiographs from a large children's hospital, focusing on images with optimized bony detail. The team employed an ordinal regression convolutional neural network to estimate fracture age, treating it as an ordinal variable. The model was trained and tested using a K-fold cross-validation procedure, achieving a mean absolute error (MAE) of 4.3 days and demonstrating high accuracy in estimating fracture ages within days of the ground truth.

This research represents a significant advance in the objective dating of infant fractures, with potential implications for diagnosing and managing suspected abuse cases. Future study could involve testing the model against pediatric radiologists and expanding its application to other tubular bones like ribs. Additionally, enhancing the model's generalizability through multicenter collaborations and automating image preprocessing could further improve its clinical utility. The study highlights the promise of deep learning as a tool for aiding radiologists in accurately dating fractures, potentially serving as a "virtual consultant" in clinical settings.

A Systematic Review and Meta-Analysis on the Diagnostic Utility of Ultrasound for Clavicle Fractures [73]

This is a machine-generated summary of:

Hassankhani, Amir; Amoukhteh, Melika; Jannatdoust, Payam; Valizadeh, Parya; Gholamrezanezhad, Ali A systematic review and meta-analysis on the diagnostic utility of ultrasound for clavicle fractures [73]

Published in: Skeletal Radiology (2023)
Link to original: https://doi.org/10.1007/s00256-023-04396-3

Copyright of the summarized publication:
The Author(s), under exclusive licence to International Skeletal Society (ISS) 2023
Copyright comment: Springer Nature or its licensor (e.g. a society or other partner) holds exclusive rights to this article under a publishing agreement with the author(s) or other rightsholder(s); author self-archiving of the accepted manuscript version of this article is solely governed by the terms of such publishing agreement and applicable law.
All rights reserved.

If you want to cite the papers, please refer to the original.

For technical reasons we could not place the page where the original quote is coming from.

Research Highlights

Ultrasound imaging has become increasingly important in medical diagnostics due to its accessibility and lack of ionizing radiation, making it a preferred choice in various specialties, including orthopedics. Traditionally, X-rays have been the primary imaging modality for diagnosing fractures, but ultrasound offers unique advantages by providing detailed images of both bone and soft tissue structures. Despite its potential, the role of ultrasound in diagnosing clavicle fractures remains underexplored. Now, a new study by Amir Hassankhani and colleagues systematically reviews and analyzes the diagnostic utility of ultrasound for clavicle fractures, assessing its sensitivity, specificity, and other accuracy measures.

The study conducted a comprehensive literature search across multiple databases to identify relevant studies on the diagnostic accuracy of ultrasound for clavicle fractures. Using the Preferred Reporting Items for Systematic Review and Meta-analyses (PRISMA) guidelines, the authors included studies that reported at least one diagnostic accuracy measure such as sensitivity or specificity. The analysis involved calculating true positive, true negative, false positive, and false negative values to generate sensitivity and specificity data. A bivariate random effects model was used to obtain summary effect estimates and assess heterogeneity among studies. The Quality Assessment of Diagnostic Accuracy Studies (QUADAS-2) tool was employed to evaluate the methodological quality of included studies.

The meta-analysis revealed that ultrasonography demonstrates high sensitivity in detecting clavicle fractures, particularly in pediatric patients due to their anatomical characteristics. However, specificity varied significantly among studies, with lower values observed in pediatric populations. This variability suggests that while ultrasonography is a valuable diagnostic tool, it may not always be definitive. Future study could focus on larger sample sizes and diverse populations to confirm these findings and explore ultrasonography's utility in different clinical settings. Additionally, addressing observer bias through blinded assessments could enhance the reliability of ultrasound as a diagnostic modality for clavicle fractures.

Nonoperative Versus Surgical Treatment of Displaced Midshaft Clavicle Fractures in Adolescents: A Systematic Review and Meta-Analysis of Comparative Studies [74]

This is a machine-generated summary of:

Galán-Olleros, María; Stitzman-Wengrowicz, Melisa L.; Martínez-Álvarez, Sergio; Molina-Corbacho, Matilde; Manzarbeitia-Arroba, Paloma; Pulido García, María del Carmen; Lopiz, Yaiza Nonoperative versus surgical treatment of displaced midshaft clavicle fractures in adolescents: a systematic review and meta-analysis of comparative studies [74]
Published in: International Orthopaedics (2025)

Link to original: https://doi.org/10.1007/s00264-025-06589-y
Copyright of the summarized publication:
The Author(s) under exclusive licence to SICOT aisbl 2025
Copyright comment: Springer Nature or its licensor (e.g. a society or other partner) holds exclusive rights to this article under a publishing agreement with the author(s) or other rightsholder(s); author self-archiving of the accepted manuscript version of this article is solely governed by the terms of such publishing agreement and applicable law.
All rights reserved.

If you want to cite the papers, please refer to the original.

For technical reasons we could not place the page where the original quote is coming from.

Research Highlights

Clavicle fractures, particularly midshaft clavicle fractures (MCFs), are common in children and adolescents, with nonoperative treatment traditionally favored due to excellent healing potential. However, in adults, there is a growing preference for surgical intervention, which has shown better functional outcomes and patient satisfaction. This shift raises questions about the optimal treatment approach for adolescents, who are physiologically between children and adults. The literature on treating displaced MCFs in adolescents is limited and less conclusive than in adults. Now a new study by María Galán-Olleros and colleagues aims to bridge this gap by comparing the outcomes and complications of nonoperative versus surgical treatment for displaced MCFs in adolescents.

The study conducted a systematic review and meta-analysis following PRISMA guidelines, focusing on original studies that compared surgical and nonoperative treatments for acute displaced MCFs in adolescents. The researchers searched PubMed, Embase, and Cochrane databases up to July 2023, identifying seven comparative studies for inclusion. Data were extracted on study characteristics, fracture details, treatment specifics, and follow-up data. Primary outcomes included radiological nonunion, malunion, and refractures, while secondary outcomes covered functional measures and complication rates. Statistical analyses were performed using Review Manager software to pool data from the included studies.

The meta-analysis revealed no significant difference in subjective functional outcomes between nonoperative and surgical treatments for displaced MCFs in adolescents. Nonoperative treatment was associated with fewer revision surgeries and complications compared to surgery. Although surgery did not offer substantial benefits in preventing nonunion or malunion compared to nonoperative treatment, it was linked to higher risks of revision surgeries due to pain or hardware irritation. Future study directions include high-quality prospective research with larger sample sizes to provide more definitive guidance on managing MCFs in adolescents. The findings suggest that nonoperative treatment should generally be recommended as the first-line approach for this population.

Operative Versus Non-operative Management of Mid-Diaphyseal Clavicle Fractures in the Skeletally Immature Population: A Systematic Review and Meta-Analysis [32]

This is a machine-generated summary of:

Nawar, Khaled; Eliya, Yousif; Burrow, Sarah; Peterson, Devin; Ayeni, Olufemi; de SA, Darren Operative Versus Non-operative Management of Mid-diaphyseal Clavicle Fractures in the Skeletally Immature Population: A Systematic Review and Meta-analysis [32]
Published in: Current Reviews in Musculoskeletal Medicine (2020)
Link to original: https://doi.org/10.1007/s12178-020-09604-4
Copyright of the summarized publication:
Springer Science+Business Media, LLC, part of Springer Nature 2020
All rights reserved.

If you want to cite the papers, please refer to the original.

For technical reasons we could not place the page where the original quote is coming from.

Research Highlights

Clavicle fractures are the most common type of fracture in skeletally immature patients, with the mid-diaphyseal region being the most frequently affected area. This is due to the unique osseous shape of the clavicle, which changes from concave to convex in the frontal plane and from round to flat on cross-section. Despite their prevalence, there is a lack of consensus on the optimal management of mid-diaphyseal clavicle fractures in children and adolescents, particularly regarding operative versus non-operative treatment. Now, a new study by Khaled Nawar and colleagues addresses this gap by comparing outcomes and complications associated with these two management strategies in skeletally immature patients.

The study utilized systematic review and meta-analysis methodologies, adhering to PRISMA guidelines, to evaluate existing literature on the topic. The researchers included studies that compared operative and non-operative management of mid-diaphyseal clavicle fractures in children and adolescents. They excluded non-original articles and studies involving patients with medical comorbidities or genetic abnormalities. Data were extracted from seven eligible studies involving 491 patients, with outcomes such as time to union, return to activity, functional scores, and complications being analyzed. The results indicated no significant differences between operative and non-operative management regarding time to union, return to activity, or overall complication rates. Functional outcome scores also showed high levels of satisfaction in both groups.

The findings suggest that there is no clear advantage of operative over non-operative management for mid-diaphyseal clavicle fractures in skeletally immature patients. Given the lack of significant differences in outcomes and complications, non-operative management should remain the standard approach unless extreme cases necessitate surgery. Future study could involve a prospective, randomized controlled trial to further explore these findings and potentially identify the most cost-effective treatment strategy. This could provide valuable guidance for families and caregivers when making treatment decisions for young patients with clavicle fractures.

Increase in Surgical Fixation of Pediatric Midshaft Clavicle Fractures Since 2008 [59]

This is a machine-generated summary of:

Sassi, Elina; Hannonen, Juuli; Serlo, Willy; Sinikumpu, Juha-Jaakko Increase in surgical fixation of pediatric midshaft clavicle fractures since 2008 [59]
Published in: BMC Musculoskeletal Disorders (2022)
Link to original: https://doi.org/10.1186/s12891-021-04918-x
Copyright of the summarized publication:
The Author(s) 2022
License: OpenAccess CC BY + CC0 4.0

This article is licensed under a Creative Commons Attribution 4.0 International License, which permits use, sharing, adaptation, distribution and reproduction in any medium or format, as long as you give appropriate credit to the original author(s) and the source, provide a link to the Creative Commons licence, and indicate if changes were made. The images or other third party material in this article are included in the article's Creative Commons licence, unless indicated otherwise in a credit line to the material. If material is not included in the article's Creative Commons licence and your intended use is not permitted by statutory regulation or exceeds the permitted use, you will need to obtain permission directly from the copyright holder. To view a copy of this licence, visit http://creativecommons.org/licenses/by/4.0/. The Creative Commons Public Domain Dedication waiver (http://creativecommons.org/publicdomain/zero/1.0/) applies to the data made available in this article, unless otherwise stated in a credit line to the data.

If you want to cite the papers, please refer to the original.

For technical reasons we could not place the page where the original quote is coming from.

Research Highlights

Clavicle fractures are a common injury in children, often resulting from falls during recreational activities like ice hockey and football. Traditionally, these fractures have been treated non-operatively due to the low rates of complications such as nonunion or delayed union. However, recent concerns have emerged regarding the potential negative outcomes of clavicle malunion in adolescents, which can affect shoulder biomechanics and long-term function. Now, a new study by Elina Sassi and colleagues investigates the trends and factors influencing the shift towards surgical fixation of clavicle fractures in children and adolescents over the past decade.

The study was conducted in a single institution within the Northern Finland Ostrobothnia Hospital District, focusing on children under 18 years old with mid-shaft clavicle fractures. Researchers utilized hospital registry data to identify cases using specific diagnostic codes and confirmed diagnoses through radiographic review. The study analyzed changes in the incidence of surgical treatment over time using linear regression analysis and evaluated patient characteristics, injury details, and radiographic findings. The researchers also assessed factors associated with an increased likelihood of surgical intervention, such as age and fracture displacement, using logistic regression analysis.

The study found a significant increase in the incidence of surgical fixation for pediatric clavicle fractures over the study period. This trend aligns with similar changes observed in adult populations, suggesting that adult-type surgical decision-making is being applied to children. The increase in sports-related injuries and higher average age of patients at the end of the study period may contribute to this shift. Future studies should focus on long-term outcomes to better understand the benefits of surgical versus non-operative treatment in pediatric patients. Additionally, randomized controlled trials are needed to determine which patients would benefit most from operative intervention, given that non-operative care remains the standard approach for most cases.

Adolescent Clavicle Fractures: Is There a Role for Open Reduction and Internal Fixation [75]

This is a machine-generated summary of:

Pandya, Nirav K. Adolescent Clavicle Fractures: Is There a Role for Open Reduction and Internal Fixation [75]
Published in: Current Reviews in Musculoskeletal Medicine (2019)
Link to original: https://doi.org/10.1007/s12178-019-09553-7
Copyright of the summarized publication:
Springer Science+Business Media, LLC, part of Springer Nature 2019
All rights reserved.

If you want to cite the papers, please refer to the original.

For technical reasons we could not place the page where the original quote is coming from.

Research Highlights

The treatment of clavicle fractures has evolved significantly in both adult and pediatric orthopedic practices over the past few decades. This shift is particularly notable in the adolescent population, where increased demands from sports and expectations for rapid recovery have led to a rise in operative fixation. However, there is a lack of high-quality studies comparing the complications and functional outcomes of operative versus non-operative management in adolescents. Now, a new study by Nirav K. Pandya and colleagues addresses this gap by examining the outcomes of different treatment approaches for adolescent clavicle fractures.

Pandya and his team conducted a comprehensive analysis using data from multiple high-volume children's hospitals to compare non-operative and operative treatments for adolescent clavicle fractures. The study employed a prospective, age-matched, pattern-matched, parallel group comparison to assess differences in healing, complications, and functional outcomes. The researchers found that while operative fixation may offer quicker return to activity, it does not necessarily lead to superior functional outcomes compared to non-operative treatment. Additionally, the study highlighted a significant complication rate associated with surgical intervention, including issues such as implant prominence and need for hardware removal.

The findings suggest that while operative fixation can facilitate faster return to sports, especially in high-demand athletes, it should not be universally applied without careful consideration of individual patient factors. Future study could focus on identifying specific cases where surgical intervention may be beneficial, such as patients at risk for refracture or non-union. The study emphasizes the importance of shared decision-making between clinicians and families, taking into account the high complication rates associated with surgery and the generally favorable healing outcomes with non-operative management. Further multi-center research is needed to refine treatment indications and optimize care for adolescent patients with clavicle fractures.

Elastic Stable Intramedullary Nailing (ESIN) for Displaced Midshaft Clavicle Fractures in Adolescents (12–18 Years): A Study of Early Functional Outcomes and Safety [76]

This is a machine-generated summary of:

Zhang, Wenbing; Chen, Jun Elastic stable intramedullary nailing (ESIN) for displaced midshaft clavicle fractures in adolescents (12–18 Years): a study of early functional outcomes and safety [76]
Published in: Journal of Orthopaedic Surgery and Research (2025)
Link to original: https://doi.org/10.1186/s13018-025-05923-9
Copyright of the summarized publication:
The Author(s) 2025
License: OpenAccess CC BY-NC-ND 4.0

This article is licensed under a Creative Commons Attribution-NonCommercial-NoDerivatives 4.0 International License, which permits any non-commercial use, sharing, distribution and reproduction in any medium or format, as long as you give appropriate credit to the original author(s) and the source, provide a link to the Creative Commons licence, and indicate if you modified the licensed material. You do not have permission under this licence to share adapted material derived from this article or parts of it. The images or other third party material in this article are included in the article's Creative Commons licence, unless indicated otherwise in a credit line to the material. If material is not included in the article's Creative Commons licence and your intended use is not permitted by statutory regulation or exceeds the permitted use, you will need to obtain permission directly from the copyright holder. To view a copy of this licence, visit http://creativecommons.org/licenses/by-nc-nd/4.0/.

If you want to cite the papers, please refer to the original.

For technical reasons we could not place the page where the original quote is coming from.

Research Highlights

Clavicle fractures are among the most common orthopedic injuries in children, with a significant number occurring in the midshaft region. Traditionally, nonoperative management has been the standard treatment for these fractures, but it poses challenges for older children due to their stronger shoulder musculature and reduced skeletal plasticity. The risk of clavicle deformity and shortening is a concern in nonoperative treatment, especially in adolescents who have limited bone remodeling capacity. Now, a new study by Wenbing Zhang and colleagues systematically evaluates the early clinical efficacy of closed reduction and percutaneous elastic intramedullary nailing (CR-PEIN) for displaced midshaft clavicle fractures in older children aged 10–16 years.

The study involved a retrospective review of medical records for patients treated between April 2018 and September 2020. Inclusion criteria focused on patients aged 10.5 to 15.5 years with closed, completely displaced midshaft clavicle fractures. The surgical procedure was performed by an experienced surgeon using CR-PEIN under general anesthesia. A small incision was made to insert an elastic stable intramedullary nail (ESIN) into the medullary cavity of the clavicle, providing biomechanical stability through three-point fixation while preserving the periosteal blood supply. Postoperative care included immobilization with an arm sling and regular follow-up visits until fracture union was confirmed. Functional outcomes were assessed using the Disabilities of the Arm, Shoulder and Hand (DASH) score at the final follow-up.

The study reported a 100% union rate with no instances of nonunion or serious complications such as infections or re-fractures. The mean operative time was 45 minutes, with minimal intraoperative blood loss and X-ray exposures. Patients experienced excellent functional outcomes as indicated by DASH scores, and cosmetic recovery was satisfactory with minimal scarring. Future study should involve multi-center collaboration to validate these findings further and explore comparisons with other surgical modalities or nonoperative treatments. This research highlights CR-PEIN as a promising minimally invasive option for managing displaced midshaft clavicle fractures in adolescents, offering advantages such as rapid recovery and ease of implant removal.

Plating Versus Elastic Stable Intramedullary Nailing for Displaced Pediatric Midshaft Clavicular Fractures [62]

This is a machine-generated summary of:

Hong, Pan; Liu, Ruikang; Rai, Saroj; Ze, Renhao; Tang, Xin; Li, Jin Plating versus elastic stable intramedullary nailing for displaced pediatric midshaft clavicular fractures [62]

Published in: Journal of Orthopaedics and Traumatology (2022)
Link to original: https://doi.org/10.1186/s10195-022-00659-2
Copyright of the summarized publication:
The Author(s) 2022
License: OpenAccess CC BY 4.0

This article is licensed under a Creative Commons Attribution 4.0 International License, which permits use, sharing, adaptation, distribution and reproduction in any medium or format, as long as you give appropriate credit to the original author(s) and the source, provide a link to the Creative Commons licence, and indicate if changes were made. The images or other third party material in this article are included in the article's Creative Commons licence, unless indicated otherwise in a credit line to the material. If material is not included in the article's Creative Commons licence and your intended use is not permitted by statutory regulation or exceeds the permitted use, you will need to obtain permission directly from the copyright holder. To view a copy of this licence, visit http://creativecommons.org/licenses/by/4.0/.

If you want to cite the papers, please refer to the original.

For technical reasons we could not place the page where the original quote is coming from.

Research Highlights

Clavicle fractures are among the most common fractures in the pediatric population, with the midshaft being the most frequently affected area. While operative interventions have become more prevalent in adults due to improved functional outcomes, the management of displaced midshaft clavicle fractures in adolescents remains underexplored. There is ongoing debate regarding surgical intervention for these fractures in adolescents, who typically exhibit rapid healing and significant remodeling potential. Now, a new study by Pan Hong and colleagues aims to address this gap by comparing the clinical outcomes of elastic stable intramedullary nail (ESIN) versus plate fixation for displaced midshaft clavicle fractures in adolescents.

The study was conducted as a retrospective cohort analysis at Tongji Medical College, Huazhong University of Science and Technology, with ethical approval and consent from patients' legal guardians. Participants were divided into two groups based on the surgical technique used: ESIN or plate fixation. The inclusion criteria required fully displaced midshaft clavicle fractures with significant bone shortening, while exclusion criteria included neuromuscular disorders and previous ipsilateral clavicle fractures. The study collected preoperative and postoperative data, including clinical outcomes assessed through various scales such as the visual analogue scale for pain and the American Shoulder and Elbow Surgeons score. The ESIN group underwent a minimally invasive procedure with a single nail insertion, while the plate group received a more extensive incision for plate fixation. Statistical analyses were performed using SPSS software to compare outcomes between groups.

The findings revealed that both ESIN and plate fixation provided satisfactory clinical outcomes for adolescent patients with displaced midshaft clavicle fractures. However, ESIN demonstrated advantages such as shorter operative time, reduced hospital stay, less esthetic concern, and easier implant removal compared to plate fixation. Despite these benefits, ESIN was associated with a higher risk of implant prominence. The study suggests that while nonoperative management should remain the standard for pediatric clavicle fractures, surgical options like ESIN offer viable alternatives for adolescents requiring early functional recovery. Future studies could focus on addressing allocation bias and exploring long-term outcomes to further refine treatment strategies for this population.

Conclusion

Clavicle fractures can be safely treated without surgery. Since there are no significant differences in outcomes or complications between surgical and non-surgical treatment, the latter should be the standard treatment for clavicle fractures in children and adolescents, unless extreme cases require surgery.

Bibliography

1. Cumming WA. Neonatal skeletal fractures. Birth trauma or child abuse? J Can Assoc Radiol. 1979;30:30–3.
2. O'Connor JF, Cohen J. Dating fractures. In: Kleinman PK, editor. Diagnostic imaging of child abuse. Baltimore: Williams & Wilkins; 1987. p. 103–13.
3. Yeo LI, Reed MH. Staging of healing of femoral fractures in children. Can Assoc Radiol J. 1994;45:16–9.
4. Islam O, Soboleski D, Symons S, et al. Development and duration of radiographic signs of bone healing in children. AJR Am J Roentgenol. 2000;175:75–8.
5. Malone CA, Sauer NJ, Fenton TW. A radiographic assessment of pediatric fracture healing and time since injury. J Forensic Sci. 2011;56:1123–30.
6. Halliday K, Broderick N, Somers J, Hawkes R. Dating fractures in infants. Clin Radiol. 2011;66:1049–54.
7. Prosser I, Lawon Z, Evans A, et al. A timetable for the radiologic features of fracture healing in young children. AJR Am J Roentgenol. 2012;198:1014–120.
8. Sanchez TR, Nguyen H, Palacios W, et al. Retrospective evaluation and dating of non-accidental rib fractures in infants. Clin Radiol. 2013;68:e467–71.
9. Warner C, Maguire S, Trefan L, et al. A study of radiological features of healing in long bone fractures among infants less than a year. Skeletal Radiol. 2017;46:333–41.
10. Walters MM, Forbes PW, Buonomo C, Kleinman PK. Healing patterns of clavicular birth injuries as a guide to fracture dating in cases of possible infant abuse. Pediatr Radiol. 2014;44:1224–9.

11. Fadell M, Miller A, Trefan L, et al. Radiological features of healing in newborn clavicular fractures. Eur Radiol. 2017;27:2180–7.
12. Chiu YH, Shyu SG. Utilization of diagnostic ultrasound in the detection of hip fracture. Med Ultrason. 2021;23(2):240–1.
13. Litrenta J, Masrouha K, Wasterlain A, Castaneda P. Ultrasound evaluation of pediatric orthopaedic patients. J Am Acad Orthop Surg. 2020;28(16):e696–705.
14. Kozaci N, Avcı M, Ararat E, et al. Comparison of ultrasonography and computed tomography in the determination of traumatic thoracic injuries. Am J Emerg Med. 2019;37(5):864–8.
15. Liu J, Zhang L, Qiu RX. Ultrasound instead of x-ray to diagnose neonatal fractures: a feasibility study based on a case series. Front Pediatr. 2022;10:847776.
16. Weinberg ER, Tunik MG, Tsung JW. Accuracy of clinician-performed point-of-care ultrasound for the diagnosis of fractures in children and young adults. Injury. 2010;41(8):862–8.
17. Moritz JD, Berthold LD, Soenksen SF, Alzen GF. Ultrasound in diagnosis of fractures in children: unnecessary harassment or useful addition to X-ray? Ultraschall Med. 2008;29(3):267–74.
18. Chien M, Bulloch B, Garcia-Filion P, Youssfi M, Shrader MW, Segal LS. Bedside ultrasound in the diagnosis of pediatric clavicle fractures. Pediatr Emerg Care. 2011;27(11):1038–41.
19. Karacabey S, Sanrı E. Use of ultrasound for diagnosis of clavicle fractures in the emergency department. Signa Vitae. 2021;17(1):139–42.
20. Cross KP, Warkentine FH, Kim IK, Gracely E, Paul RI. Bedside ultrasound diagnosis of clavicle fractures in the pediatric emergency department. Acad Emerg Med. 2010;17(7):687–93.
21. Schulz J, Moor M, Roocroft J, Bastrom TP, Pennock AT. Functional and radiographic outcomes of nonoperative treatment of displaced adolescent clavicle fractures. J Bone Joint Surg Am. 2013;95(13):1159–65. https://doi.org/10.2106/JBJS.L.01390.
22. Parry JA, Van Straaten M, Luo TD, et al. Is there a deficit after nonoperative versus operative treatment of shortened midshaft clavicular fractures in adolescents? J Pediatr Orthop. 2017;37(4):227–33. https://doi.org/10.1097/BPO.0000000000000627.
23. Bae DS, Shah AS, Kalish LA, et al. Shoulder motion, strength, and functional outcomes in children with established malunion of the clavicle. J Pediatr Orthop. 2013;33(5):544–50. https://doi.org/10.1097/BPO.0b013e3182857d9e.
24. Randsborg PH, Fuglesang HF, Røtterud JH, et al. Long-term patient-reported outcome after fractures of the clavicle in patients aged 10 to 18 years. J Pediatr Orthop. 2014;34(4):393–9. https://doi.org/10.1097/BPO.0000000000000082.
25. Robinson L, Gargoum R, Auer R, et al. Sports participation and radiographic findings of adolescents treated nonoperatively for displaced clavicle fractures. Injury. 2015;46(7):1372–6. https://doi.org/10.1016/j.injury.2015.04.019.
26. Kubiak R, Slongo T. Operative treatment of clavicle fractures in children: a review of 21 years. J Pediatr Orthop. 2002;22:736–9.
27. Vander Have KL, Perdue AM, Caird MS, Farley FA. Operative versus nonoperative treatment of midshaft clavicle fractures in adolescents. J Pediatr Orthop. 2010;30(4):307–12. https://doi.org/10.1097/BPO.0b013e3181db3227.
28. Namdari S, Ganley TJ, Baldwin K, et al. Fixation of displaced midshaft clavicle fractures in skeletally immature patients. J Pediatr Orthop. 2011;31(5):507–11. https://doi.org/10.1097/BPO.0b013e318220ba48.
29. Slim K, Nini E, Forestier D, et al. Methodological index for non-randomized studies (minors): development and validation of a new instrument. ANZ J Surg. 2003;73(9):712–6. https://doi.org/10.1046/j.1445-2197.2003.02748.x.
30. Hozo SP, Djulbegovic B, Hozo I. Estimating the mean and variance from the median, range, and the size of a sample. BMC Med Res Methodol. 2005;5:13. https://doi.org/10.1186/1471-2288-5-13.
31. Gao B, Dwivedi S, Patel SA, et al. Operative versus nonoperative management of displaced midshaft clavicle fractures in pediatric and adolescent patients: a systematic review and meta-analysis. J Orthop Trauma. 2019;33(11):e439–46. https://doi.org/10.1097/BOT.0000000000001580.

32. Nawar K, Eliya Y, Burrow S, et al. Operative versus non-operative management of mid-diaphyseal clavicle fractures in the skeletally immature population: a systematic review and meta-analysis. Curr Rev Musculoskelet Med. 2020;13(1):38–49. https://doi.org/10.1007/s12178-020-09604-4.
33. Hagstrom LS, Ferrick M, Galpin R. Outcomes of operative versus nonoperative treatment of displaced pediatric clavicle fractures. Orthopedics. 2015;38(2):e135–8. https://doi.org/10.3928/01477447-20150204-62.
34. Mukhtar IA, Yaghmour KM, Ahmed AF, Ibrahim T. Flexible intramedullary nailing versus nonoperative treatment for paediatric displaced midshaft clavicle fractures. J Child Orthop. 2018;12:104–10. https://doi.org/10.1302/1863-2548.12.170185.
35. Herzog MM, Whitesell R, Mac LM, et al. Functional outcomes following nonoperative versus operative treatment of clavicle fractures in adolescents. Pediatrics. 2016;137:593A. https://doi.org/10.1542/peds.137.supplement_3.593a.
36. Song MH, Yun YH, Kang K, et al. Nonoperative versus operative treatment for displaced midshaft clavicle fractures in adolescents: a comparative study. J Pediatr Orthop B. 2019;28(1):45–50. https://doi.org/10.1097/BPB.0000000000000535.
37. Canadian Orthopaedic Trauma Society. Nonoperative treatment compared with plate fixation of displaced midshaft clavicular fractures. A multicenter, randomized clinical trial. J Bone Joint Surg Am. 2007;89(1):1–10. https://doi.org/10.2106/JBJS.F.00020.
38. van der Meijden OA, Gaskill TR, Millett PJ. Treatment of clavicle fractures: current concepts review. J Shoulder Elb Surg. 2012;21:423–9. https://doi.org/10.1016/j.jse.2011.08.053.
39. Carry PM, Koonce R, Pan Z, Polousky JD. A survey of physician opinion: adolescent midshaft clavicle fracture treatment preferences among POSNA members. J Pediatr Orthop. 2011;31(1):44–9. https://doi.org/10.1097/BPO.0b013e3181ff67ce.
40. Shannon EG, Hart ES, Grottkau BE. Clavicle fractures in children: the essentials. Orthop Nurs. 2009;28:210–4. https://doi.org/10.1097/NOR.0b013e3181b57a27.
41. Neer CS. Nonunion of the clavicle. JAMA J Am Med Assoc. 1960; https://doi.org/10.1001/jama.1960.03020100014003.
42. McKee MD. Clavicle fractures in 2010: sling/swathe or open reduction and internal fixation? Orthop Clin North Am. 2010;41:225–31.
43. Robinson MM, Court-Brown CM, McQueen MM, Wakefield AE. Estimating the risk of nonunion following nonoperative treatment of a clavicular fracture. J Bone Joint Surg Am. 2004; https://doi.org/10.2106/00004623-200407000-00002.
44. Nowak J, Holgersson M, Larsson S. Can we predict long-term sequelae after fractures of the clavicle based on initial findings? A prospective study with nine to ten years of follow-up. J Shoulder Elb Surg. 2004;13(5):479–86. https://doi.org/10.1016/j.jse.2004.01.026.
45. Hill JM, McGuire MH, Crosby LA. Closed treatment of displaced middle-third fractures of the clavicle gives poor results. J Bone Joint Surg Br. 1997;79-B:537–8. https://doi.org/10.1302/0301-620X.79B4.0790537.
46. Brudvik C, Hove LM. Childhood fractures in Bergen, Norway: identifying high-risk groups and activities. J Pediatr Orthop. 2003;23:629–34. https://doi.org/10.1097/00004694-200309000-00010.
47. Mayranpaa MK, Makitie O, Kallio PE. Decreasing incidence and changing pattern of childhood fractures: a population-based study. J Bone Miner Res. 2010;25:2476–83. https://doi.org/10.1002/jbmr.155.
48. Randsborg P. Fractures in children: aspects on health service, epidemiology and risk factors. Acta Orthop. 2013;84:1–24. https://doi.org/10.3109/17453674.2013.789731.
49. Robinson CM. Fractures of the clavicle in the adult: epidemiology and classification. J Bone Joint Surg Br. 1998;80:476–84. https://doi.org/10.1302/0301-620x.80b3.8079.
50. Suppan CA, Bae DS, Donohue KS, et al. Trends in the volume of operative treatment of midshaft clavicle fractures in children and adolescents: a retrospective, 12-year, single-institution analysis. J Pediatr Orthop B. 2016;25(4):305–9. https://doi.org/10.1097/BPB.0000000000000301.

51. Li Y, Helvie P, Farley FA, et al. Complications after plate fixation of displaced pediatric midshaft clavicle fractures. J Pediatr Orthop. 2018;38(7):350–3. https://doi.org/10.1097/BPO.0000000000000832.
52. Kehr PH, Karger C. Tachdjian's pediatric orthopaedics. In: Herring J, editor. , vol. 19. 4th ed. Eur J Orthop Surg Traumatol; 2009. p. 605.
53. Strauss BJ, Carey TP, Seabrook JA, Lim R. Pediatric clavicular fractures: assessment of fracture patterns and predictors of complicated outcome. J Emergency Med. 2012;43:29–35. https://doi.org/10.1016/j.jemermed.2011.06.132.
54. Mehlman CT, Yihua G, Bochang C, et al. Operative treatment of completely displaced clavicle shaft fractures in children. J Pediatr Orthop. 2009;29(8):851–5. https://doi.org/10.1097/BPO.0b013e3181c29c9c.
55. McIntosh AL. Surgical treatment of adolescent clavicle fractures: results and complications. J Pediatr Orthop. 2016;36(Suppl 1):S41–3. https://doi.org/10.1097/BPO.0000000000000757.
56. Yang S, Werner BC, Gwathmey FW Jr. Treatment trends in adolescent clavicle fractures. J Pediatr Orthop. 2015;35(3):229–33. https://doi.org/10.1097/BPO.0000000000000258.
57. Tamaoki MJS, Matsunaga FT, Costa ARFD, Netto NA, Matsumoto MH, Belloti JC. Treatment of displaced midshaft clavicle fractures: figure-of-eight harness versus anterior plate osteosynthesis: a randomized controlled trial. J Bone Joint Surg Am. 2017;99(14):1159–65. This study demonstrates a change from prior adult studies which demonstrated superior outcomes with operative intervention compared with non-operative intervention
58. Hubbard EW, Riccio AI. Pediatric orthopedic trauma: an evidence-based approach. Orthop Clin North Am. 2018;49(2):195–210.
59. Sassi E, Hannonen J, Serlo W, Sinikumpu JJ. Increase in surgical fixation of pediatric midshaft clavicle fractures since 2008. BMC Musculoskelet Disord. 2022;23(1):173. https://doi.org/10.1186/s12891-021-04918-x.
60. Genena A, Abouelela A, Mohamed R, Nagi A. Clinical outcome of percutaneous intramedullary fixation for midshaft clavicular fractures using elastic stable nails. Ortop Traumatol Rehabil. 2021;23(1):15–20.
61. Yadav S, Phalak MO, Shevate I, Salunkhe R, Khandge A, Deshmukh A, Patel S, Patil GL. Comparative study of postoperative outcomes of clavicle midshaft fracture treated by nailing vs. Plat. Cureus. 2022;14(3):e22862.
62. Hong P, Liu R, Rai S, Ze R, Tang X, Li J. Plating versus elastic stable intramedullary nailing for displaced pediatric midshaft clavicular fractures. J Orthop Traumatol. 2022;23(1):42. https://doi.org/10.1186/s10195-022-00659-2.
63. Eisenstein ED, Misenhimer JJ, Kotb A, Thabet AM, Abdelgawad AA. Management of displaced midshaft clavicle fractures in adolescent patients using intramedullary flexible nails: a case series. J Clin Orthop Trauma. 2018;9(Suppl 1):S97–S102.
64. Park JS, Ko SH, Hong TH, Ryu DJ, Kwon DG, Kim MK, Jeon YS. Plate fixation versus titanium elastic nailing in midshaft clavicle fractures based on fracture classifications. J Orthop Surg (Hong Kong). 2020;28(3):2309499020972204.
65. Luo TD, Ashraf A, Larson AN. Complications in the treatment of adolescent clavicle fractures. Orthopedics. 2015;38(4):e287–91. https://doi.org/10.3928/01477447-20150402-56.
66. Yang S, Andras L. Clavicle shaft fractures in adolescents. Orthop Clin North Am. 2017;48(1):47–58. https://doi.org/10.1016/j.ocl.2016.08.007.
67. Meinberg EG, Agel J, Roberts CS, Karam MD, Kellam JF. Fracture and dislocation classification compendium—2018. J Orthop Trauma. 2018;32(Suppl 1):S1–S170. https://doi.org/10.1097/BOT.0000000000001063.
68. Richards RR, An K-N, al Bigliani LU e. A standardized method for the assessment of shoulder function. J Bone Joint Surg. 2009;3:347–52. https://doi.org/10.1016/S1058-2746(09)80019-0.
69. Woltz S, Stegeman SA, Krijnen P, et al. Plate fixation compared with nonoperative treatment for displaced midshaft clavicular fractures: a multicenter randomized controlled trial. J Bone Joint Surg Am. 2017;99(2):106–12. https://doi.org/10.2106/JBJS.15.01394.
70. Rapp M, Prinz K, Kaiser MM. Elastic stable intramedullary nailing for displaced pediatric clavicle midshaft fractures: a prospective study of the results and patient satisfaction in 24

children and adolescents aged 10 to 15 years. J Pediatr Orthop. 2013;33(6):608–13. https://doi.org/10.1097/BPO.0b013e31829d1a76.
71. Ode GE, Larson TB, Connor PM, Fleischli JE, D'Alessandro DF. Intramedullary fixation for displaced clavicle fractures in the adolescent athlete. J Surg Orthop Adv. 2020;29(2):81–7.
72. Tsai A, Grant PE, Warfield SK, Ou Y, Kleinman PK. Deep learning of birth-related infant clavicle fractures: a potential virtual consultant for fracture dating. Pediatr Radiol. 2022; https://doi.org/10.1007/s00247-022-05380-0.
73. Hassankhani A, Amoukhteh M, Jannatdoust P, Valizadeh P, Gholamrezanezhad A. A systematic review and meta-analysis on the diagnostic utility of ultrasound for clavicle fractures. Skeletal Radiol. 2023; https://doi.org/10.1007/s00256-023-04396-3.
74. Galán-Olleros M, Stitzman-Wengrowicz ML, Martínez-Álvarez S, Molina-Corbacho M, Manzarbeitia-Arroba P, Pulido García M d C, Lopiz Y. Nonoperative versus surgical treatment of displaced midshaft clavicle fractures in adolescents: a systematic review and meta-analysis of comparative studies. Int Orthop. 2025; https://doi.org/10.1007/s00264-025-06589-y.
75. Pandya NK. Adolescent clavicle fractures: is there a role for open reduction and internal fixation. Curr Rev Musculoskelet Med. 2019; https://doi.org/10.1007/s12178-019-09553-7.
76. Zhang W, Chen J. Elastic stable intramedullary nailing (ESIN) for displaced midshaft clavicle fractures in adolescents (12–18 years): a study of early functional outcomes and safety. J Orthop Surg Res. 2025; https://doi.org/10.1186/s13018-025-05923-9.

Proximal Humerus Fracture

2

Introduction by the Author

Fractures of the proximal humerus account for only a small percentage of all pediatric fractures, making up approximately 2% to 6% of the total. These fractures are typically the result of sports injuries, motor vehicle accidents, or birth trauma.

Proximal humerus fractures are classified based on their severity and location. The Salter-Harris classification system categorizes fractures involving the growth plate. Other classifications, such as the one by Neer and Horowitz, consider the amount of displacement.

Preadolescents and adolescents are more prone to epiphyseal fractures of the proximal humerus, which are primarily Salter-Harris type 2 and type 1 (about 30% of all proximal humerus fractures). Proximal humerus epiphyseal fractures account for 4% to 7% of all pediatric epiphyseal fractures. Metaphyseal fractures (about 70% of all proximal humerus fractures), on the other hand, are more frequent than epiphyseal fractures and are more common in younger patients, typically under the age of 10 years.

Non-operative treatment is generally preferred because children have an excellent ability to heal and remodel. Additionally, the proximal humerus growth plate is responsible for approximately 80% of humeral growth. However, surgical intervention may be necessary for significantly displaced fractures or those involving nerve or artery injuries.

Although the incidence of proximal humerus fractures has remained stable over the past two decades, there has been an increase in surgical interventions in the last decade. Despite the growing number of surgical indications for treating proximal humerus fractures, there are still no accepted guidelines for determining when to perform surgery based on minimal angulation and translation.

© The Author(s), under exclusive license to Springer Nature Switzerland AG 2026
F. Canavese, *Advances in Pediatric Extremity Fracture Management*,
https://doi.org/10.1007/978-3-032-33306-3_2

Though less common than other upper limb fractures, proximal humeral fractures in children can also be treated surgically using different techniques. These include Kirschner wires, elastic stable intramedullary nailing, and Shanz screws. In recent years, elastic stable intramedullary nailing has become the preferred method for treating significantly displaced proximal humerus fractures. This minimally invasive method is widely used because it is easy to learn, has a low risk of postoperative complications, and allows for early mobilization and good functional outcomes.

Other surgical techniques have been described, such as the use of a double-Schanz screw external fixator combined with an anti-rotating Kirschner wire, which has demonstrated advantages, including early postoperative mobility without prolonged immobilization, thereby enhancing recovery quality. However, pin tract infection was noted as a common complication. With similar goals in mind, plate and screw fixation has also been described, especially in cases where other treatment options have failed. While plate fixation is more invasive than methods like Kirschner wire fixation or elastic stable intramedullary nailing, it allows for early rehabilitation and stable outcomes. However, its use is not universally accepted, given the excellent remodeling potential of such injuries, especially in younger patients.

2.1 Machine Generated Summaries

Disclaimer: The summaries in this chapter were generated from Springer Nature publications using abstractive AI auto-summarization: An abstraction-based summarizer creates new text based on deep learning. New phrases are created to summarize the content. As the constituted sentences are machine selected, they may not fully reflect the body of the work, so we strongly advise that the original content is read and cited. The auto-generated summaries were curated by the author(s) to meet Springer Nature publication standards.

The Incidence and Treatment Trends of Pediatric Proximal Humerus Fractures [33]

This is a machine-generated summary of:

Hannonen, Juuli; Hyvönen, Hanna; Korhonen, Linda; Serlo, Willy; Sinikumpu, Juha-Jaakko The incidence and treatment trends of pediatric proximal humerus fractures [33]
Published in: BMC Musculoskeletal Disorders (2019)
Link to original: https://doi.org/10.1186/s12891-019-2948-7

Copyright of the summarized publication:
The Author(s). 2019
License: OpenAccess CC BY + CC0 4.0

This article is distributed under the terms of the Creative Commons Attribution 4.0 International License (http://creativecommons.org/licenses/by/4.0/), which permits unrestricted use, distribution, and reproduction in any medium, provided you give appropriate credit to the original author(s) and the source, provide a link to the Creative Commons license, and indicate if changes were made. The Creative Commons Public Domain Dedication waiver (http://creativecommons.org/publicdomain/zero/1.0/) applies to the data made available in this article, unless otherwise stated.

If you want to cite the papers, please refer to the original.

For technical reasons we could not place the page where the original quote is coming from.

Research Highlights

Proximal humerus fractures in children account for a small percentage of all pediatric fractures, typically resulting from sports injuries, motor vehicle accidents, or birth trauma. These fractures are classified based on their severity and location, with the Salter-Harris classification used for growth plate involvement. While non-operative treatment is generally preferred due to the excellent healing and remodeling potential in children, surgical intervention is considered when fractures are significantly displaced or involve complications such as nerve or artery injuries. Now, a new study by Juuli Hannonen and colleagues investigates the local incidence and treatment trends of proximal humerus fractures in children within the Oulu University Hospital district from 2005 to 2015.

The study was population-based, including children under 16 years old diagnosed with proximal humerus fractures. Researchers reviewed hospital charts and radiographs to confirm diagnoses and gather data on fracture types, treatments, and outcomes. Fractures were classified using the AO-classification system, and treatment was categorized as operative or non-operative. Statistical analyses were conducted to assess trends in fracture incidence and treatment approaches over time. The study found that while the annual incidence of these fractures remained stable at approximately 29 per 100,000 children, there was an increasing trend in operative treatments, particularly among boys. The most common causes of injury were horse riding and winter sports like skiing.

Despite the stable incidence of proximal humerus fractures, the study highlights a shift towards more frequent surgical interventions over the past decade. This trend aligns with broader patterns observed in pediatric fracture management but lacks robust evidence supporting its necessity for proximal humerus fractures specifically. Future study could focus on understanding the reasons behind this shift and evaluating long-term outcomes of operative versus non-operative treatments. The study's strengths include its comprehensive population-based design; however, limitations such as a lack of long-term follow-up data suggest areas for further research to better inform clinical practice.

Functional Results of Displaced Proximal Humerus Fractures in Children Treated by Elastic Stable Intramedullary Nail [34]

This is a machine-generated summary of:

Khan, A.; Athlani, L.; Rousset, M.; Samba, A.; Canavese, F. Functional results of displaced proximal humerus fractures in children treated by elastic stable intramedullary nail [34]
Published in: European Journal of Orthopaedic Surgery & Traumatology (2013)
Link to original: https://doi.org/10.1007/s00590-013-1177-2
Copyright of the summarized publication:
Springer-Verlag France 2013
All rights reserved.

If you want to cite the papers, please refer to the original.

For technical reasons we could not place the page where the original quote is coming from.

Research Highlights

In pediatric orthopedic surgery, displaced diaphyseal or metaphyseal fractures of long bones in the limbs are often treated using elastic stable intramedullary nailing (ESIN), a technique initially described by Métaizeau. This minimally invasive method is widely adopted due to its ease of learning and low risk of post-operative complications. Proximal humeral fractures in children, though less common than other upper limb fractures, can also be treated with ESIN when significantly displaced. However, previous studies evaluating the outcomes of such treatments have lacked standardized evaluation methods, complicating comparisons across studies. Now, a new study by A. Khan and colleagues addresses this gap by using a standardized evaluation scale to assess the functional outcomes of displaced proximal humeral fractures treated with ESIN in pediatric patients.

The study involved consecutive children who underwent ESIN for displaced proximal humeral fractures at a single medical center from March to December. All patients were treated using the Métaizeau technique by the same surgical team. Inclusion criteria included closed fractures without neurovascular injury and the presence of a physeal plate, while pathological fractures and poly-traumatized patients were excluded. Fractures were classified according to the AO pediatric comprehensive classification system, and displacement was assessed via radiographs. Post-operatively, patients were followed up with regular clinical evaluations and radiographs to monitor healing and detect any complications. Functional outcomes were assessed using the QuickDASH® score after hardware removal, providing a standardized measure of patient recovery.

The study found that all patients achieved good functional outcomes without significant complications, as evidenced by low QuickDASH® scores. The results showed no significant differences in functional outcomes between epiphyseal and metaphyseal fractures or between age groups under and over years old. All children returned to their daily activities and sports without difficulty or pain. The use of a standardized evaluation scale like QuickDASH® allowed for consistent assessment across patients, highlighting its value in future studies. Future study could focus on comparing these surgical outcomes with those from conservatively treated cases to further refine treatment protocols for pediatric proximal humeral fractures.

Efficacy Analysis of a Double-Schanz Screw External Fixator Combined with Anti-rotating Kirschner Wire in the Treatment of Proximal Humerus Fractures in Skeletally Immature Patients [35]

This is a machine-generated summary of:

Wang, Qian; Wang, Yu; Zhao, Huai; Kong, Qingzhu; Zhao, Jingxin; jin, Yu Efficacy analysis of a double-Schanz screw external fixator combined with anti-rotating Kirschner wire in the treatment of proximal humerus fractures in skeletally immature patients [35]
Published in: Journal of Orthopaedic Surgery and Research (2022)
Link to original: https://doi.org/10.1186/s13018-022-03434-5
Copyright of the summarized publication:
The Author(s) 2022
License: OpenAccess CC BY + CC0 4.0

This article is licensed under a Creative Commons Attribution 4.0 International License, which permits use, sharing, adaptation, distribution and reproduction in any medium or format, as long as you give appropriate credit to the original author(s) and the source, provide a link to the Creative Commons licence, and indicate if changes were made. The images or other third party material in this article are included in the article's Creative Commons licence, unless indicated otherwise in a credit line to the material. If material is not included in the article's Creative Commons licence and your intended use is not permitted by statutory regulation or exceeds the permitted use, you will need to obtain permission directly from the copyright holder. To view a copy of this licence, visit http://creativecommons.org/licenses/by/4.0/. The Creative Commons Public Domain Dedication waiver (http://creativecommons.org/publicdomain/zero/1.0/) applies to the data made available in this article, unless otherwise stated in a credit line to the data.

Copyright comment: corrected publication 2023

If you want to cite the papers, please refer to the original.

For technical reasons we could not place the page where the original quote is coming from.

Research Highlights

Proximal humeral fractures, though less common than other pediatric fractures, represent a significant concern in children and adolescents, typically occurring between certain age ranges. These fractures are often classified using the Neer–Horowitz and Salter–Harris systems, with Salter–Harris type II being prevalent in older children and adolescents. While younger children benefit from conservative treatment due to the strong remodeling capacity of their bones, the optimal surgical approach for adolescents remains debated. Now, a new study by Qian Wang and colleagues explores the efficacy of using a double-Schanz screw external fixator combined with an anti-rotating Kirschner wire for treating Salter–Harris II proximal humeral fractures in older children and adolescents.

The study conducted by Wang et al. involved a retrospective analysis of skeletally immature patients over 10 years old treated at the Affiliated Hospital of Chengde Medical College between June 2015 and April 2020. The researchers included patients with Neer–Horowitz type II, III, and IV fractures, excluding those with open fractures or additional injuries. The surgical procedure involved placing patients under general anesthesia, achieving fracture reduction through abduction confirmed by C-arm fluoroscopy, and securing the fracture with Schanz screws and Kirschner wires. Postoperative follow-ups assessed fracture healing and shoulder function using DASH and Constant scores. Statistical analysis was performed to compare limb lengths and evaluate outcomes.

The study found that all fractures healed successfully, allowing patients to resume pain-free shoulder movement. The double-Schanz screw external fixator combined with anti-rotating Kirschner wire demonstrated advantages such as early postoperative mobility without prolonged immobilization, enhancing recovery quality. However, pin tract infection was noted as a common complication. The authors acknowledge limitations due to the small sample size and retrospective nature of the study but suggest that future studies could compare this method with other surgical techniques to establish more comprehensive treatment guidelines for proximal humeral fractures in adolescents.

Open Plate Fixation in Displaced Pediatric Proximal Humerus Fractures Is Safe and Leads to Very Good Functional Outcomes [36]

This is a machine-generated summary of:

Oenning, Sebastian; Michel, Philipp A.; Vehring, Imke; Heilmann, Lukas; Katthagen, J. Christoph; Raschke, Michael J. Open plate fixation in displaced pediatric proximal humerus fractures is safe and leads to very good functional outcomes [36]

Published in: Archives of Orthopaedic and Trauma Surgery (2024)
Link to original: https://doi.org/10.1007/s00402-024-05526-9
Copyright of the summarized publication:
The Author(s) 2024
License: OpenAccess CC BY 4.0

This article is licensed under a Creative Commons Attribution 4.0 International License, which permits use, sharing, adaptation, distribution and reproduction in any medium or format, as long as you give appropriate credit to the original author(s) and the source, provide a link to the Creative Commons licence, and indicate if changes were made. The images or other third party material in this article are included in the article's Creative Commons licence, unless indicated otherwise in a credit line to the material. If material is not included in the article's Creative Commons licence and your intended use is not permitted by statutory regulation or exceeds the permitted use, you will need to obtain permission directly from the copyright holder. To view a copy of this licence, visit http://creativecommons.org/licenses/by/4.0/.

If you want to cite the papers, please refer to the original.

For technical reasons we could not place the page where the original quote is coming from.

Research Highlights

Fractures of the proximal humerus in pediatric patients are relatively rare, comprising a small percentage of all pediatric fractures. These injuries predominantly occur during early adolescence and can vary from metaphyseal to physeal fractures, with the latter often being Salter-Harris types I and II. The treatment of these fractures remains a topic of debate due to the diverse fracture patterns and the significant remodeling potential of the proximal humeral growth plate. Now, a new study by Sebastian Oenning and colleagues investigates the efficacy of open reduction and plate fixation in treating pediatric proximal humerus fractures (PHFs) with severe displacement or failed closed reduction.

The study was conducted as a retrospective, single-center series involving skeletally immature patients who underwent open reduction and internal plate fixation for dislocated PHFs. The researchers included patients who met specific criteria, excluding those with pathological fractures or polytrauma. Surgical procedures were performed using either a deltopectoral or delta-split approach, depending on the case, with temporary K-wire fixation followed by final retention using various plates. Postoperative care emphasized early functional treatment without immobilizers. Clinical assessments included range of motion (ROM) evaluations and subjective satisfaction surveys, while radiographs were used to monitor implant positioning and fracture consolidation.

The study found that open reduction and plate fixation provided a reliable treatment option for pediatric PHFs with severe displacement or when other methods failed. All patients achieved good to excellent functional outcomes, regardless of age, gender, or fracture morphology. The authors noted that while plate fixation is more invasive than other methods like K-wire fixation, it allows for early rehabilitation and stable outcomes. Future studies with larger cohorts are needed to further validate these findings and explore comparisons between different surgical techniques. Additionally, considerations such as cosmetic concerns from scarring and the necessity for implant removal highlight areas for further investigation in optimizing treatment strategies for pediatric PHFs.

Conclusion

Due to their significant remodeling potential, proximal humerus fractures in pediatric patients can be safely treated conservatively. Since there are no significant differences in outcomes or complications between surgical and non-surgical treatment, the non-surgical approach should remain the standard. However, due to the diverse fracture patterns and significant remodeling potential of the proximal humeral growth plate, surgery remains a topic of debate without widely accepted guidelines.

Bibliography

1. Mayranpaa MK, Makitie O, Kallio PE. Decreasing incidence and changing pattern of childhood fractures: a population-based study. J Bone Miner Res. 2010;25:2476–83. https://doi.org/10.1002/jbmr.155.
2. Fernandez FF, Eberhardt O, Langendorfer M, Wirth T. Treatment of severely displaced proximal humeral fractures in children with retrograde elastic stable intramedullary nailing. Injury. 2008;39(12):1453–9.
3. Dameron TB, Reibel DB. Fractures involving the proximal humeral epiphyseal plate. J Bone Joint Surg Am. 1969;51(2):289–97.
4. Shrader MW. Proximal humerus and humeral shaft fractures in children. Hand Clin. 2007;23(4):431–5.
5. Beringer DC, Weiner DS, Noble JS, Bell RH. Severely displaced proximal humeral epiphyseal fractures: a follow-up study. J Pediatr Orthop. 1998;18(1):31–7.
6. Larsen CF, Kiaer T, Lindequist S. Fractures of the proximal humerus in children: nine-year follow-up of 64 unoperated on cases. Acta Orthop Scand. 1990;61(3):255–7.
7. Dobbs MB, Luhmann SL, Gordon JE, Strecker WB, Schoenecker PL. Severely displaced proximal humeral epiphyseal fractures. J Pediatr Orthop. 2003;23(2):208–15.
8. Bahrs C, Zipplies S, Ochs BG, et al. Proximal humeral fractures in children and adolescents. J Pediatr Orthop. 2009;29(3):238–42.
9. Sinikumpu JJ, Lautamo A, Pokka T, Serlo W. The increasing incidence of pediatric diaphyseal both-bone forearm fractures and their internal fixation during the last decade. Injury. 2012;43(3):362–6.
10. Cruz AI Jr, Kleiner JE, Gil JA, Goodman AD, Daniels AH, Eberson CP. Inpatient surgical treatment of pediatric proximal humerus fractures between 2000 and 2012. J Child Orthop. 2018;12(2):111–6.
11. Chaus G, Carry P, Pishkenari A, Hadley-Miller N. Operative versus nonoperative treatment of displaced proximal humeral physeal fractures: a matched cohort. J Pediatr Orthop. 2015;35(3):234–9.
12. Ligier JN, Métaizeau JP, Prévot J. Closed flexible medullary nailing in pediatric traumatology. Chir Pediatr. 1983;24:383–5.
13. Sessa S, Lascombes P, Prevot J, et al. Centro-medullary nailing in fractures of the upper end of the humerus in children and adolescents. Chir Pediatr. 1990;31:43–6.
14. Beringer DC, Weiner DS, Noble JS, Bell RH. Severely displaced proximal humeral epiphyseal fractures: a follow-up study. J Pediatr Orthop. 1998;18:31–7.
15. Métaizeau JP. Ostéosynthèse chez l'enfant: embrochage centromédullaire élastique stable. Montpellier: Ed. Sauramps Médical; 1988.

16. Lascombes P, Prévot J, Ligier JN, Métaizeau JP, Poncelet T. Elastic stable intramedullary nailing in forearm shaft fractures in children: 85 cases. J Pediatr Orthop. 1990;10:167–71.
17. Slongo T, Audigé L, Schlickewei W, Clavert JM, Hunter J. Development and validation of the AO pediatric comprehensive classification of long bone fractures by the pediatric expert group of the AO foundation in collaboration with AO clinical investigation and documentation and the international association for pediatric traumatology. J Pediatr Orthop. 2006;26:43–9.
18. Slongo T, Audigé L, Clavert JM, Nicolas L, Frick S, Hunter J. The AO comprehensive classification of pediatric long-bone fractures: a web-based multicenter agreement study. J Pediatr Orthop. 2007;27:171–80.
19. Xie F, Wang S, Jiao Q, Shen Y, Ni XY, Ying H. Minimally invasive treatment for severely displaced proximal humeral fractures in children using titanium elastic nails. J Pediatr Orthop. 2011;31:839–46.
20. Sidor ML, Zuckerman JD, Lyon T, Cuomo F, Shoenberg N. The Neer classification system for proximal humeral fractures. J Bone Joint Surg Am. 1992;75:1745–50.
21. Karatosun V, Unver B, Alici E, Serin E. Treatment of displaced, proximal, humeral, epiphyseal fractures with a two-prong splint. J Orthop Trauma. 2003;17:578–81.
22. Lucas JC, Mehlman CT, Laor T. The location of the biceps tendon in completely displaced proximal humerus fractures in children. J Pediatr Orthopaed. 2004;24:249–53.
23. Lefevre Y, Journeau P, Angelliaume A, Bouty A, Dobremez E. Proximal humerus fractures in children and adolescents. Orthop Traumatol Surg Res. 2014;100(1 Suppl):S149–56.
24. Kraus T, Hoermann S, Ploder G, Zoetsch S, Eberl R, Singer G. Elastic stable intramedullary nailing versus Kirschner wire pinning: outcome of severely displaced proximal humeral fractures in juvenile patients. J Shoulder Elb Surg. 2014;23:1462–7.
25. Li J, Rai S, Qian H, Tang X, Liu R, Hong P. Operative choice for displaced proximal humeral fractures in adolescents with open visible physis: a comparative study of external fixator vs Kirschner wire. Injury. 2021;52:2279–84.
26. Lähdeoja T, Pakkasjärvi N, Aronen P, Willamo P, Aronniemi J, Sintonen H, et al. Outcomes at a mean of 13 years after proximal humeral fracture during adolescence. J Bone Jt Surg. 2023;105:839–48. https://doi.org/10.2106/JBJS.22.01131.
27. Shahriar R, Hosseinzadeh P. Proximal humerus fractures: what alignment is acceptable in children 10 and up? J Pediatr Orthopaed. 2021;41:S20–3.
28. Binder H, Tiefenboeck T, Payr S, Schurz M, Aldrian S, Sarahrudi K. Treatment of proximal humerus fractures in children and young adolescents. Wien Klin Wochenschr. 2016;128(3–4):120–4.
29. Hohloch L, Eberbach H, Wagner FC, Strohm PC, Reising K, Südkamp NP, et al. Age- and severity-adjusted treatment of proximal humerus fractures in children and adolescents – a systematical review and meta-analysis. PLoS One. 2017;12:e0183157.
30. Pavone V, de Cristo C, Cannavò L, Testa G, Buscema A, Condorelli G, et al. Midterm results of surgical treatment of displaced proximal humeral fractures in children. Eur J Orthop Surg Traumatol. 2016;26:461–7. https://doi.org/10.1007/s00590-016-1773-z.
31. Freislederer F, Bensler S, Specht T, Magerkurth O, Eid K. Plate fixation for irreducible proximal humeral fractures in children and adolescents-a single-center case series of six patients. Children. 2021; https://doi.org/10.3390/children8080635.
32. Schwendenwein E, Hajdu S, Gaebler C, Stengg K, Vécsei V. Displaced fractures of the proximal humerus in children require open/closed reduction and internal fixation. Eur J Pediatr Surg. 2004;14(1):51–5.
33. Hannonen J, Hyvönen H, Korhonen L, Serlo W, Sinikumpu J-J. The incidence and treatment trends of pediatric proximal humerus fractures. BMC Musculoskelet Disord. 2019; https://doi.org/10.1186/s12891-019-2948-7.

34. Khan A, Athlani L, Rousset M, Samba A, Canavese F. Functional results of displaced proximal humerus fractures in children treated by elastic stable intramedullary nail. Eur J Orthop Surg Traumatol. 2013; https://doi.org/10.1007/s00590-013-1177-2.
35. Wang Q, Wang Y, Zhao H, Kong Q, Zhao J, Jin Y. Efficacy analysis of a double-Schanz screw external fixator combined with anti-rotating Kirschner wire in the treatment of proximal humerus fractures in skeletally immature patients. J Orthop Surg Res. 2022; https://doi.org/10.1186/s13018-022-03434-5.
36. Oenning S, Michel PA, Vehring I, Heilmann L, Katthagen JC, Raschke MJ. Open plate fixation in displaced pediatric proximal humerus fractures is safe and leads to very good functional outcomes. Arch Orthop Trauma Surg. 2024; https://doi.org/10.1007/s00402-024-05526-9.

Diaphyseal Humerus Fracture

3

Introduction by the Author

Diaphyseal humeral fractures in children are relatively uncommon, accounting for only a small percentage of pediatric fractures. Approximately 20% of humeral fractures in children are humeral shaft fractures. The estimated incidence is between 12 and 30 fractures per 100,000 children per year. Such injuries exhibit a bimodal distribution. Most occur in children younger than 3 or older than 12 years of age.

Birth-related diaphyseal humeral fractures in infants are rare and are often only reported in small case series. The most recent data report an incidence rate of 0.1 fractures per 1000 children, primarily affecting boys.

Diaphyseal humeral fractures can occur in older infants. However, most of these fractures in older children are caused by high-energy trauma.

These fractures are traditionally managed conservatively due to the humerus's remodeling ability, especially in younger children. Older children, however, may require surgery due to their reduced remodeling capacity and increased risk of secondary displacement. Open diaphyseal humeral fractures and polytrauma also indicate the need for surgery in children.

Diaphyseal humeral fractures can injure the radial nerve. If radial nerve injury is suspected, exploration is generally recommended immediately; however, this is only necessary if the deficit does not recover after 10–12 weeks.

Elastic stable intramedullary nailing is a viable treatment option for displaced diaphyseal humeral fractures in older children and adolescents. This method provides stable fixation and has low complication rates. This method allows for early mobilization, reduces postoperative pain, and poses a lower risk of direct radial nerve injury than an external fixator does.

© The Author(s), under exclusive license to Springer Nature Switzerland AG 2026
F. Canavese, *Advances in Pediatric Extremity Fracture Management*,
https://doi.org/10.1007/978-3-032-33306-3_3

Though the current evidence is limited, elastic stable intramedullary nailing demonstrates favorable clinical and functional outcomes, even with mild residual deformities. Future studies could examine long-term outcomes and compare elastic stable intramedullary nailing with conservative treatments for managing diaphyseal humeral fractures to further validate its efficacy in pediatric populations.

3.1 Machine Generated Summaries

Disclaimer: The summaries in this chapter were generated from Springer Nature publications using abstractive AI auto-summarization: An abstraction-based summarizer creates new text based on deep learning. New phrases are created to summarize the content. As the constituted sentences are machine selected, they may not fully reflect the body of the work, so we strongly advise that the original content is read and cited. The auto-generated summaries were curated by the author(s) to meet Springer Nature publication standards.

The Epidemiology of Infant Shaft Fractures of Femur or Humerus by Incidence, Birth, Accidents, and Other Causes [26]

This is a machine-generated summary of:

von Heideken, Johan; Thiblin, Ingemar; Högberg, Ulf The epidemiology of infant shaft fractures of femur or humerus by incidence, birth, accidents, and other causes [26]
Published in: BMC Musculoskeletal Disorders (2020)
Link to original: https://doi.org/10.1186/s12891-020-03856-4
Copyright of the summarized publication:
The Author(s) 2020
License: OpenAccess CC BY + CC0 4.0

This article is licensed under a Creative Commons Attribution 4.0 International License, which permits use, sharing, adaptation, distribution and reproduction in any medium or format, as long as you give appropriate credit to the original author(s) and the source, provide a link to the Creative Commons licence, and indicate if changes were made. The images or other third party material in this article are included in the article's Creative Commons licence, unless indicated otherwise in a credit line to the material. If material is not included in the article's Creative Commons licence and your intended use is not permitted by statutory regulation or exceeds the permitted use, you will need to obtain permission directly from the copyright holder. To view a copy of this licence, visit http://creativecommons.org/

licenses/by/4.0/. The Creative Commons Public Domain Dedication waiver (http://creativecommons.org/publicdomain/zero/1.0/) applies to the data made available in this article, unless otherwise stated in a credit line to the data.

If you want to cite the papers, please refer to the original.

For technical reasons we could not place the page where the original quote is coming from.

Research Highlights

Shaft fractures of the femur and humerus in infants can occur during birth or later in infancy, with birth-related cases being rare and often reported only in small case series. Previous studies have documented the incidence of these fractures, but there is limited data on the relationship between maternal conditions like obesity or pre-eclampsia and these fractures. Now, a new study by Johan von Heideken and colleagues investigates both birth-related and later-occurring shaft fractures of the femur and humerus during infancy, using a comprehensive population-based registry from Sweden.

The study utilized data from over 1.3 million infants born in Sweden between 1997 and 2014, tracking them until they reached 1 year of age. Researchers identified cases of femur and humerus shaft fractures using diagnostic codes from national health registers. They categorized fractures as birth-related if diagnosed without reported accidents or abuse within the first days of life. The study analyzed associations with prenatal exposures, birth complications, and other diagnoses during infancy. Statistical analyses were conducted to assess differences in incidence rates by sex, age at diagnosis, and associated risk factors such as maternal obesity, pre-eclampsia, and delivery methods.

The findings reveal that birth-related shaft fractures are more common than previously reported in hospital case studies, suggesting potential underestimation in past research. The study highlights the importance of considering both accidental and non-accidental causes when diagnosing these fractures. Future study could focus on improving diagnostic precision through double coding practices and further exploring the role of bone fragility disorders. This research provides valuable insights into the epidemiology of infant shaft fractures, emphasizing the need for thorough risk factor analysis to guide clinical practice and inform future investigations.

Upper Limb Pediatric Fractures in 22 Tertiary Children's Hospitals, China: A Multicenter Epidemiological Investigation and Economic Factor Analysis of 32,832 Hospitalized Children [27]

This is a machine-generated summary of:

Qiu, Xin; Deng, Hansheng; Zhao, Zhenhui; Zeng, Shuaidan; Zeng, Yueping; Wang, Xinyu; Xu, Hui; Li, Weiqing; Chen, Xiaodi; Yang, Qisong; Zhao, Jiaxin; Li, Shicheng; Cui, Zhiwen; Tang, Yu; Cui, Shuting; Liu, Min; Sun, Yiyuan; Feng, Guoshuang; Tang, Gen; Xiong, Zhu; Tang, Shengping Upper limb pediatric frac-

tures in 22 tertiary children's hospitals, China: a multicenter epidemiological investigation and economic factor analysis of 32,832 hospitalized children [27]
Published in: Journal of Orthopaedic Surgery and Research (2022)
Link to original: https://doi.org/10.1186/s13018-022-03159-5
Copyright of the summarized publication:
The Author(s) 2022
License: OpenAccess CC BY + CC0 4.0

This article is licensed under a Creative Commons Attribution 4.0 International License, which permits use, sharing, adaptation, distribution and reproduction in any medium or format, as long as you give appropriate credit to the original author(s) and the source, provide a link to the Creative Commons licence, and indicate if changes were made. The images or other third party material in this article are included in the article's Creative Commons licence, unless indicated otherwise in a credit line to the material. If material is not included in the article's Creative Commons licence and your intended use is not permitted by statutory regulation or exceeds the permitted use, you will need to obtain permission directly from the copyright holder. To view a copy of this licence, visit http://creativecommons.org/licenses/by/4.0/. The Creative Commons Public Domain Dedication waiver (http://creativecommons.org/publicdomain/zero/1.0/) applies to the data made available in this article, unless otherwise stated in a credit line to the data.

If you want to cite the papers, please refer to the original.

For technical reasons we could not place the page where the original quote is coming from.

Research Highlights

Childhood unintentional injuries, particularly fractures, are a significant global public health concern, with fractures being the most common type of injury among children. These injuries not only result in substantial morbidity but also impose a considerable economic burden. In China, which has the second-largest child population globally, there is a lack of comprehensive data on the epidemiology and economic impact of upper limb fractures in children. Now, a new study by Xin Qiu and colleagues addresses this gap by presenting detailed epidemiological data on hospitalized children with upper limb fractures in China and analyzing the associated economic costs.

The study retrospectively reviewed medical records of children hospitalized with recent or old upper limb fractures across tertiary children's hospitals in China from December 2016 to December 2020. Data were extracted on demographics, fracture types, causes, treatment methods, and hospital costs. The researchers categorized fractures by anatomical site and age group and analyzed the causes of injuries, which included falls and traffic accidents. The study found that distal humerus fractures were the most common type across all age groups, with boys being more frequently affected than girls. The majority of fresh fractures were treated with closed surgical reduction, while old fractures often required open reduction. Hospital costs varied significantly depending on fracture type and treatment method.

The findings highlight the need for targeted preventive strategies to reduce the incidence of upper limb fractures in children. Future study could focus on improving safety education for parents and guardians to prevent falls and traffic-related injuries. Additionally, enhancing medical insurance coverage for children could alleviate the financial burden on families. The study suggests that establishing more specialized pediatric trauma centers could improve diagnosis and treatment outcomes for childhood fractures. These measures could ultimately enhance children's quality of life and reduce the public health burden associated with pediatric upper limb fractures.

Displaced Humeral Shaft Fractures in Children and Adolescents: Results and Adverse Effects in Patients Treated by Elastic Stable Intramedullary Nailing [28]

This is a machine-generated summary of:

Marengo, Lorenza; Rousset, Marie; Paonessa, Matteo; Vanni, Stefania; Dimeglio, Alain; Samba, Antoine; Andreacchio, Antonio; Canavese, Federico Displaced humeral shaft fractures in children and adolescents: results and adverse effects in patients treated by elastic stable intramedullary nailing [28]
Published in: European Journal of Orthopaedic Surgery & Traumatology (2016)
Link to original: https://doi.org/10.1007/s00590-016-1758-y
Copyright of the summarized publication:
Springer-Verlag France 2016
All rights reserved.

If you want to cite the papers, please refer to the original.

For technical reasons we could not place the page where the original quote is coming from.

Research Highlights

Humeral shaft fractures in children are relatively rare, comprising a small percentage of pediatric fractures. Traditionally, these fractures have been managed conservatively due to the humerus's ability to remodel, especially in younger children. However, surgical intervention is sometimes necessary for older children due to reduced remodeling capacity and the risk of secondary displacement. Now, a new study by Lorenza Marengo and colleagues investigates the outcomes of using elastic stable intramedullary nailing (ESIN) for treating humeral shaft fractures in children under 16 years old, focusing on clinical, radiological, and functional outcomes.

The study retrospectively reviewed medical records from two pediatric institutions, identifying 106 children with humeral shaft fractures treated between September 2010 and May 2020. Of these, 38 met the inclusion criteria for surgical treatment with ESIN. The procedure involved reducing the fracture under fluoroscopic control and stabilizing it with pre-contoured titanium elastic nails.

Post-surgery, patients were immobilized in a splint for 3 weeks, with hardware removal occurring 6–12 months later. Follow-up assessments included radiographic evaluations and functional outcomes measured using the Quick Disabilities of the Arm, Shoulder and Hand (Quick DASH) questionnaire. The study found that all patients returned to daily activities within 3–6 months post-surgery, with minimal complications such as secondary displacement or re-fracture.

The study highlights that ESIN is a viable option for managing displaced humeral shaft fractures in older children and adolescents, providing stable fixation with low complication rates. Despite some limitations like its retrospective nature and lack of a non-operative control group, the research demonstrates good clinical and functional outcomes even with mild residual deformities. Future studies could explore long-term outcomes and compare ESIN with conservative treatments to further validate its efficacy in pediatric populations.

Conclusion
Although diaphyseal humeral fractures can be treated conservatively, elastic stable intramedullary nailing has been shown to provide an excellent clinical and radiographic outcome.

Bibliography

1. Morris S, Cassidy N, Stephens M, McCormack D, McManus F. Birth-associated femoral fractures: incidence and outcome. J Pediatr Orthop. 2002;22:27–30.
2. Basha A, Amarin Z, Abu-Hassan F. Birth-associated long-bone fractures. Int J Gynaecol Obstet. 2013;123:127–30.
3. Sherr-Lurie N, Bialik GM, Ganel A, Schindler A, Givon U. Fractures of the humerus in the neonatal period. Isr Med Assoc J. 2011;13:363–5.
4. Heideken J, Svensson T, Blomqvist P, Haglund-Akerlind Y, Janarv PM. Incidence and trends in femur shaft fractures in Swedish children between 1987 and 2005. J Pediatr Orthop. 2011;31:512–9.
5. Talbot C, Davis N, Majid I, Young M, Bouamra O, Lecky FE, Jones S. Fractures of the femoral shaft in children: national epidemiology and treatment trends in England following activation of major trauma networks. Bone Joint J. 2018;100-B:109–18.
6. Shaw BA, Murphy KM, Shaw A, Oppenheim WL, Myracle MR. Humerus shaft fractures in young children: accident or abuse? J Pediatr Orthop. 1997;17:293–7.
7. Högberg U, Andersson J, Högberg G, Thiblin I. Metabolic bone disease risk strongly contributing to long bone and rib fractures during early infancy: a population register study. PLoS One. 2018;13:e0208033.
8. Mitchell PD, Brown R, Wang T, Shah RD, Samworth RJ, Deakin S, Edge P, Hudson I, Hutchinson R, Stohr K, et al. Multicentre study of physical abuse and limb fractures in young children in the East Anglia region. UK Arch Dis Child. 2019;104:956–61.
9. Högberg U, Fellman V, Thiblin I, Karlsson R, Wester K. Difficult birth is the main contributor to birthrelated fracture, and accidents to other neonatal fractures. Acta Paediatr. 2020;109:2040–8.
10. Roda D, Trenchs V, Curcoy AI, Martinez AD, Pou J, Luaces C. Epidemiology of fractures in children younger than 12 months. Pediatr Emerg Care. 2019;35:256–60.

11. Jones G, Cooley HM. Symptomatic fracture incidence in those under 50 years of age in southern Tasmania. J Paediatr Child Health. 2002;38(3):278–83.
12. Hedström EM, Svensson O, Bergström U, Michno P. Epidemiology of fractures in children and adolescents. Acta Orthop. 2010;81(1):148–53. https://doi.org/10.3109/17453671003628780.
13. Wang X, et al. A brief introduction to the FUTang Updating medical REcords (FUTURE) database. Pediatr Investig. 2021;5(3):247–8.
14. Yang H, et al. Incidence patterns of traumatic upper limb fractures in children and adolescents: data from medical university-affiliated hospitals in Chongqing, China. Medicine. 2019;98(38):e17299.
15. Cheng BC, Cai QX. Statistical analysis of 3271 cases of fracture in children. Chin J Pediatr Surg. 1997;18(4):241–2.
16. Baig MN. A review of epidemiological distribution of different types of fractures in paediatric age. Cureus. 2017;9(8):e1624.
17. Hudak PL, Amadio PC, Bombardier C. Development of an upper extremity outcome measure: the DASH (disabilities of the arm, shoulder and hand) [corrected]. The upper extremity collaborative group (UECG). Am J Ind Med. 1996;29(6):602–8.
18. Beaton DE, Wright JG, Katz JN, Upper Extremity Collaborative Group. Development of the quickdash: comparison of three item-reduction approaches. J Bone Joint Surg Am. 2005;87(5):1038–46. https://doi.org/10.2106/JBJS.D.02060.
19. Beaty JH. Fractures of the proximal humerus and shaft in children. Instr Course Lect. 1992;41:369–72.
20. Marengo L, Canavese F, Cravino M, De Rosa V, Rousset M, Samba A, Mansour M, Andreacchio A. Outcome of displaced fractures of the distal metaphyseal-diaphyseal junction of the humerus in children treated with elastic stable intramedullary nails. J Pediatr Orthop. 2015;35:611–6.
21. Senes FM, Catena N. Intramedullary osteosynthesis for metaphyseal and diaphyseal humeral fractures in developmental age. J Pediatr Orthop B. 2012;21:300–4.
22. Garg S, Dobbs MB, Schoenecker PL, Luhmann SJ, Gordon JE. Surgical treatment of traumatic pediatric humeral diaphyseal fractures with titanium elastic nails. J Child Orthop. 2009;3:121–7.
23. Sahu RL. Percutaneous Kirschner wire (K-wire) fixation for humerus shaft fractures in children: a treatment concept. Niger Med J. 2013;54:356–60.
24. Ligier JN, Métaizeau JP, Prévot J. Closed flexible medullary nailing in pediatric traumatology. Chir Pediatr. 1983;24:383–5.
25. Ligier JN, Métaizeau JP, Prévot J, Lascombes P. Elastic stable intramedullary nailing of femoral shaft fractures in children. J Bone Joint Surg Br. 1988;70:74–7.
26. von Heideken J, Thiblin I, Högberg U. The epidemiology of infant shaft fractures of femur or humerus by incidence, birth, accidents, and other causes. BMC Musculoskelet Disord. 2020;21:840. https://doi.org/10.1186/s12891-020-03856-4.
27. Xin Q, Hansheng D, Zhenhui Z, Shuaidan Z, Yueping Z, Xinyu W, Hui X, Weiqing L, Xiaodi C, Qisong Y, Jiaxin Z, Shicheng L, Zhiwen C, Yu T, Shuting C, Min L, Yiyuan S, Guoshuang F, Gen T, Zhu X, Shengping T. Upper limb pediatric fractures in 22 tertiary children's hospitals, China: a multicenter epidemiological investigation and economic factor analysis of 32,832 hospitalized children. J Orthop Surg Res. 2022;17:300. https://doi.org/10.1186/s13018-022-03159-5.
28. Lorenza M, Marie R, Matteo P, Stefania V, Alain D, Antoine S, Antonio A, Federico C. Displaced humeral shaft fractures in children and adolescents: results and adverse effects in patients treated by elastic stable intramedullary nailing. Eur J Orthop Surg Traumatol. 2016;26:453–9. https://doi.org/10.1007/s00590-016-1758-y.

Supracondylar Fracture

4

Introduction by the Author

Supracondylar fractures of the humerus are the second most common type of upper extremity fracture, representing about 17% of the total. Yet, they are the primary indication for surgery in children. In particular, these fractures are the most common type of elbow injury in children, particularly affecting those aged 5–7.

A precise vascular and neurological assessment is mandatory for all children with a supracondylar fracture. Careful preoperative and postoperative radiographic evaluations are needed for diagnosis and to detect early and late complications, malrotation, and cubitus varus, respectively.

The Gartland classification system categorizes supracondylar fractures into four subtypes based on displacement and its direction. The subtypes are: extension type 1: minimally or not displaced; extension type 2: displaced with contact between fragments (subtypes A and B, with and without rotation of the distal fragment, respectively); extension type 3: displaced with loss of contact between the two fragments; and flexion type. The extension type accounts for the highest proportion of children's humeral supracondylar fractures, while the flexion type accounts for only 2%–5%.

According to the Gartland classification, non-displaced or minimally displaced fractures can be managed conservatively. The other subtypes are managed with closed reduction and percutaneous wires fixation. If stable fixation can be achieved, closed reduction and Kirschner wire fixation is an effective treatment. The outcome of these fractures depends on factors such as the quality of reduction, pin configuration, and fracture stability.

© The Author(s), under exclusive license to Springer Nature Switzerland AG 2026

F. Canavese, *Advances in Pediatric Extremity Fracture Management*,
https://doi.org/10.1007/978-3-032-33306-3_4

Non-displaced fractures can be treated conservatively. However, significantly displaced fractures often require surgery to prevent complications such as cubitus varus. The standard treatment for pediatric supracondylar fractures is closed reduction and Kirschner wire fixation. If there is no indication to operate the same night outside of regular hours and the patient is neurologically intact, treatment can be delayed until the next day without increasing the risk of complications.

There is an ongoing debate about the optimal pin construct, whether to use only lateral wires or both lateral and medial wires. From a biomechanical perspective, the construct with two lateral and one medial wire is the most stable, though lateral-only wires can also provide stable fixation if they are sufficiently divergent and do not cross at the fracture site. Overall, fixation with entry wires through the lateral and medial sides offers biomechanical stability but can cause iatrogenic ulnar nerve injury. Lateral entry wire fixation avoids this issue, but the construct may be less stable.

Supracondylar fractures are less common in adolescents and typically result from higher-energy trauma, leading to more complex fracture patterns.

Open reduction remains a viable option when technical difficulties arise or after unsuccessful closed reduction attempts. The anterior approach for open reduction is safe and reliable and yields results similar to those obtained with the lateral and medial approaches.

The specific anatomical features of the distal humerus increase the risk of requiring open reduction and internal fixation for flexion-type supracondylar fractures. Ulnar nerve injury and rotational displacement of the distal fragment are key risk factors. Several minimally invasive techniques have been described for reducing and fixing supracondylar fractures. These techniques achieve good radiographic and functional results, even for unstable flexion-type supracondylar fractures.

Despite a generally favorable prognosis and successful treatment, supracondylar fractures carry a risk of complications, including vascular and neurological injury, infection, malunion, delayed union, deformities such as cubitus varus, and functional impairment.

4.1 Machine Generated Summaries

Disclaimer: The summaries in this chapter were generated from Springer Nature publications using abstractive AI auto-summarization: An abstraction-based summarizer creates new text based on deep learning. New phrases are created to summarize the content. As the constituted sentences are machine selected, they may not fully reflect the body of the work, so we strongly advise that the original content is read and cited. The auto-generated summaries were curated by the author(s) to meet Springer Nature publication standards.

Are We Staying up Too Late? Timing of Surgery of Displaced Supracondylar Fractures in Children. Clinical Audit in a Paediatric Tertiary UK Trauma Centre and Literature Review [168]

This is a machine-generated summary of:

Abdelmalek, Amir; Towner, Matthew; Clarke, Anna Are we staying up too late? Timing of surgery of displaced supracondylar fractures in children. Clinical audit in a paediatric tertiary UK trauma centre and literature review [168]
Published in: Archives of Orthopaedic and Trauma Surgery (2022)
Link to original: https://doi.org/10.1007/s00402-021-04289-x
Copyright of the summarized publication:
The Author(s), under exclusive licence to Springer-Verlag GmbH Germany, part of Springer Nature 2021
All rights reserved.

If you want to cite the papers, please refer to the original.

For technical reasons we could not place the page where the original quote is coming from.

Research Highlights

Supracondylar humerus fractures are the most common type of fracture in children under 7 years old and are particularly susceptible to neurovascular complications and failure of closed reduction. This has sparked a debate on whether these fractures should be treated urgently to minimize risks or if treatment can be delayed until the next day. The controversy primarily concerns late-presenting patients, with some surgeons advocating for emergency treatment to reduce peri-operative complications, while others suggest that night-time operations may not always be in the patient's best interest due to limited resources and expertise. Now, a new study by Amir Abdelmalek and colleagues examines the impact of implementing British Orthopaedic Association Standards for Trauma (BOAST) guidelines on surgical timing and outcomes for these fractures.

The study conducted a retrospective audit comparing data before and after adopting BOAST guidelines at their institution. Researchers reviewed electronic records from January to December, followed by prospective data collection over two subsequent years. The audit included all patients with surgically treated type II and III supracondylar humerus fractures. Radiographs confirmed fracture types, while admission notes clarified neurovascular status and skin integrity. The study categorized surgeries into three timing groups: green (normal working hours), amber (evening), and red (overnight). The audit aimed to assess whether delaying surgery increased the rate of conversion to open reduction or led to neurovascular complications. Results showed no increase in open reduction rates or neurovascular complications with delayed surgery, aligning with BOAST guidelines that recommend urgent surgery only for specific indications.

The findings suggest that delaying surgery until the next day is safe for children with displaced supracondylar humerus fractures, provided there are no urgent indications such as absent radial pulse or impaired hand perfusion. This approach reduces unnecessary out-of-hours operations without increasing complication rates. Future studies could include randomized controlled trials to provide stronger evidence supporting these findings. The audit highlights the importance of adhering to national guidelines and demonstrates a pragmatic approach in a busy pediatric trauma center, contributing valuable insights into optimizing surgical timing for these common pediatric injuries.

Sagittal Plane Analysis of the Open and Closed Methods in Children with Displaced Supracondylar Fractures of the Humerus (a Radiological Study) [169]

This is a machine-generated summary of:

Turhan, Egemen; Aksoy, Cemalettin; Ege, Ahmet; Bayar, Ahmet; Keser, Selçuk; Alpaslan, Mümtaz Sagittal plane analysis of the open and closed methods in children with displaced supracondylar fractures of the humerus (a radiological study) [169]

Published in: Archives of Orthopaedic and Trauma Surgery (2007)
Link to original: https://doi.org/10.1007/s00402-007-0523-4
Copyright of the summarized publication:
Springer-Verlag 2007
All rights reserved.

If you want to cite the papers, please refer to the original.

For technical reasons we could not place the page where the original quote is coming from.

Research Highlights

Supracondylar humerus fractures are the most common type of elbow injury in children, often requiring surgical intervention due to their displaced nature. These fractures can lead to complications such as malunion and neurovascular issues if not properly treated. Closed reduction and percutaneous pin fixation are typically preferred to avoid complications associated with open reduction. However, there is a lack of studies evaluating the success of fracture reduction using multiple radiological criteria on the sagittal plane. Now, a new study by Egemen Turhan and colleagues addresses this gap by assessing the quality of sagittal plane reduction in pediatric supracondylar humerus fractures using various radiological criteria.

The study retrospectively evaluated pediatric patients treated for supracondylar humerus fractures at different centers between 2010 and 2020. Patients were divided into two groups based on the treatment method: open reduction-percutaneous fixation and closed reduction-percutaneous fixation. The researchers used the Gartland classification to include type IIb and type III fractures, excluding type IIa due to its lack of rotational deformity information. Radiological assessments focused on three criteria: humero-capitellar angle, anterior humeral line, and anterior coronoid line. The quality of reduction was categorized as perfect, good, intermediate, or bad based on these criteria. Statistical analyses were conducted to compare the outcomes between the two groups.

The study found no significant difference in sagittal plane reduction success between open and closed methods, suggesting that the choice of surgical technique does not impact early postoperative outcomes in this regard. The authors emphasize that achieving at least two out of three radiological criteria is crucial for adequate reduction. Future studies could focus on correlating these radiological findings with functional outcomes to better understand their clinical significance. This research highlights the importance of comprehensive radiological assessment in ensuring successful treatment outcomes for pediatric supracondylar humerus fractures.

Ultrasound Diagnosis of Supracondylar Fractures in Children [170]

This is a machine-generated summary of:

Eckert, K.; Janssen, N.; Ackermann, O.; Schweiger, B.; Radeloff, E.; Liedgens, P. Ultrasound diagnosis of supracondylar fractures in children [170]
Published in: European Journal of Trauma and Emergency Surgery (2013)
Link to original: https://doi.org/10.1007/s00068-013-0306-2
Copyright of the summarized publication:
Springer-Verlag Berlin Heidelberg 2013
All rights reserved.

If you want to cite the papers, please refer to the original.

For technical reasons we could not place the page where the original quote is coming from.

Research Highlights

Supracondylar fractures (SCFs) of the humerus are prevalent injuries in children, often resulting from falls on an extended arm. These fractures are typically classified using the Gartland system, which categorizes them based on displacement and angulation. Diagnosing SCFs can be challenging, especially in young children, due to pain and incomplete ossification of bones, which complicates radiographic assessment. Now, a new study by K. Eckert and colleagues explores the use of ultrasound (US) as an alternative imaging method to standard radiographs for diagnosing SCFs in children, aiming to reduce radiation exposure.

The study was conducted in an urban pediatric emergency department and involved children aged 1–12 years with suspected SCFs. Excluding those with obvious dislocation or severe swelling, each child underwent US followed by standard radiography. The US examinations were performed by experienced pediatric emergency physicians using a high-frequency linear scanner. The researchers assessed the presence of cortical gaps or bulging and positive dorsal fat pad signs as indicators of fractures. Radiographic findings served as the reference standard for comparison. The study found that US had a sensitivity of 95% and a specificity of 98% for detecting SCFs compared to radiographs, demonstrating its potential as a reliable diagnostic tool.

The study suggests that US could serve as a primary imaging modality for evaluating suspected SCFs in children, potentially reducing the need for radiographs when fractures are unlikely. Future studies could focus on refining US techniques to differentiate between stable and unstable fractures more accurately and assess its application across various emergency settings. As more emergency physicians gain experience with US, it may become a standard practice for initial fracture evaluation in pediatric cases, minimizing radiation exposure and improving diagnostic efficiency.

Diagnostic Accuracy of the Shaft-Condylar Angle for an Incomplete Supracondylar Fracture of Elbow in Children [171]

This is a machine-generated summary of:

Sukvanich, Pawaris; Samun, Peen; Kongmalai, Pinkawas Diagnostic accuracy of the shaft-condylar angle for an incomplete supracondylar fracture of elbow in children [171]
Published in: European Journal of Orthopaedic Surgery & Traumatology (2019)
Link to original: https://doi.org/10.1007/s00590-019-02489-1
Copyright of the summarized publication:
Springer-Verlag France SAS, part of Springer Nature 2019
All rights reserved.

If you want to cite the papers, please refer to the original.

For technical reasons we could not place the page where the original quote is coming from.

Research Highlights

Supracondylar fractures of the humerus are among the most common injuries in children, often resulting from falls onto an outstretched hand. These fractures can lead to significant complications, including nerve injuries and deformities like cubitus varus. Accurate diagnosis is crucial, especially for incomplete fractures that may not show obvious displacement on X-rays. Traditional diagnostic methods rely on signs such as the posterior fat pad sign and anterior humeral line (AHL) displacement, but these can be insufficient in certain cases. Now, a new study by Pawaris Sukvanich and colleagues explores the diagnostic potential of the shaft-condylar angle (SCA) and lateral capitellohumeral angle (LCHA) in identifying incomplete supracondylar fractures in children.

The study conducted a retrospective review of pediatric patients with elbow injuries at MSMC hospital over a 2-year period. Excluding those with complete fractures or other elbow injuries, the researchers focused on patients with incomplete fractures and those without fractures. Two orthopedic surgeons measured the SCA and LCHA on lateral elbow films to assess their diagnostic accuracy. The SCA was evaluated using a cut-off point of 40°, while the LCHA was assessed with a cut-off point of 30°. The study calculated sensitivity, specificity, positive predictive value (PPV), and negative predictive value (NPV) for both angles. Results showed that while the SCA had moderate sensitivity, it demonstrated high specificity and accuracy, suggesting its utility in diagnosing incomplete supracondylar fractures.

The findings indicate that the SCA could serve as a valuable diagnostic tool for identifying incomplete supracondylar fractures when traditional methods fall short. With high specificity and accuracy, the SCA may help guide treatment decisions by identifying cases likely to involve displacement. Future study could focus on prospective analyses to confirm these results and explore inter- and intra-observer reliability further. Additionally, integrating SCA measurements into routine diagnostic protocols could enhance early detection and improve outcomes for pediatric patients with elbow injuries.

Long-Arm Splinting Versus Above-Elbow Casting for Type 1 Supracondylar Fractures of the Humerus in Children: A Randomized Controlled Trial [172]

This is a machine-generated summary of:

Siu, Caitlyn; Farrell, Sarah; Schaeffer, Emily K.; Doan, Quynh; Dobbe, Ashlee; Bone, Jeffrey; Reilly, Christopher W.; Mulpuri, Kishore Long-Arm Splinting Versus Above-Elbow Casting for Type 1 Supracondylar Fractures of the Humerus in Children: a Randomized Controlled Trial [172]

Published in: SN Comprehensive Clinical Medicine (2023)
Link to original: https://doi.org/10.1007/s42399-023-01417-z
Copyright of the summarized publication:
The Author(s), under exclusive licence to Springer Nature Switzerland AG 2023
Copyright comment: Springer Nature or its licensor (e.g. a society or other partner) holds exclusive rights to this article under a publishing agreement with the author(s) or other rightsholder(s); author self-archiving of the accepted manuscript version of this article is solely governed by the terms of such publishing agreement and applicable law.
All rights reserved.

If you want to cite the papers, please refer to the original.

For technical reasons we could not place the page where the original quote is coming from.

Research Highlights

Supracondylar fractures of the humerus are the most common type of elbow fracture in children, accounting for a significant portion of pediatric elbow injuries. These fractures are typically stable and can be effectively treated with immobilization methods such as long-arm splinting or above-elbow casting. Despite the prevalence of these fractures, there is a lack of studies directly comparing the efficacy of these two treatment methods. Now, a new study by Caitlyn Siu and colleagues addresses this gap by conducting a randomized controlled trial (RCT) to compare long-term outcomes between long-arm splinting and above-elbow casting for Gartland type I supracondylar humerus (SCH) fractures in children.

The study was conducted at BC Children's Hospital and involved children aged 3–10 years diagnosed with type I SCH fractures. Participants were randomized into two groups: one receiving above-elbow casting and the other receiving long-arm splinting. Due to visible differences between treatments, blinding was not feasible; however, outcome assessors were blinded to treatment allocation. The primary outcome was the change in Baumann's angle from initial to 6-month follow-up radiographs, with secondary outcomes including functional limb scores and complication rates. The study faced challenges in recruitment and follow-up, leading to its treatment as a pilot study. Despite these limitations, preliminary results suggested that long-arm splinting might offer comparable radiographic and functional outcomes to above-elbow casting.

The study highlights potential advantages of long-arm splinting, such as at-home removal, which reduces hospital visits—a benefit particularly relevant during the COVID-19 pandemic. However, due to the small sample size and incomplete follow-up data, definitive conclusions could not be drawn. Future studies with larger cohorts and comprehensive follow-up are needed to validate these findings. The insights gained from this pilot study can inform the design of future trials aimed at establishing non-inferiority of long-arm splinting compared to traditional casting for pediatric type I SCH fractures.

Operative Management of Type III Extension Supracondylar Fractures in Children [173]

This is a machine-generated summary of:

Kazimoglu, Cemal; Çetin, Murat; Şener, Muhittin; Aguş, Haluk; Kalanderer, Önder
Operative management of type III extension supracondylar fractures in children [173]
Published in: International Orthopaedics (2008)
Link to original: https://doi.org/10.1007/s00264-008-0605-0
Copyright of the summarized publication:
Springer-Verlag 2008
All rights reserved.

If you want to cite the papers, please refer to the original.

For technical reasons we could not place the page where the original quote is coming from.

Research Highlights

Supracondylar fractures of the humerus are a common injury in children, particularly before the age of seven, and present significant challenges in surgical treatment, especially for type III fractures. These fractures, classified by Gartland's criteria, can lead to complications such as malunion, elbow stiffness, and neurovascular injuries. Despite established guidelines for type I and II fractures, there remains controversy over the optimal treatment for type III fractures. Now, a new study by Cemal Kazimoglu and colleagues evaluates the outcomes of two different treatment approaches—closed reduction with percutaneous pinning (CRPF) and open reduction with internal fixation (ORIF)—for type III supracondylar humerus fractures in children.

The study involved children treated at two different institutes, each employing distinct protocols for managing displaced Gartland type III extension fractures. At one institute, patients underwent primarily open reduction through a lateral incision with various pin configurations based on fracture stability. In contrast, the other institute utilized closed reduction with percutaneous cross-pinning. The researchers assessed medical records for fracture details, surgical timing, and postoperative complications such as infection and nerve injury. Patients were followed up radiologically and clinically to evaluate functional and cosmetic outcomes using Flynn's criteria. Statistical analysis revealed no significant differences between the two groups in terms of cosmetic and functional results, although each method had its own set of complications.

The study advances our understanding of treatment options for type III supracondylar humerus fractures by demonstrating that both CRPF and ORIF can yield satisfactory outcomes. While closed reduction with cross-pinning is effective if stable fixation is achieved, open reduction remains a viable alternative when technical difficulties arise or after unsuccessful closed attempts. Future study could focus on refining pin configurations to minimize complications like ulnar nerve palsy while maintaining fracture stability. The findings suggest that surgeons should consider their experience and the specific fracture characteristics when choosing between these treatment methods.

Minimally Invasive Techniques Utilizing the "Joy Stick" Method for Managing Irreducible Flexion-Type Supracondylar Fractures of the Humerus in Older Children [174]

This is a machine-generated summary of:

Li, Yang; Feng, Yongyi; Chu, XiangJun; Yuan, Yue; Yuan, Yi; Sun, Jun Minimally invasive techniques utilizing the "Joy Stick" method for managing irreducible flexion-type supracondylar fractures of the humerus in older children [174]

Published in: Journal of Orthopaedic Surgery and Research (2024)
Link to original: https://doi.org/10.1186/s13018-024-04922-6
Copyright of the summarized publication:
The Author(s) 2024
License: OpenAccess CC BY + CC0 4.0

This article is licensed under a Creative Commons Attribution-NonCommercial-NoDerivatives 4.0 International License, which permits any non-commercial use, sharing, distribution and reproduction in any medium or format, as long as you give appropriate credit to the original author(s) and the source, provide a link to the Creative Commons licence, and indicate if you modified the licensed material. You do not have permission under this licence to share adapted material derived from this article or parts of it. The images or other third party material in this article are included in the article's Creative Commons licence, unless indicated otherwise in a credit line to the material. If material is not included in the article's Creative Commons licence and your intended use is not permitted by statutory regulation or exceeds the permitted use, you will need to obtain permission directly from the copyright holder. To view a copy of this licence, visit http://creativecommons.org/licenses/by-nc-nd/4.0/.

If you want to cite the papers, please refer to the original.

For technical reasons we could not place the page where the original quote is coming from.

Research Highlights

Supracondylar fractures of the humerus are the most common type of elbow injury in children, with extension-type fractures being more prevalent than flexion-type. However, flexion-type supracondylar fractures pose significant treatment challenges due to their higher complication rates and difficulty in achieving closed reduction, especially in older children with increased body weight. Traditional treatment methods, such as open reduction and Kirschner wire fixation, often result in significant surgical trauma and suboptimal recovery. Now, a new study by Yang Li and colleagues explores a minimally invasive technique using percutaneous poking reduction and Kirschner wire fixation to address these challenges effectively.

In this retrospective study conducted at Anhui Provincial Children's Hospital, Yang Li and colleagues analyzed cases of non-reducible flexion-type supracondylar humerus fractures in older children treated between September 2019 and September 2021. The study included patients aged 7 years or older who sustained Gartland type III-IV flexion-type fractures from falls. When traditional closed reduction methods failed, the team employed the "Joy-stick technique," using a Kirschner wire as a lever to achieve fracture reduction under C-arm fluoroscopy guidance. The procedure involved inserting Kirschner wires into the humeral epicondyles for cross fixation while avoiding nerve damage. Postoperative care included immobilization with a plaster cast for 4 weeks, followed by functional exercises to restore elbow joint function.

The study demonstrated that percutaneous poking reduction combined with Kirschner wire fixation offers a minimally invasive alternative for treating irreducible flexion-type supracondylar fractures in older children. This approach resulted in high rates of excellent and good outcomes according to the Flynn criteria, with no observed complications such as fracture re-displacement or nerve injury during follow-ups. Future studies could explore the long-term outcomes of this technique compared to other minimally invasive methods or investigate its application in different patient populations. The findings suggest that this method could be clinically promoted due to its simplicity, minimal trauma, and rapid recovery benefits.

Minimally Invasive Technique Combined with External Fixator in the Treatment of Pediatric Flexion-Type Humeral Supracondylar Fractures [175]

This is a machine-generated summary of:

Zhu, ChengMing; Feng, QiYuan; Ou, ZiXuan; Zhong, HaoBo; Tang, Xin Minimally invasive technique combined with external fixator in the treatment of pediatric flexion-type humeral supracondylar fractures [175]
Published in: Scientific Reports (2023)
Link to original: https://doi.org/10.1038/s41598-023-48158-6
Copyright of the summarized publication:
The Author(s) 2023
License: OpenAccess CC BY 4.0

This article is licensed under a Creative Commons Attribution 4.0 International License, which permits use, sharing, adaptation, distribution and reproduction in any medium or format, as long as you give appropriate credit to the original author(s) and the source, provide a link to the Creative Commons licence, and indicate if changes were made. The images or other third party material in this article are included in the article's Creative Commons licence, unless indicated otherwise in a credit line to the material. If material is not included in the article's Creative Commons licence and your intended use is not permitted by statutory regulation or exceeds the permitted use, you will need to obtain permission directly from the copyright holder. To view a copy of this licence, visit http://creativecommons.org/licenses/by/4.0/.

If you want to cite the papers, please refer to the original.

For technical reasons we could not place the page where the original quote is coming from.

Research Highlights

Supracondylar humeral fractures (SHF) are the most common elbow injuries in children, with the flexion-type being particularly rare and challenging to treat. These fractures often result from direct impact to the elbow, leading to a reverse angulation compared to the more common extension-type SHF. The standard treatment involves closed reduction with percutaneous pinning, but this can be difficult in severely displaced cases due to potential nerve damage and soft tissue interposition. Now, a new study by ChengMing Zhu and colleagues introduces a minimally invasive reduction technique combined with external fixation as an alternative approach for treating displaced flexion-type SHF in children.

The study retrospectively reviewed pediatric patients treated for displaced flexion-type SHF at the authors' institution. Patients were divided into two groups: Group A received traditional closed reduction, while Group B underwent the new minimally invasive technique after unsuccessful attempts at closed reduction. The minimally invasive method involved making a small incision at the fracture site and using mosquito forceps to separate soft tissues and achieve reduction. This was followed by stabilization with Schanz pins and percutaneous K-wire fixation under fluoroscopic guidance. The study evaluated outcomes based on operation time, radiographic results, and functional recovery using the MEPS and Flynn criteria.

The findings suggest that the minimally invasive technique offers comparable clinical outcomes to traditional methods but with shorter operation times and less carrying angle loss. The use of an external fixator provided stable fracture stabilization, allowing early mobilization and potentially reducing complications associated with repeated K-wire insertions. While promising, the study acknowledges limitations such as a small sample size and potential selection bias. Future studies with larger samples are needed to further validate these findings and refine the technique for broader clinical application.

Predictive Factors for Open Reduction of Flexion-Type Supracondylar Fracture of Humerus in Children [176]

This is a machine-generated summary of:

Sun, Jun; Shan, Jing; Meng, Lian; Liu, Tianjing; Wang, Enbo; Jia, Guoqiang
Predictive factors for open reduction of flexion-type supracondylar fracture of humerus in children [176]
Published in: BMC Musculoskeletal Disorders (2022)
Link to original: https://doi.org/10.1186/s12891-022-05798-5
Copyright of the summarized publication:
The Author(s) 2022
License: OpenAccess CC BY + CC0 4.0

This article is licensed under a Creative Commons Attribution 4.0 International License, which permits use, sharing, adaptation, distribution and reproduction in any medium or format, as long as you give appropriate credit to the original author(s) and the source, provide a link to the Creative Commons licence, and indicate if changes were made. The images or other third party material in this article are included in the article's Creative Commons licence, unless indicated otherwise in a credit line to the material. If material is not included in the article's Creative Commons licence and your intended use is not permitted by statutory regulation or exceeds the permitted use, you will need to obtain permission directly from the copyright holder. To view a copy of this licence, visit http://creativecommons.org/licenses/by/4.0/. The Creative Commons Public Domain

Dedication waiver (http://creativecommons.org/publicdomain/zero/1.0/) applies to the data made available in this article, unless otherwise stated in a credit line to the data.

If you want to cite the papers, please refer to the original.

For technical reasons we could not place the page where the original quote is coming from.

Research Highlights

Flexion-type supracondylar humerus fractures (SCHF) in children are uncommon, representing a small percentage of all SCHF cases. These fractures are classified by the degree of displacement, with Wilkins type III being the most severe, characterized by complete loss of cortical integrity. Traditional treatment involves closed reduction and internal fixation (CRIF), but this often fails in flexion-type SCHF, necessitating open reduction and internal fixation (ORIF). The factors contributing to CRIF failure in these cases remain poorly understood. Now, a new study by Jun Sun and colleagues retrospectively analyzes medical records to identify independent risk factors for ORIF in children with Wilkins type III flexion-type SCHF.

The study was conducted at a tertiary pediatric hospital in Anhui province, China, analyzing data from children treated for SCHF over several years. Patients were divided into ORIF and CRIF groups based on surgical outcomes. The researchers collected data on various factors, including age, sex, injury side, obesity, fracture deviation and level, rotation of the distal fragment, ulnar nerve injury, and time from injury to surgery. Statistical analyses were performed using SPSS software to identify associations between these factors and the likelihood of requiring ORIF. The study found that ulnar nerve injury and rotation of the distal fracture fragment were significant predictors of CRIF failure.

The findings suggest that specific anatomical features increase the risk of requiring ORIF in flexion-type SCHF. Ulnar nerve injury and rotational displacement of the distal fragment emerged as key risk factors. These insights can aid surgeons in preoperative planning by identifying patients at higher risk for CRIF failure. Future study could focus on refining surgical techniques or developing new strategies to address these risk factors effectively. Additionally, further research might explore whether similar patterns exist in other populations or settings to validate these findings across diverse clinical environments.

Dual Tension Band Wiring for Adolescent Supracondylar Fractures of the Humerus: Mechanical Assessment and a Clinical Series [177]

This is a machine-generated summary of:

Jitprapaikulsarn, Surasak; Chantarapanich, Nattapon; Apivatthakakul, Theerachai; Lertvilai, Pasin; Wanchat, Sujin; Gromprasit, Arthit; Sengpanich, Pasit; Mahaisavariya, Chantas; Saramas, Yotakarn; Simonet, Louis Paul Dual tension band wiring for adolescent supracondylar fractures of the humerus: mechanical assessment and a clinical series [177]

Published in: European Journal of Orthopaedic Surgery & Traumatology (2025)
Link to original: https://doi.org/10.1007/s00590-025-04454-7

Copyright of the summarized publication:
The Author(s), under exclusive licence to Springer-Verlag France SAS, part of Springer Nature 2025
Copyright comment: Springer Nature or its licensor (e.g. a society or other partner) holds exclusive rights to this article under a publishing agreement with the author(s) or other rightsholder(s); author self-archiving of the accepted manuscript version of this article is solely governed by the terms of such publishing agreement and applicable law.
All rights reserved.

If you want to cite the papers, please refer to the original.

For technical reasons we could not place the page where the original quote is coming from.

Research Highlights

Supracondylar fractures of the humerus (SCFH) are the most common elbow injuries in children, particularly affecting those aged 5–7 years. While non-displaced fractures can be treated conservatively, significantly displaced fractures often require surgical intervention to prevent complications such as cubitus varus. The standard treatment for pediatric SCFH is closed reduction and Kirschner-wire (K-wire) fixation, but there is ongoing debate about the optimal pinning construct. In adolescents, SCFH is less common and typically results from higher-energy trauma, leading to more complex fracture patterns. The literature on surgical options for adolescent SCFH (A-SCFH) is limited, with no consensus on the best treatment approach. Now, a new study by Surasak Jitprapaikulsarn and colleagues explores the efficacy of Dual Tension Band Wiring (DTBW) in A-SCFH through mechanical testing and clinical evaluation.

The study involved creating a synthetic model of an adolescent distal humerus fracture using 3D printing technology based on CT data from a 14-year-old patient. The researchers compared the mechanical performance of different fixation constructs, including Lateral Divergent Pinning (LDP) and DTBW, through bending and torsion tests. The DTBW construct demonstrated superior mechanical strength and stiffness compared to other pinning methods. Additionally, a retrospective clinical case series was conducted involving patients aged 10–16 years with displaced non-comminuted A-SCFH treated with DTBW. The surgical procedure involved open reduction via a paratricipital approach with K-wires and tension band wires applied to achieve stable fixation. Postoperative outcomes were assessed through radiographic evaluations and clinical scores such as MEPS and DASH.

The study's findings suggest that DTBW offers a mechanically robust alternative for managing non-comminuted A-SCFH, providing stable fixation while minimizing injury to the open physis compared to dual plating. Future study could focus on larger clinical trials comparing DTBW with other fixation techniques to validate its effectiveness in clinical practice further. Additionally, longer follow-up periods are necessary to assess potential late deformities in this transitional age group. Despite some limitations, such as the small sample size and retrospective nature of the clinical series, this research provides valuable insights into optimizing surgical treatment for adolescent humeral fractures.

A Comparative Study of Two Percutaneous Pinning Techniques (Lateral vs Medial–Lateral) for Gartland Type III Pediatric Supracondylar Fracture of the Humerus [178]

This is a machine-generated summary of:

Prashant, Kumar; Lakhotia, Devendra; Bhattacharyya, Tulsi Das; Mahanta, Anil Kumar; Ravoof, Aakhil A comparative study of two percutaneous pinning techniques (lateral vs medial–lateral) for Gartland type III pediatric supracondylar fracture of the humerus [178]
Published in: Journal of Orthopaedics and Traumatology (2016)
Link to original: https://doi.org/10.1007/s10195-016-0410-2
Copyright of the summarized publication:
The Author(s) 2016
License: OpenAccess CC BY 4.0

This article is distributed under the terms of the Creative Commons Attribution 4.0 International License (http://creativecommons.org/licenses/by/4.0/), which permits unrestricted use, distribution, and reproduction in any medium, provided you give appropriate credit to the original author(s) and the source, provide a link to the Creative Commons license, and indicate if changes were made.

If you want to cite the papers, please refer to the original.

For technical reasons we could not place the page where the original quote is coming from.

Research Highlights

Supracondylar humerus fractures are common injuries in children, particularly affecting the elbow joint, with peak incidence occurring between certain ages. These fractures can lead to complications such as malunion, ischemic contracture, and neurovascular damage. The preferred treatment method for displaced extension-type supracondylar humeral fractures is closed reduction with percutaneous pin stabilization. However, there is ongoing debate regarding the optimal pinning technique—whether lateral or crossed medial-lateral pin fixation is more effective. Now, a new study by Kumar Prashant and colleagues investigates the efficacy of these two pinning techniques in terms of stability, functional outcomes, and risk of iatrogenic ulnar nerve injury.

The study was conducted as a prospective, single-blinded randomized control trial at Gauhati Medical College and Hospital in India over 1 year. Participants included children aged between specific years with closed Gartland type III supracondylar humeral fractures. The researchers randomly assigned patients to either lateral entry or medial-lateral entry pin fixation groups using a computer-generated randomization table. Surgical techniques were standardized across both groups, with procedures performed by an experienced orthopedic surgeon under general anesthesia. Postoperative care included radiographic evaluations and regular follow-ups to assess fracture stability and functional outcomes. The study found no significant differences between the two groups regarding major loss of reduction or iatrogenic ulnar nerve injury.

The findings suggest that both lateral and medial-lateral pinning techniques provide satisfactory outcomes for treating supracondylar humerus fractures in children, with no significant difference in functional results or complication rates. However, the study's small sample size limits the generalizability of these results. Future studies involving larger patient populations and long-term follow-up are necessary to further elucidate the differences between these techniques and optimize treatment protocols for pediatric supracondylar humerus fractures.

A New Technique of Intramedullary Elastic Reduction of the "De-sharpened" Kirschner Wire for the Treatment of Gartland Type III Posterolateral Displaced Supracondylar Fracture of the Humerus in Children [179]

This is a machine-generated summary of:

Lin, Yudong; Hua, Zhongtuo; Zhou, Cheng; Chen, Saiwen; Sun, Xiwei; Liu, Fang; Meng, Ge; Zhang, Sicheng; Sun, Jun A new technique of intramedullary elastic reduction of the "de-sharpened" Kirschner wire for the treatment of Gartland type III posterolateral displaced supracondylar fracture of the humerus in children [179]
Published in: European Journal of Medical Research (2024)
Link to original: https://doi.org/10.1186/s40001-024-01671-4
Copyright of the summarized publication:
The Author(s) 2024
License: OpenAccess CC BY + CC0 4.0

This article is licensed under a Creative Commons Attribution 4.0 International License, which permits use, sharing, adaptation, distribution and reproduction in any medium or format, as long as you give appropriate credit to the original author(s) and the source, provide a link to the Creative Commons licence, and indicate if changes were made. The images or other third party material in this article are included in the article's Creative Commons licence, unless indicated otherwise in a credit line to the material. If material is not included in the article's Creative Commons licence and your intended use is not permitted by statutory regulation or exceeds the permitted use, you will need to obtain permission directly from the copyright holder. To view a copy of this licence, visit http://creativecommons.org/licenses/by/4.0/. The Creative Commons Public Domain Dedication waiver (http://creativecommons.org/publicdomain/zero/1.0/) applies to the data made available in this article, unless otherwise stated in a credit line to the data.

If you want to cite the papers, please refer to the original.

For technical reasons we could not place the page where the original quote is coming from.

Research Highlights

Supracondylar fractures of the humerus are the most common type of elbow fracture in children, with extension fractures being particularly prevalent. Gartland type III fractures, characterized by severe displacement, typically require closed reduction and percutaneous Kirschner wire fixation. However, traditional three-dimensional reduction methods can be challenging, especially for posterolateral displaced fractures, due to difficulties in correcting coronal and rotational deformities and maintaining fracture stability. Now, a new study by Yudong Lin and colleagues explores the use of intramedullary elastic reduction with a "de-sharpened" Kirschner wire as an alternative treatment for these complex fractures.

In this study, patients with posterolateral displaced supracondylar fractures were divided into two groups: one treated with the novel intramedullary elastic reduction technique using a de-sharpened Kirschner wire, and the other with traditional three-dimensional reduction methods. The researchers employed general anesthesia and brachial plexus block anesthesia during surgery. The de-sharpened Kirschner wire was inserted into the medullary cavity of the humerus to aid in fracture reduction. This method aimed to correct sagittal displacement using the posterior periosteal hinge and adjust coronal deformities through the elastic force of the wire. The study compared operation time, intraoperative fluoroscopy frequency, clinical healing time, and postoperative outcomes between the two groups.

The findings suggest that intramedullary elastic reduction with a de-sharpened Kirschner wire offers several advantages over traditional methods. It reduces operation time and intraoperative fluoroscopy frequency while effectively correcting coronal and rotational deformities. The technique also minimizes soft tissue injury and potential complications such as osteomyelitis or nerve damage. Future studies could focus on larger sample sizes and biomechanical testing to further validate these results and refine the technique's application in clinical practice. This approach may represent a promising advancement in treating complex pediatric elbow fractures.

A Prospective Randomised, Controlled Clinical Trial Comparing Medial and Lateral Entry Pinning with Lateral Entry Pinning for Percutaneous Fixation of Displaced Extension Type Supracondylar Fractures of the Humerus in Children [180]

This is a machine-generated summary of:

Maity, Abhijan; Saha, Debasish; Roy, Debasis Sinha A prospective randomised, controlled clinical trial comparing medial and lateral entry pinning with lateral entry pinning for percutaneous fixation of displaced extension type supracondylar fractures of the humerus in children [180]
Published in: Journal of Orthopaedic Surgery and Research (2012)
Link to original: https://doi.org/10.1186/1749-799x-7-6
Copyright of the summarized publication:
Maity et al.; licensee BioMed Central Ltd. 2012
License: OpenAccess CC BY 2.0

This article is published under license to BioMed Central Ltd. This is an Open Access article distributed under the terms of the Creative Commons Attribution License (http://creativecommons.org/licenses/by/2.0), which permits unrestricted use, distribution, and reproduction in any medium, provided the original work is properly cited.

If you want to cite the papers, please refer to the original.

For technical reasons we could not place the page where the original quote is coming from.

Research Highlights

Supracondylar fractures of the humerus are the most common type of elbow fracture in children, often leading to complications such as neurovascular injuries and malunion. The standard treatment involves closed reduction and percutaneous pin fixation, but there is ongoing debate about the optimal pinning method. Crossed medial-lateral pinning offers greater biomechanical stability but poses a risk of iatrogenic ulnar nerve injury, while lateral pinning is safer for the nerve but less stable. Now, a new study by Abhijan Maity and colleagues compares these two methods to determine their efficacy and safety in treating displaced extension-type supracondylar fractures in children.

The study was a single-center, prospective, randomized controlled trial conducted at the Department of Orthopaedics and Traumatology. Children with unilateral displaced Gartland type II and III fractures were randomly assigned to receive either crossed medial-lateral or two-lateral pin fixation. Surgery was performed under general anesthesia with fluoroscopic guidance, following standardized techniques for each pinning method. Postoperative care included specific protocols for pin site management and follow-up assessments at 3 weeks, 6 weeks, and 3 months post-surgery. The primary outcome measure was the major loss of reduction, defined by changes in the Baumann angle between intraoperative and 3-month follow-up radiographs.

The study found no significant differences between the two groups regarding iatrogenic ulnar nerve injury or loss of reduction grading. These findings align with previous studies that also reported no significant differences between the two methods in terms of safety and efficacy. The prospective randomized design is a major strength of this study, ensuring uniformity in surgical technique and follow-up assessments. However, limitations include the lack of blinding for surgeons and patients and a notable number of participants lost to follow-up. Future studies could focus on larger sample sizes or explore alternative techniques to further refine treatment strategies for these common pediatric fractures.

Treatment of Supracondylar Fractures of the Humerus in Children through an Anterior Approach Is a Safe and Effective Method [181]

This is a machine-generated summary of:

Ersan, Onder; Gonen, Emel; Arik, Ahmet; Dasar, Uygar; Ates, Yalim Treatment of supracondylar fractures of the humerus in children through an anterior approach is a safe and effective method [181]
Published in: International Orthopaedics (2008)
Link to original: https://doi.org/10.1007/s00264-008-0668-y
Copyright of the summarized publication:
Springer-Verlag 2008
All rights reserved.

If you want to cite the papers, please refer to the original.

For technical reasons we could not place the page where the original quote is coming from.

Research Highlights

Supracondylar humerus fractures are the most common type of pediatric elbow fractures, often requiring surgical intervention when displaced. While closed reduction and percutaneous pinning are standard treatments, open reduction is necessary in cases with neurovascular compromise or when closed methods fail. Now, a new study by Onder Ersan and colleagues explores the anterior approach for open reduction in pediatric supracondylar humerus fractures, a method that has been less frequently documented in clinical literature.

In this prospective study, Ersan and his team operated on children with displaced supracondylar humerus fractures using the anterior approach. The procedure involved making an incision along the anterior skin crease of the elbow to access the fracture site, allowing for direct visualization and manipulation of the fracture fragments. The fractures were stabilized using two Kirschner wires inserted from the medial and lateral epicondyles. The study included detailed clinical and radiological examinations pre- and post-operation, with follow-ups scheduled to monitor recovery. The operations were performed by residents under close supervision, ensuring adherence to protocol and minimizing complications.

The study demonstrated that the anterior approach is a viable option for treating these fractures, offering excellent visibility of the fracture site and surrounding structures. Patients showed satisfactory recovery with no significant complications such as ulnar nerve damage or loss of fixation. The aesthetic outcome of the incision was also favorable. Future studies could focus on randomized trials across multiple centers to further validate these findings and potentially recommend the anterior approach as a standard practice for cases requiring open reduction. This research contributes valuable insights into surgical techniques for pediatric elbow fractures, emphasizing safety and efficacy in treatment outcomes.

Reduction and Stabilization of Acute, Displaced Supracondylar Fractures of Distal Humerus in Children Using the Sauvé-Kapandji Technique [182]

This is a machine-generated summary of:

Saeed, Muhammad Zahid; Aktselis, Ioannis; Mann, H. A.; Kumar, K. H. Sunil; Goddard, Nicholas Reduction and stabilization of acute, displaced supracondylar fractures of distal humerus in children using the Sauvé-Kapandji technique [182]
Published in: European Orthopaedics and Traumatology (2015)
Link to original: https://doi.org/10.1007/s12570-015-0309-z
Copyright of the summarized publication:
EFORT 2015
All rights reserved.

If you want to cite the papers, please refer to the original.

For technical reasons we could not place the page where the original quote is coming from.

Research Highlights

Supracondylar fractures are among the most common fracture types in children, particularly those under the age of 10, accounting for a significant percentage of pediatric fractures. These fractures are classified into four types according to the Gartland classification, with type III being completely displaced and prone to complications such as neurovascular injury. Achieving and maintaining reduction is crucial for proper healing and functional outcomes. Now, a new study by Muhammad Zahid Saeed and colleagues explores a closed method of reducing and stabilizing displaced supracondylar fractures using the Sauvé-Kapandji technique.

The study involved 13 children, aged 5–12 years, who sustained displaced Gartland type III supracondylar fractures from falls during sports activities. All patients underwent surgery within 24 h of admission. The procedure was performed with the patient in a supine position under general anesthesia. The Sauvé-Kapandji technique was employed, involving the insertion of a K-wire to lever and reduce the distal fragment without compromising neurovascular structures. Additional cross Kirschner wires were used for stabilization. Postoperative care included immobilization in an above-elbow back-slab and follow-up assessments over several months to evaluate healing and function.

The study demonstrated that the Sauvé-Kapandji technique is effective in achieving stable reduction of supracondylar fractures with minimal complications. All patients achieved full range of motion within weeks postoperatively, except one who had a minor extension loss that resolved by 1 year. The authors suggest that this method offers a reliable alternative when initial closed reduction attempts fail, avoiding open surgery's potential complications. Future study could focus on comparing this technique with other methods in larger cohorts to further validate its efficacy and safety profile.

Locking Plate Versus External Fixation in the Treatment of Displaced Femoral Supracondylar Fracture in Children [183]

This is a machine-generated summary of:

Li, Jin; Guo, Xikai; Wang, Hai Qiang; Yue, Changjie; Chen, Kailei; Ma, Jiewen; Wang, Jing; Tang, Xin Locking plate versus external fixation in the treatment of displaced femoral supracondylar fracture in children [183]
Published in: Journal of Orthopaedic Surgery and Research (2020)
Link to original: https://doi.org/10.1186/s13018-020-01759-7
Copyright of the summarized publication:
The Author(s) 2020
License: OpenAccess CC BY + CC0 4.0

This article is licensed under a Creative Commons Attribution 4.0 International License, which permits use, sharing, adaptation, distribution and reproduction in any medium or format, as long as you give appropriate credit to the original author(s) and the source, provide a link to the Creative Commons licence, and indicate if changes were made. The images or other third party material in this article are included in the article's Creative Commons licence, unless indicated otherwise in a credit line to the material. If material is not included in the article's Creative Commons licence and your intended use is not permitted by statutory regulation or exceeds the permitted use, you will need to obtain permission directly from the copyright holder. To view a copy of this licence, visit http://creativecommons.org/licenses/by/4.0/. The Creative Commons Public Domain Dedication waiver (http://creativecommons.org/publicdomain/zero/1.0/) applies to the data made available in this article, unless otherwise stated in a credit line to the data.

If you want to cite the papers, please refer to the original.

For technical reasons we could not place the page where the original quote is coming from.

Research Highlights

Supracondylar femoral fractures (SFF) are rare but serious injuries in children, often leading to complications such as growth arrest, angular deformity, and joint motion limitations. Despite the availability of various surgical interventions like external fixation and locking plate fixation, the optimal treatment method for pediatric SFF remains unclear. Now, a new study by Jin Li and colleagues evaluates the clinical outcomes of locking plate versus external fixation in treating SFF in children, aiming to provide clarity on the most effective approach.

The study involved a retrospective review of medical records from patients treated for SFF at the authors' institution between April and August. Patients were included if they had confirmed SFF on radiographs and underwent surgical procedures with either locking plate or external fixation, with follow-up until complete clinical and radiographic union or at least 6 months. The study excluded cases with intra-articular fractures, knee ligament tears, neurovascular injuries, congenital anomalies, or significant comorbidities. In the locking plate group, open reduction was performed under general anesthesia with careful placement of the plate to avoid damage to surrounding structures. In contrast, the external fixation group underwent traction reduction with pins inserted to stabilize the fracture without spanning the knee joint. Both groups received postoperative care including antibiotics and rehabilitation exercises.

The study found that both treatment methods resulted in satisfactory radiographic union and functional recovery without significant differences in postoperative knee range of motion or complications. However, external fixation had advantages such as shorter operation time, less intraoperative blood loss, and faster union time compared to locking plate fixation. Despite these benefits, external fixation did not show superior outcomes in terms of knee flexion range of motion compared to locking plates. Future studies could explore long-term outcomes and refine treatment protocols to further optimize care for pediatric SFF patients.

Open Versus Closed Reduction and K-Wire Fixation for Displaced Supracondylar Fracture of the Humerus in Children [184]

This is a machine-generated summary of:

Hussein al-Algawy, Alaa A.; Aliakbar, Adil Hasan; Witwit, Ibrahim H. N. Open versus closed reduction and K-wire fixation for displaced supracondylar fracture of the humerus in children [184]

Published in: European Journal of Orthopaedic Surgery & Traumatology (2018)
Link to original: https://doi.org/10.1007/s00590-018-2305-9
Copyright of the summarized publication:
Springer-Verlag France SAS, part of Springer Nature 2018
All rights reserved.

If you want to cite the papers, please refer to the original.

For technical reasons we could not place the page where the original quote is coming from.

Research Highlights

Supracondylar humerus fractures in children are the second most common type of fracture in young patients, accounting for a significant percentage of elbow fractures. Despite their prevalence, the optimal management of severely displaced supracondylar fractures remains controversial, with debates centering on whether closed reduction and percutaneous k-wire fixation or open reduction and internal fixation (ORIF) is more effective. Now, a new study by Alaa A. Hussein al-Algawy and colleagues aims to address this knowledge gap by comparing these two treatment methods in terms of outcomes, hospitalization duration, healing time, and complications.

The study was a retrospective comparative analysis involving pediatric patients with type III supracondylar fractures treated at two hospitals between September and October. Patients were divided into two groups based on the treatment protocol followed by each hospital: one group received ORIF, while the other underwent closed reduction with k-wire fixation. The study excluded cases with open fractures, neurovascular injuries, or unsuccessful initial closed reductions. Surgical techniques varied between groups; ORIF involved a posterolateral approach with triceps splitting and ulnar nerve protection, while closed reduction used an elbow support device for stabilization during k-wire insertion. Post-operative care included monitoring for complications such as nerve injury and assessing fracture union and range of motion using Flynn et al.'s criteria.

The study found no significant difference in final outcomes between the two groups according to Flynn et al.'s evaluation criteria. Both treatment methods yielded similar rates of excellent and good results, suggesting that closed reduction should be considered the first choice due to its shorter hospitalization time and lack of surgical scars. However, ORIF remains a viable option when closed reduction is not feasible. Future studies could explore larger sample sizes or different patient demographics to further validate these findings and refine treatment protocols for displaced supracondylar humerus fractures in children.

Peripheral Nerve Injuries Associated with Dislocated Supracondylar Fractures of Distal Humerus in Children: Incidence and Need of Surgical Treatment [185]

This is a machine-generated summary of:

Chrenko, Robert; Hanko, Martin; Grega, Marek; Sýkora, Ľubomír; Jáger, René
Peripheral nerve injuries associated with dislocated supracondylar fractures of distal humerus in children: incidence and need of surgical treatment [185]
Published in: Child's Nervous System (2024)
Link to original: https://doi.org/10.1007/s00381-024-06497-3
Copyright of the summarized publication:

The Author(s), under exclusive licence to Springer-Verlag GmbH Germany, part of Springer Nature 2024
Copyright comment: Springer Nature or its licensor (e.g. a society or other partner) holds exclusive rights to this article under a publishing agreement with the author(s) or other rightsholder(s); author self-archiving of the accepted manuscript version of this article is solely governed by the terms of such publishing agreement and applicable law.
All rights reserved.

If you want to cite the papers, please refer to the original.

For technical reasons we could not place the page where the original quote is coming from.

Research Highlights

Supracondylar fractures (SCFs) of the humerus are the most common type of pediatric fracture, often requiring surgical intervention due to potential complications such as arterial injuries and peripheral nerve damage. These nerve injuries can result from the initial trauma or as complications during surgical procedures like closed reduction and pinning with K-wires. Now, a new study by Robert Chrenko and colleagues at the Department of Pediatric Neurosurgery of the National Institute of Children's Diseases addresses the management of post-traumatic peripheral nerve injuries in children with SCFs, highlighting their experience and findings.

The study retrospectively analyzed clinical records of children treated for dislocated SCFs at their institution over a 1-year period. Patients were assessed preoperatively using X-rays to classify the fractures, and surgical techniques were chosen accordingly. Postoperative evaluations included neurological exams to identify any peripheral nerve injuries. In cases where nerve injury was confirmed, further assessments such as conduction studies and electromyography were conducted. If no significant improvement was observed after 3 months, neurosurgical revision was considered. This involved procedures like nerve deliberation or reconstruction using a sural nerve graft. The study found that 19% of patients experienced some form of peripheral nerve injury, with the ulnar nerve being most commonly affected.

The findings suggest that while most peripheral nerve injuries associated with SCFs are neurapraxias and recover spontaneously, a subset of patients may require surgical intervention to prevent permanent deficits. The study emphasizes the importance of regular neurological monitoring and a proactive approach in managing stagnant neurological deficits. Future study could explore alternative surgical techniques to minimize nerve injury risk or refine criteria for surgical intervention timing. The authors advocate for close collaboration between pediatric trauma surgeons, neurologists, and neurosurgeons to optimize outcomes for children with SCFs and associated nerve injuries.

The Fate of the Malrotated Elbow Supracondylar Fractures in Children: Is Varus Really a Problem? [186]

This is a machine-generated summary of:

Sanpera, Ignacio; Salom, Marta; Fenandez-Ansorena, Ana; Frontera-Juan, Guillem; Pizà-Vallespir, Gabriel The fate of the malrotated elbow supracondylar fractures in children: is varus really a problem? [186]
Published in: International Orthopaedics (2024)
Link to original: https://doi.org/10.1007/s00264-024-06153-0
Copyright of the summarized publication:
The Author(s) under exclusive licence to SICOT aisbl 2024
Copyright comment: Springer Nature or its licensor (e.g. a society or other partner) holds exclusive rights to this article under a publishing agreement with the author(s) or other rightsholder(s); author self-archiving of the accepted manuscript version of this article is solely governed by the terms of such publishing agreement and applicable law.
All rights reserved.

If you want to cite the papers, please refer to the original.

For technical reasons we could not place the page where the original quote is coming from.

Research Highlights

Extension supracondylar elbow fractures account for a significant portion of pediatric fractures, with their incidence remaining steady over time. These fractures, classified as type III according to the Gartland classification, are typically managed through closed reduction and percutaneous pin fixation. The outcome of these fractures is influenced by factors such as the quality of reduction, pin configuration, and fracture stability. Malrotation alignment, characterized by a mismatch between fracture sites on lateral radiographs, is a common issue that can lead to complications like cubitus varus deformity (CVD). Now, a new study by Ignacio Sanpera and colleagues investigates the effects of residual malrotation after supracondylar elbow fractures and its impact on arm function.

The study involved a retrospective review of postoperative radiographs from children who underwent surgical treatment for type III supracondylar fractures between 2015 and 2017. Patients with evidence of malrotation were identified based on metaphyseal overhang observed in X-rays. Exclusions were made for those with incomplete follow-up or additional injuries. Participants were invited for follow-up assessments, which included clinical and radiological evaluations. The study measured rotation using lateral rotation percentage techniques and assessed outcomes using Flynn's criteria and QuickDASH scores. Statistical analyses were conducted to explore associations between variables such as fracture type, rotation amount, and clinical outcomes.

The findings suggest that moderate malrotation does not significantly compromise functional outcomes in patients with supracondylar elbow fractures. While some patients exhibited asymmetry in shoulder rotation, this did not adversely affect their clinical results. The study highlights that most patients with malrotation achieve good or excellent outcomes according to Flynn's criteria. Future studies could focus on larger sample sizes to further elucidate the role of malrotation in these fractures and explore long-term complications such as posterolateral elbow instability or tardy ulnar palsy. Additionally, understanding the remodeling capacity in younger patients could provide insights into managing rotational deformities more effectively.

Postoperative Brachial Artery Entrapment Associated with Pediatric Supracondylar Fracture of the Humerus: A Case Report [187]

This is a machine-generated summary of:

Latz, David; Grassmann, Jan; Schiffner, Erik; Gehrmann, Sebastian; Duran, Mansur; Windolf, Joachim; Jungbluth, Pascal Postoperative brachial artery entrapment associated with pediatric supracondylar fracture of the humerus: a case report [187]
Published in: Journal of Medical Case Reports (2017)
Link to original: https://doi.org/10.1186/s13256-017-1240-4
Copyright of the summarized publication:
The Author(s). 2017
License: OpenAccess CC BY + CC0 4.0

This article is distributed under the terms of the Creative Commons Attribution 4.0 International License (http://creativecommons.org/licenses/by/4.0/), which permits unrestricted use, distribution, and reproduction in any medium, provided you give appropriate credit to the original author(s) and the source, provide a link to the Creative Commons license, and indicate if changes were made. The Creative Commons Public Domain Dedication waiver (http://creativecommons.org/publicdomain/zero/1.0/) applies to the data made available in this article, unless otherwise stated.

If you want to cite the papers, please refer to the original.

For technical reasons we could not place the page where the original quote is coming from.

Research Highlights

Supracondylar fractures of the humerus are common in children and are often classified using Gartland's system, which assesses the degree of displacement. These fractures, particularly when completely displaced, can lead to complications such as neurovascular injuries or compartment syndrome. Preoperative neurovascular assessment scores have been developed to improve evaluation in emergency settings. However, a new study by David Latz and colleagues highlights a rare vascular complication that occurred despite an unremarkable preoperative neurovascular examination, underscoring the importance of thorough postoperative assessments.

In this case study, a young boy presented with a severely displaced right elbow after a fall. Initial examinations showed no neurovascular deficits, and surgical intervention was promptly initiated. Closed reduction attempts failed, necessitating open reduction and internal fixation with K-wires. Post-surgery, the boy's arterial pulses were initially palpable, but he later experienced acute forearm pain and absent pulses while immobilized in a cast. A Doppler ultrasound revealed pulse absence in flexion but faint pulses in extension. Revision surgery identified brachial artery kinking due to entrapment by the fracture's tunica externa, which was resolved through microsurgical arteriolysis.

The case concluded with successful recovery following implant removal and physical therapy. At final follow-up, the boy exhibited excellent elbow function with full range of motion and no loss of carrying angle. This study highlights the potential for delayed neurovascular complications even when initial assessments appear normal. It suggests that future studies should focus on standardized postoperative neurovascular assessments across full elbow motion ranges to detect possible artery entrapments early. This approach could improve outcomes by ensuring timely intervention for circulatory failures post-surgery.

Spontaneous Humeral Torsion Deformity Correction after Displaced Supracondylar Fractures in Children [188]

This is a machine-generated summary of:

Hell, Anna K.; Gadomski, Claudia; Braunschweig, Lena Spontaneous humeral torsion deformity correction after displaced supracondylar fractures in children [188]
Published in: BMC Musculoskeletal Disorders (2021)
Link to original: https://doi.org/10.1186/s12891-021-04909-y
Copyright of the summarized publication:
The Author(s) 2021
License: OpenAccess CC BY + CC0 4.0

This article is licensed under a Creative Commons Attribution 4.0 International License, which permits use, sharing, adaptation, distribution and reproduction in any medium or format, as long as you give appropriate credit to the original author(s) and the source, provide a link to the Creative Commons licence, and indicate if changes were made. The images or other third party material in this article are included in the article's Creative Commons licence, unless indicated otherwise in a credit line to the material. If material is not included in the article's Creative Commons licence and your intended use is not permitted by statutory regulation or exceeds the permitted use, you will need to obtain permission directly from the copyright holder. To view a copy of this licence, visit http://creativecommons.org/licenses/by/4.0/. The Creative Commons Public Domain Dedication waiver (http://creativecommons.org/publicdomain/zero/1.0/) applies to the data made available in this article, unless otherwise stated in a credit line to the data.

If you want to cite the papers, please refer to the original.

For technical reasons we could not place the page where the original quote is coming from.

Research Highlights

Supracondylar humeral fractures (SCHF) are the most common type of pediatric elbow fractures, often resulting from falls onto an outstretched hand. These fractures are typically diagnosed through clinical evaluation and radiography, with unstable or displaced fractures requiring surgical intervention. The standard treatment involves closed reduction and percutaneous crossed pin fixation, which is generally effective but can lead to complications such as neurovascular lesions and cubitus varus (CV) deformity. CV is a complex deformity that can cause cosmetic and functional issues, yet there is no simple clinical method to measure humeral torsion deformity, which may contribute to CV. Now, a new study by Anna K. Hell and colleagues investigates the incidence of humeral torsion differences in children with displaced SCHF and their spontaneous changes over time using ultrasound.

The study was conducted as a prospective cohort analysis at a University Pediatric Trauma Centre, involving children with displaced SCHF who underwent surgical treatment. Participants were followed from the time of injury up to 12 months post-accident. The researchers used sonographic measurements to assess humeral torsion at multiple follow-up points: 6 weeks, 4 months, 6 months, and 12 months after the injury. Radiographic evaluations were also performed at various stages to assess fracture consolidation and potential rotational deformities. The sonographic method employed involved a standardized positioning device for accurate measurement of humeral torsion. Statistical analyses were conducted using Student's t-test and ANOVA to evaluate changes over time.

The study found that rotational deformity was present in 40% of the children 6 weeks post-injury, with significant improvements observed by 4 months. Younger children showed the most pronounced changes in humeral torsion, suggesting a higher correction potential due to growth-related factors. Despite these findings, the study acknowledges limitations such as a small sample size and variability in individual measurements. Future studies could explore larger populations to establish age-dependent normal values for humeral torsion and investigate whether athletic activity influences torsion development post-SCHF. This research provides valuable insights into the natural correction mechanisms of post-traumatic rotational deformities in children, highlighting the potential for spontaneous recovery facilitated by growth dynamics.

Evaluation and Management of Pulseless Pink/Pale Hand Syndrome Coexisting with Supracondylar Fractures of the Humerus in Children [116]

This is a machine-generated summary of:

Matuszewski, Łukasz Evaluation and management of pulseless pink/pale hand syndrome coexisting with supracondylar fractures of the humerus in children [116]
Published in: European Journal of Orthopaedic Surgery & Traumatology (2013)
Link to original: https://doi.org/10.1007/s00590-013-1337-4
Copyright of the summarized publication:
The Author(s) 2013
License: OpenAccess CC BY 2.0

This article is distributed under the terms of the Creative Commons Attribution License which permits any use, distribution, and reproduction in any medium, provided the original author(s) and the source are credited.

If you want to cite the papers, please refer to the original.

For technical reasons we could not place the page where the original quote is coming from.

Research Highlights

Supracondylar fractures of the humerus are the most common elbow injuries in children, often resulting from high-energy impacts that cause significant displacement of the bone. These fractures can lead to severe soft tissue injuries, including damage to arteries and nerves, particularly the brachial artery and median nerve. Despite seemingly straightforward diagnosis and treatment, errors or oversights can have irreversible consequences. Now, a new study by Łukasz Matuszewski and colleagues at the Medical University of Lublin explores treatment approaches for supracondylar fractures with associated vascular injuries in children, emphasizing the management of cases with a "pink pulseless hand."

The study involved a retrospective analysis of pediatric patients treated for supracondylar humeral fractures at the Clinic of Pediatric Surgery and Traumatology. Researchers classified fractures using Gartland's scale and assessed vascular status through clinical examination, capillary refill tests, oxygen saturation measurements, and Doppler ultrasound. The study focused on patients with Grade III extension-type injuries. Closed reduction and stabilization with K-wires were performed under general anesthesia for most cases. In instances where closed reduction failed to restore radial pulse or proper perfusion, surgical exploration was conducted using a standard anterior approach. The study found that conservative treatment led to good outcomes in cases where anatomical reduction restored perfusion despite an absent radial pulse.

The findings suggest that children with well-perfused hands but absent radial pulses after closed reduction do not necessarily require routine brachial artery exploration. Instead, anatomical fracture reduction is crucial, and conservative management should be prioritized unless additional vascular compromise signs appear. Future studies could further refine diagnostic criteria and treatment protocols to optimize outcomes for pediatric patients with these complex injuries. The study underscores the importance of timely intervention and highlights advances in diagnostic tools and surgical techniques that have improved management outcomes for supracondylar fractures with vascular involvement.

Treatment of Pink Pulseless Hand Following Supracondylar Fractures of the Humerus in Children [189]

This is a machine-generated summary of:

Korompilias, A. V.; Lykissas, M. G.; Mitsionis, G. I.; Kontogeorgakos, V. A.; Manoudis, G.; Beris, A. E. Treatment of pink pulseless hand following supracondylar fractures of the humerus in children [189]
Published in: International Orthopaedics (2008)
Link to original: https://doi.org/10.1007/s00264-007-0509-4
Copyright of the summarized publication:
Springer-Verlag 2007
All rights reserved.

If you want to cite the papers, please refer to the original.
For technical reasons we could not place the page where the original quote is coming from.

Research Highlights

Supracondylar fractures of the humerus are prevalent among children, accounting for a significant percentage of elbow fractures in this demographic. These injuries typically result from falls on an outstretched arm and can lead to neurovascular complications, including brachial artery and nerve injuries. The management of a pulseless but well-perfused hand following such fractures remains contentious. Now, a new study by A. V. Korompilias and colleagues addresses this issue by exploring therapeutic approaches for children with supracondylar humeral fractures and a pink yet pulseless hand.

The study involved a retrospective review of displaced supracondylar humeral fractures in children, focusing on those with type III fractures according to Gartland's classification. The researchers assessed neurovascular injuries using physical examinations and Doppler sonography. For patients with a pink pulseless hand, emergency surgical treatment was performed if closed reduction did not restore the radial pulse. Surgical exploration included vascular reconstruction using microsurgical techniques when necessary. The study found that while some patients regained pulse after closed reduction, others required further surgical intervention to address brachial artery occlusions or spasms.

The findings suggest that immediate surgical exploration may be beneficial in cases where the radial pulse does not return after fracture reduction, even if the hand appears well-perfused. This approach could prevent potential complications associated with relying solely on collateral circulation. Future study could focus on long-term outcomes of surgical versus conservative management in similar cases to better inform treatment protocols. The study highlights the importance of timely intervention and thorough evaluation in managing these complex pediatric injuries.

Kirschner Wire Reconstruction of Medial and Lateral Column Periosteal Hinge in the Treatment of Multidirectionally Unstable Supracondylar Fracture of the Humerus in Children [190]

This is a machine-generated summary of:

Ma, Hai-Long; Sun, Xi-Wei; Liu, Fang; Hua, Zhong Tuo; Sun, Jun; Zhang, Si-Cheng Kirschner wire reconstruction of medial and lateral column periosteal hinge in the treatment of multidirectionally unstable supracondylar fracture of the humerus in children [190]
Published in: European Journal of Medical Research (2023)
Link to original: https://doi.org/10.1186/s40001-023-01560-2
Copyright of the summarized publication:
The Author(s) 2023
License: OpenAccess CC BY + CC0 4.0

This article is licensed under a Creative Commons Attribution 4.0 International License, which permits use, sharing, adaptation, distribution and reproduction in any medium or format, as long as you give appropriate credit to the original author(s) and the source, provide a link to the Creative Commons licence, and indicate if changes were made. The images or other third party material in this article are included in the article's Creative Commons licence, unless indicated otherwise in a credit line to the material. If material is not included in the article's Creative Commons licence and your intended use is not permitted by statutory regulation or exceeds the permitted use, you will need to obtain permission directly from the copyright holder. To view a copy of this licence, visit http://creativecommons.org/licenses/by/4.0/. The Creative Commons Public Domain Dedication waiver (http://creativecommons.org/publicdomain/zero/1.0/) applies to the data made available in this article, unless otherwise stated in a credit line to the data.

If you want to cite the papers, please refer to the original.

For technical reasons we could not place the page where the original quote is coming from.

Research Highlights

Supracondylar fractures of the humerus are the most common type of elbow fracture in children, with the extended fracture being particularly prevalent. The Gartland classification is widely used to guide treatment, with types I and IIA typically managed through outpatient manual reduction and plaster fixation, while types IIB and III often require closed reduction and percutaneous pinning. However, a subset of these fractures, known as modified Gartland type IV or multidirectionally unstable supracondylar fractures, present significant challenges due to their instability and the difficulty in achieving stable reduction before Kirschner wire placement. Now, a new study by Hai-Long Ma and colleagues explores a novel surgical technique involving Kirschner wire reconstruction of internal and lateral column periosteal hinges to improve outcomes for these complex fractures.

The study involved patients with multidirectionally unstable supracondylar fractures who were divided into two groups based on the surgical technique used. The study group underwent Kirschner wire reconstruction of the periosteal hinge assisted by closed reduction and internal fixation, while the control group received conventional closed reduction and Kirschner wire internal fixation. All surgeries were performed by the same team of surgeons using standardized procedures. The researchers compared operation time, intraoperative fluoroscopy times, fracture healing time, and functional outcomes between the two groups. Statistical analyses were conducted to determine the significance of differences observed in these parameters.

The findings indicate that both surgical methods achieved satisfactory results in terms of appearance and function postoperatively. However, the novel technique demonstrated advantages such as reduced operation time and fewer intraoperative fluoroscopy times compared to conventional methods. This approach also showed a lower rate of conversion to open reduction, suggesting improved stability during closed reduction attempts. Future study could focus on larger sample sizes to confirm these findings and explore long-term outcomes further. This research contributes valuable insights into optimizing surgical strategies for challenging pediatric elbow fractures, potentially guiding future clinical practice improvements.

Conclusion

In children, undisplaced supracondylar fractures can be treated conservatively, while displaced fractures require closed reduction and Kirschner wire fixation. If these methods fail, open reduction can be performed without compromising the final functional outcome. Despite the favorable prognosis, supracondylar fractures can still result in early and late complications.

Bibliography

1. Association BO. BOAST–Supracondylar Fractures in the Humerus in Children. https://www.boa.ac.uk/resources/knowledge-hub/boast-11-pdf.html. Accessed 9 Jan 2021.
2. Bales JG, Spencer HT, Wong MA, Fong Y-J, Zionts LE, Silva M. The effects of surgical delay on the outcome of pediatric supracondylar humeral fractures. J Pediatr Orthop. 2010;30(8):785–91.
3. Carmichael KD, Joyner K. Quality of reduction versus timing of surgical intervention for pediatric supracondylar humerus fractures. Orthopedics. 2006;29(7):628–32.
4. Cashman JP, Guerin SM, Hemsing M, McCormack D. Effect of deferred treatment of supracondylar humeral fractures. Surgeon. 2010;8(2):71–3.
5. Gupta N, Kay RM, Leitch K, Femino JD, Tolo VT, Skaggs DL. Effect of surgical delay on perioperative complications and need for open reduction in supracondylar humerus fractures in children. J Pediatr Orthop. 2004;24(3):245–8.
6. Han Q-L, Wang Y-H, Liu F. Comparison of complications and results of early versus delayed surgery for Gartland type III supracondylar humeral fractures in pediatric patients. Orthop Surg. 2011;3(4):242–6.
7. Iyengar SR, Hoffinger SA, Townsend DR. Early versus delayed reduction and pinning of type III displaced supracondylar fractures of the humerus in children: a comparative study. J Orthop Trauma. 1999;13(1):51–5.
8. Kronner JM Jr, Legakis JE, Kovacevic N, Thomas RL, Reynolds RAK, Jones ET. An evaluation of supracondylar humerus fractures: is there a correlation between postponing treatment and the need for open surgical intervention? J Child Orthop. 2013;7(2):131–7.
9. Kwiatkowska M, Dhinsa BS, Mahapatra AN. Does the surgery time affect the final outcome of type III supracondylar humeral fractures? J Clin Orthop Trauma. 2018;9(Suppl 1):S112–5.
10. Larson AN, Garg S, Weller A, Fletcher ND, Schiller JR, al Kwon M e. Operative treatment of type II supracondylar humerus fractures: does time to surgery affect complications? J Pediatr Orthop. 2014;34(4):382–7.
11. Leet AI, Frisancho J, Ebramzadeh E. Delayed treatment of type 3 supracondylar humerus fractures in children. J Pediatr Orthop. 2002;22(2):203–7.
12. Mayne AIW, Perry DC, Bruce CE. Delayed surgery in displaced paediatric supracondylar fractures: a safe approach? Results from a large UK tertiary paediatric trauma centre. Eur J Orthop Surg Traumatol. 2014;24(7):1107–10.
13. Mehlman CT, Strub WM, Roy DR, Wall EJ, Crawford AH. The effect of surgical timing on the perioperative complications of treatment of supracondylar humeral fractures in children. J Bone Jt Surg Am. 2001;83(3):323–7.
14. Murnaghan ML, Slobogean BL, Byrne A, Tredwell SJ, Mulpuri K. The effect of surgical timing on operative duration and quality of reduction in Type III supracondylar humeral fractures in children. J Child Orthop. 2010;4(2):153–8.
15. Prabhakar P, Ho CA. Delaying surgery in type III supracondylar humerus fractures does not lead to longer surgical times or more difficult reduction. J Orthop Trauma. 2019;33(8):e285–90.
16. Pullagura M, Odak S, Pratt R. Managing supracondylar fractures of the distal humerus in children in a district general hospital. Ann R Coll Surg Engl. 2013;95(8):582–5.
17. Schmid T, Joeris A, Slongo T, Ahmad SS, Ziebarth K. Displaced supracondylar humeral fractures: influence of delay of surgery on the incidence of open reduction, complications and outcome. Arch Orthop Trauma Surg. 2015;135(7):963–9.
18. Sibinski M, Sharma H, Bennet GC. Early versus delayed treatment of extension type-3 supracondylar fractures of the humerus in children. J Bone Jt Surg Br. 2006;88(3):380–1.
19. Yaokreh JB, Odehouri-Koudou TH, Tembely S, Dieth AG, Kouame DB, Ouattara O, et al. Delayed treatment of supracondylar elbow fractures in children. Orthop Traumatol Surg Res OTSR. 2012;98(7):808–12.

20. Walmsley PJ, Kelly MB, Robb JE, Annan IH, Porter DE. Delay increases the need for open reduction of type-III supracondylar fractures of the humerus. J Bone Jt Surg Br. 2006;88(4):528–30.
21. Farrow L, Ablett AD, Mills L, Barker S. Early versus delayed surgery for paediatric supracondylar humeral fractures in the absence of vascular compromise: a systematic review and meta-analysis. Bone Jt J. 2018;100(12):1535–41.
22. Silberstein MJ, Brodeur AE, Graviss ER, Atchawee L. Some vagaries of the capitellum. J Bone Joint Surg. 1981;A63:524–8.
23. de las Heras J, Duran D, de la Cerda J, Romanillos O, Martinez-Miranda J, Rodriguez-Merchan EC. Supracondylar fractures of the humerus in children. Clin Orthop Relat Res. 2005;432:57–64.
24. Biyani A, Gupta SP, Sharma JC. Determination of medial epicondylar epiphyseal angle for supracondylar humeral fractures in children. J Pediatr Orthop. 1993;13:94–7.
25. Roberts PH. Dislocation of the elbow. Br J Surg. 1969;56:806–15.
26. Rathfelder FJ, Paar O. Ultrasound as an alternative diagnostic measure for fractures during the growth phase. Unfallchirurg. 1995;98:645–9.
27. Moritz JD, Berthold LD, Soenksen SF, Alzen GF. Ultrasound in diagnosis of fractures in children: unnecessary harassment or useful addition to X-ray? Ultraschall Med. 2008;29(3):267–74.
28. Moritz JD, Hoffmann B, Meuser SH, et al. Is ultrasound equal to X-ray in pediatric fracture diagnosis? Rofo. 2010;182:706–14.
29. Ackermann O, Liedgens P, Eckert K, et al. Sonographische Diagnostik von metaphysären Wulstbrüchen. Unfallchirurg. 2009;112:706–11.
30. Williamson D, Watura R, Cobby M. Ultrasound imaging of forearm fractures in children: a viable alternative? J Accid Emerg Med. 2000;17:22–4.
31. Cheng JC, Lam TP, Maffulli N. Epidemiological features of supracondylar fractures of the humerus in Chinese children. J Pediatr Orthop B. 2001;10(1):63–7.
32. Suangyanon P, Chalayon O, Worawuthangkul K, Kaewpornsawan K, Ariyawatkul T, Eamsobhana P. Pediatric elbow measurement parameters: evaluation of the six angles in inter- and intra-observer reliability. J Clin Orthop Trauma. 2018; https://doi.org/10.1016/j.jcot.2018.07.019.
33. Skaggs DL, Flynn JM. Supracondylar fractures of the distal humerus. In: Beaty JH, Kasser JR, editors. Rockwood & Wilkins' fractures in children. 7th ed. Philadelphia: Lippincott Williams & Wilkins; 2010. p. 487–532.
34. Herring JA, Rathjen KE, Carter PR. Upper extremity injuries. In: Herring JA, editor. Tachdjian's pediatric orthopedics. 4th ed. Philadelphia: Saunders; 2007. p. 3152.
35. Price CT, Flynn JM. Management of fractures. In: Morrissy RT, Weinstein SL, editors. Lovell and Winter's pediatric orthopaedics. 6th ed. Philadelphia: Lippincott Williams & Wilkins; 2006. p. 1430–63.
36. Cuomo AV, Howard A, Hsueh S, Boutis K. Gartland type I supracondylar humerus fractures in children: is splint immobilization enough? Pediatr Emerg Care. 2012;28(11):1150–3.
37. Battagila TC, Armstrong DG, Schwend RM. Factors affecting forearm compartment pressures in children with supracondylar fractures of the humerus. J Pediatr Orthop. 2002;22:431–9.
38. Gartland JJ. Management of supracondylar fractures of the humerus in children. Surg Gynecol Obstet. 1959;109:145–54.
39. Rockwood CA Jr, Wilkins KE, Beaty JH. Fractures in children, vol. 3. Philadelphia: Lippincott-Raven; 1996.
40. Agus H, Kalanderer O, Kayalı C, Eryanılmaz G. Skeletal traction and delayed percutaneous fixation of complicated supracondylar humerus fractures due to delayed or unsuccessful reductions and extensive swelling in children. J Pediatr Orthop B. 2002;11(2):150–4.
41. Mulhall KJ, Abuzakuk T, Curtin W, O'Sullivan M. Displaced supracondylar fractures of the humerus in children. Int Orthop. 2000;24(4):221–3.
42. Sadiq MZ, Syed T, Travlos J. Management of grade III supracondylar fracture of the humerus by straight-arm lateral traction. Int Orthop. 2007;31(2):155–8.

43. Xiong Z, Zeng SD, Han S, Li SQ, Zeng QR, Wang L, et al. Regional epidemiological investigation of supracondylar fracture of humerus in children. Chin J Bone Joint. 2021;10(3):210–4.
44. Slongo T, Schmid T, Wilkins K, Joeris A. Lateral external fixation—a new surgical technique for displaced unreducible supracondylar humeral fractures in children. J Bone Joint Surg Am. 2008;90:1690–7.
45. Wei YS, Liu WL, Cui PF, Bai R, Li DH, Zhao ZQ, et al. Comparative study of ulna olecranon needle joystick technique in the treatment of multi-directional unstable supracondylar fractures of humerus in children. Chin J Pediatr Surg. 2020;41:542–9.
46. Green BM, Stone JD, Bruce RW Jr, Fletcher ND. The use of a transolecranon pin in the treatment of pediatric flexion-type supracondylar humerus fractures. J Pediatr Orthop. 2017;37(6):e347–52. https://doi.org/10.1097/BPO.0000000000000904. PMID: 27824796.
47. Kao HK, Lee WC, Yang WE, Chang CH. Treatment of displaced flexion-type pediatric supracondylar humeral fractures in the prone position. J Orthop Surg (Hong Kong). 2017;25(1):2309499016684412. https://doi.org/10.1177/2309499016684412. PMID: 29185384.
48. Kim KY, Conaway W, Schell R, Hennrikus WL. Prevalence of ulnar nerve palsy with flexion-type supracondylar fractures of the humerus. J Pediatr Orthop B. 2020;29(2):133–6. https://doi.org/10.1097/BPB.0000000000000702. PMID: 31856042.
49. Kazimoglu C, Cetin M, Sener M, Aguş H, Kalanderer O. Operative management of type III extension supracondylar fractures in children. Int Orthop. 2009;33(4):1089–94.
50. Flynn JC, Matthews JG, Benoit RL. Blind pinning of displaced supracondylar fractures of the humerus in children sixteen years' experience with long-term followup. J Bone Joint Surg Am. 1974;56(2):263–72.
51. De Boeck H. Flexion-type supracondylar elbow fractures in children. J Pediatr Orthop. 2001;21(4):460–3.
52. Chukwunyerenwa C, Orlik B, El-Hawary R, Logan K, Howard JJ. Treatment of flexion-type supracondylar fractures in children: the 'push-pull' method for closed reduction and percutaneous K-wire fixation. J Pediatr Orthop B. 2016;25(5):412–6. https://doi.org/10.1097/BPB.0000000000000241. PMID: 26517762
53. Havránek P, Pešl T, Hendrych J, Kučerová M. Supracondylar fracture of the humerus in childhood. Rozhl Chir. 2018;97(3):122–7.
54. Hart GM, Wilson DW, Arden GP. The operative management of the difficult supracondylar fracture of the humerus in the child. Injury. 1977;9(1):30–4.
55. Yen YM, Kocher MS. Lateral entry compared with medial and lateral entry pin fixation for completely displaced supracondylar humeral fractures in children. Surgical technique. J Bone Joint Surg Am. 2008;90(Suppl2):20–30.
56. Bashyal RK, et al. Complications after pinning of supracondylar distal humerus fractures. J Pediatr Orthop. 2009;29(7):704–8.
57. Wang R, et al. Closed reduction percutaneous intramedullary fixation with Kirschner wires in 4 children with displaced fractures of the distal humerus. Med Sci Monit: Int Med J Exp Clin Res. 2022;28:e935448.
58. Lee HY, Kim SJ. Treatment of displaced supracondylar fractures of the humerus in children by a pin leverage technique. J Bone Joint Sur Br. 2007;89(5):646–50.
59. Pei X, Mo Y, Huang P. Leverage application on Gartland type IV supracondylar humeral fracture in children. Int Orthop. 2016;40(11):2417–22.
60. Basaran SH, et al. A new joystick technique for unsuccessful closed reduction of supracondylar humeral fractures: minimum trauma. Eur J Orthop Surg Traumatol: Orthop Traumatol. 2015;25(2):297–303.
61. Das R, Borthakur B, Agarwala V, Ghosh S. Evaluation of anterior approach in failed closed reduction and delayed presentation of supracondylar humerus fractures in children. J Orthop. 2022;30:51–8.
62. Wilkins KE. The operative management of supracondylar fractures. Orthop Clin North Am. 1990;21(2):269–89.

63. Flynn K, Shah AS, Brusalis CM, et al. Flexion-type supracondylar humeral fractures: ulnar nerve injury increases risk of open reduction. J Bone Joint Surg Am. 2017;99(17):1485–7. https://doi.org/10.2106/JBJS.17.00068.
64. Kuoppala E, Parviainen R, Pokka T, Sirviö M, Serlo W, Sinikumpu JJ. Low incidence of flexion-type supracondylar humerus fractures but high rate of complications. Acta Orthop. 2016;87(4):406–11. https://doi.org/10.1080/17453674.2016.1176825. Epub 2016 May 11. PMID: 27168001; PMCID: PMC4967285.
65. Steinman S, Bastrom TP, Newton PO, Mubarak SJ. Beware of ulnar nerve entrapment in flexion-type supracondylar humerus fractures. J Child Orthop. 2007;1(3):177–80. https://doi.org/10.1007/s11832-007-0034-4. Epub 2007 Sep 1. PMID: 19308492; PMCID: PMC2656725.
66. Novais EN, Carry PM, Mark BJ, et al. Posterolaterally displaced and flexion-type supracondylar fractures are associated with a higher risk of open reduction. J Pediatr Orthop B. 2016;25(5):406–11. https://doi.org/10.1097/BPB.0000000000000314.
67. Çabuk H, Dedeoğlu SS, Adaş M, et al. Medial spike and obesity associate with open reduction in type III supracondylar humeral fracture. Acta Chir Orthop Traumatol Cechoslov. 2016;83(2):102–5.
68. Li NY, Bruce WJ, Joyce C, et al. Obesity's influence on operative management of pediatric supracondylar humerus fractures. J Pediatr Orthop. 2018;38(3):e118–21. https://doi.org/10.1097/BPO.0000000000001126.
69. Prusick VW, Gibian JT, Ross KE, et al. Surgical technique: closed reduction and percutaneous pinning of posterolaterally displaced supracondylar humerus fractures. J Orthop Trauma. 2021;35(3):e108–15. https://doi.org/10.1097/BOT.0000000000001854.
70. Bekmez S, Camp MW, Ling R, et al. Supracondylar humerus fractures in older children: success of closed reduction and percutaneous pinning. J Pediatr Orthop. 2021;41(4):242–8. https://doi.org/10.1097/BPO.0000000000001732.
71. Okkaoglu MC, Ozdemir FE, Ozdemir E, et al. Is there an optimal timing for surgical treatment of pediatric supracondylar humerus fractures in the first 24 hours? J Orthop Surg Res. 2021;16(1):484. https://doi.org/10.1186/s13018-021-02638-5.
72. Yang J, Sun LJ, Du S, et al. Risk factors of failure in closed reduction for supracondylar fractures of humerus in children. Chin J Pediat Surg. 2013;34(12):904–6. https://doi.org/10.3760/cma.j.issn.0253-3006.2013.12.008.
73. Beck JD, Riehl JT, Moore BE, et al. Risk factors for failed closed reduction of pediatric supracondylar humerus fractures. Orthopedics. 2012;35(10):1492–6. https://doi.org/10.3928/01477447-20120919-18.
74. Fletcher ND, Schiller JR, Garg S, Weller A, Larson AN, Kwon M, Browne R, Copley L, Ho C. Increased severity of type III supracondylar humerus fractures in the preteen population. J Pediatr Orthop. 2012;32(6):567–72.
75. Li M, Xu J, Hu T, Zhang M, Li F. Surgical management of Gartland type III supracondylar humerus fractures in older children: a retrospective study. J Pediatr Orthop B. 2019;28(6):530–5.
76. Bell P, Scannell BP, Loeffler BJ, Brighton BK, Gaston RG, Casey V, Peters ME, Frick S, Cannada L, Vanderhave KL. Adolescent distal humerus fractures: ORIF versus CRPP. J Pediatr Orthop. 2017;37(8):511–20.
77. Marengo L, Andreacchio A, Alberghina F, Dimeglio A, Canavese F. Functional outcome of displaced intercondylar fractures of the humerus in children and adolescents. J Pediatr Orthop B. 2018;27(2):121–7.
78. Julfiqar PA, Huda N, Ahmed W. Closed reductions and percutaneus 'k' wire fixation for adolescent intercondylar fractures of the distal humerus. J Clin Diagn Res. 2013;7(8):1666–8.
79. Slongo T, Schmid T, Wilkins K, Joeris A. Lateral external fixation–a new surgical technique for displaced unreducible supracondylar humeral fractures in children. J Bone Joint Surg Am. 2008;90(8):1690–7.

80. Beck NA, Ganley TJ, McKay S, Tomlinson L, Ahn J, Flynn JM, Baldwin K. T-condylar fractures of the distal humerus in children: does early motion affect final range of motion? J Child Orthop. 2014;8(2):161–5.
81. Cook JB, Riccio AI, Anderson T, Chen W, Shaha SH, Wimberly RL. Outcomes after surgical treatment of adolescent intra-articular distal humerus fractures. J Pediatr Orthop. 2016;36(8):773–9.
82. Dreyfuss D, Eidelman M. Treatment of complex intercondylar humeral fractures in adolescents by open reduction and internal fixation through the transolecranon approach. J Pediatr Orthop B. 2014;23(4):364–8.
83. He M, Wang Q, Zhao J, Jin Y, Wang Y. Lateral entry pins and Slongo's external fixation: which method is more ideal for older children with supracondylar humeral fractures? J Orthop Surg Res. 2021;16(1):396.
84. Kokly S, Castagna A, Mohamadreza M. Modified tension band wiring in adult distal humeral fracture types A2 and C1. Arch Bone Jt Surg. 2019;7(4):325–30.
85. Munde SL, Bhatti MJ, Siwach RC, Gulia A, Kundu ZS, Bansal S, Middha S, Kamra HT. Double tension band osteosynthesis in inter-condylar humeral fractures. J Clin Diagn Res. 2015;9(12):RC08-11.
86. Allende C, Gutierrez N, Fernandez Savoy I, Allende BT. Double tension band osteosynthesis in transverse supracondylar distal humerus fractures and nonunions. Int Orthop. 2012;36(12):2565–9.
87. Houben PFJ, Bongers KJ, Wildenberg F. Double tension band osteosynthesis in supra-and transcondylar humeral fractures. Injury. 1994;25(5):305–9.
88. Kocher MS, Kasser JR, Waters PM, Bae D, Snyder BD, Hresko MT, et al. Lateral entry compared with medial and lateral entry pin fixation for completely displaced supracondylar humeral fractures in children. A randomized clinical trial. J Bone Jt Surg Am. 2007;89(4):706–12.
89. Brauer CA, Lee BM, Bae DS, Waters PM, Kocher MS. A systematic review of medial and lateral entry pinning versus lateral entry pinning for supracondylar fractures of the humerus. J Pediatr Orthop. 2007;27(2):181–6.
90. Zionts LE, McKellop HA, Hathaway R. Torsional strength of pin configurations used to fix supracondylar fractures of the humerus in children. J Bone Jt Surg Am. 1994;76(2):253–6.
91. Shannon FJ, Mohan P, Chacko J, D'Souza LG. "Dorgan's" percutaneous lateral cross-wiring of supracondylar fractures of the humerus in children. J Pediatr Orthop. 2004;24(4):376–9.
92. Skaggs DL, Cluck MW, Mostofi A, Flynn JM, Kay RM. Lateral-entry pin fixation in the management of supracondylar fractures in children. J Bone Jt Surg Am. 2004;86-A(4):702–7.
93. Topping RE, Blanco JS, Davis TJ. Clinical evaluation of crossed-pin versus lateral-pin fixation in displaced supracondylar humerus fractures. J Pediatr Orthop. 1995;15(4):435–9.
94. Omid R, Choi PD, Skaggs DL. Supracondylar humeral fractures in children. J Bone Jt Surg Am. 2008;90(5):1121–32.
95. Sibinski M, Sharma H, Sherlock DA. Lateral versus crossed wire fixation for displaced extension supracondylar humeral fractures in children. Injury. 2006;37(10):961–5.
96. Zenios M, Ramachandran M, Milne B, Little D, Smith N. Intraoperative stability testing of lateral-entry pin fixation of pediatric supracondylar humeral fractures. J Pediatr Orthop. 2007;27(6):695–702.
97. Kalenderer O, Reisoglu A, Surer L, Agus H. How should one treat iatrogenic ulnar injury after closed reduction and percutaneous pinning of paediatric supracondylar humeral fractures? Injury. 2008;39(4):463–6.
98. Rasool MN. Ulnar nerve injury after K-wire fixation of supracondylar humerus fractures in children. J Pediatr Orthop. 1998;18(5):686–90.
99. Low L, Barry ME, Condell R, et al. Single-surgeon perspective: is there ever a need to open extension-type supracondylar fractures. Ir J Med Sci. 2023;192(6):2845–9.
100. Hou P, Liu W, Zhao Z. The, "hand as foot" teaching method in three-dimensional manual reduction of the supracondylar fracture of humerus in children. Asian J Surg. 2022;45:934–5.

101. Smuin D, Hatch M, Winthrop Z, Gidvani S, Hennrikus W. The reduction maneuver for pediatric extension type 3 supracondylar humerus fractures. Cureus. 2020;12(7):e9213. https://doi.org/10.7759/cureus.9213.
102. Chai KK. A prospective study on supracondylar fractures of the humerus in children: comparing the results of closed manipulation and plaster cast with closed manipulation and percutaneous cross K wiring for the treatment of displaced fractures. Master Thesis, University of Malaya; 2000. PMID:11200043.
103. Skaggs DL, Hale JM, Bassett J, Kaminsky C, Kay RM, Tolo VT. Operative treatment of supracondylar fractures of the humerus in children. The consequences of pin placement. J Bone Joint Surg Am. 2001;83:735–40. PMID:11379744
104. Gordon JE, Patton CM, Luhmann SJ, Bassett GS, Schoenecker PL. Fracture stability after pinning of displaced supracondylar distal humerus fractures in children. J Pediatr Orthop. 2001;21:313–8. PMID: 11371812
105. Davis RT, Gorczyca JT, Pugh K. Supracondylar humerus fractures in children. Comparison of operative treatment methods. Clin Orthop Relat Res. 2000;376:49–55.
106. Celiker O, Pestilci FI, Tuzuner M. Supracondylar fractures of the humerus in children: analysis of results in 142 patients. J Orthop Trauma. 1990;4:265–9.
107. Koudstaal MJ, De Ridder VA, De Lange S, Ulrich C. Pediatric supracondylar humerus fractures: the anterior approach. J Orthop Trauma. 2002;16:409–12.
108. Otsuka NY, Kasser JR. Supracondylar fractures of the humerus in children. J Am Acad Orthop Surg. 1997;5:19–26.
109. Skaggs DL, Hale JM, Basset J, Kaminsky C, Kay RM, Tolo VT. Operative treatment of supracondylar fractures of the humerus in children. The consequences of pin placement. J Bone Joint Surg Am. 2001;83-A:735–40.
110. Wilkins KE, Aroojis AJ. Incidence of fractures in children. In: Beaty JH, Kasser JR, editors. Rockwood and Wilkins' fractures in children. 6th ed. Philadelphia: Lippincott Williams and Wilkins; 2005. p. 10–1.
111. Meling T, Harboe K, Søreide K. Incidence of traumatic long-bone fractures requiring in-hospital management: a prospective age- and gender-specific analysis of 4890 fractures. Injury. 2009;40(11):1212–9.
112. Christopher CB, Eduard BH. Supracondylar fractures of the femur in children. J Pediatr Orthop. 2005;25:145–8.
113. Nicholas CS, David P, David M. Supracondylar fractures of the femur in children. J Pediatr Orthop. 2001;21:600–3.
114. Anup KG, Chinenye ON. Management of distal femur fractures in adults an overview of options. Orthop Clin N Am. 2016;47:85–96.
115. Battaglia TC, Armstrong DG, Schwend RM. Factors affecting forearm compartment pressures in children with supracondylar fractures of the humerus. J Pediatr Orthop. 2002;22(22):431–9. https://doi.org/10.1097/01241398-200207000-00004.
116. Matuszewski Ł. Evaluation and management of pulseless pink/pale hand syndrome coexisting with supracondylar fractures of the humerus in children. Eur J Orthop Surg Traumatol. 2014;24:1401–6. https://doi.org/10.1007/s00590-013-1337-4.
117. Bulut G, Sarıoğlu E, Mık G, Ofluoğlu Ö, Bekler Hİ. Posterior bilaterotricipital approach for surgical treatment of children's Gartland Type III supracondylar humeral fractures. Eur J Orthop Surg Traumatol. 2012;22:457–65. https://doi.org/10.1007/s00590-011-0862-2.
118. Houshian S, Mehdi B, Larsen MS. The epidemiology of elbow fracture in children: analysis of 355 fractures, with special reference to supracondylar humerus fractures. J Orthop Sci. 2001;6(4):312–5.
119. Haddad RJ Jr, Saer JK, Riordan DC. Percutaneous pinning of displaced supracondylar fractures of the elbow in children. Clin Orthop Relat Res. 1970;71:112–7.
120. Hadlow AT, Devane P, Nicol RO. A selective treatment approach to supracondylar fracture of the humerus in children. J Pediatr Orthop. 1996;16:104–6. https://doi.org/10.1097/01241398-199601000-00021.

121. Abebneh M, Shannak A, Agabi S, Hadidi S. The treatment of dispalced supracondylar fractures of the humerus in children. A comparison of three methods. Int Orthop. 1998;22:263–5.
122. Nacht JL, Ecker ML, Chung SMK, Lotke PA, Das M. Supracondylar fractures of the humerus in children treated by closed reduction and percutaneous pinning. Clin Orthop Relat Res. 1983;177:203–9. https://doi.org/10.1097/00003086-198307000-00031.
123. Campbell C, Waters P, Emans J, et al. Neurovascular injury and displacement in type III supracondylar humerus fractures. J Pediatr Orthop. 1995;25:47.
124. Wang SI, Kwon TY, Hwang HP, Kim JR. Functional outcomes of Gartland III supracondylar humerus fractures with early neurovascular complications in children: a retrospective observational study. Medicine (Baltimore). 2017;96(25):e7148. https://doi.org/10.1097/MD.0000000000007148.
125. Vaquero-Picado A, González-Morán G, Moraleda L. Management of supracondylar fractures of the humerus in children. EFORT Open Rev. 2018;3(10):526–40. https://doi.org/10.1302/2058-5241.3.170049.
126. Joiner ER, Skaggs DL, Arkader A, Andras LM, Lightdale-Miric NR, Pace JL, Ryan DD. Iatrogenic nerve injuries in the treatment of supracondylar humerus fractures: are we really just missing nerve injuries on preoperative examination? J Pediatr Orthop. 2014;34(4):388–92. https://doi.org/10.1097/BPO.0000000000000171.
127. Gosens T, Bongers KJ. Neurovascular complications and functional outcome in displaced supracondylar fractures of the humerus in children. Injury. 2003;34(4):267–73. https://doi.org/10.1016/s0020-1383(02)00312-1.
128. Kwok IH, Silk ZM, Quick TJ, Sinisi M, MacQuillan A, Fox M. Nerve injuries associated with supracondylar fractures of the humerus in children: our experience in a specialist peripheral nerve injury unit. Bone Joint J. 2016;98-B(6):851–6. https://doi.org/10.1302/0301-620X.98B6.35686.
129. Ramachandran M, Birch R, Eastwood DM. Clinical outcome of nerve injuries associated with supracondylar fractures of the humerus in children: the experience of a specialist referral Centre. J Bone Joint Surg Br. 2006;88(1):90–4. https://doi.org/10.1302/0301-620X.88B1.16869.
130. Štichhauer R, Preis J, Kanta M, Krobot J. Poranění periferních nervů při suprakondylických zlomeninách humeru u dětí. Cesk Slov Neurol N. 2017;80/13(4):440–4. https://doi.org/10.14735/amcsnn2017440.
131. Greve F, Müller M, Wurm M, Biberthaler P, Singer G, Till H, et al. Standalone axial malrotation after pediatric supracondylar fracture does not seem to be an indication for immediate postoperative revision surgery. Children. 2022;9(7):13.
132. Skaggs DL, Flynn JM. Supracondylar fractures of the distal humerus. In: Waters PM, Skaggs DL, Flynn JM, editors. Rockwood and Wilkin's fractures in children. 9th ed. Philadelphia: Wolters Kluwer; 2020. p. 478–526.
133. Ege T, Turkkan S, Gunay C, et al. Late onset brachial artery thrombosis and total temporary peripheral neuropathy in a child with humerus supracondylar fracture: a case report. Ulus Travma Acil Cerrahi Derg. 2015;21:75–8. https://doi.org/10.5505/tjtes.2015.92072.
134. Reigstad O, Thorkildsen R, Grimsgaard C, et al. Supracondylar fractures with circulatory failure after reduction, pinning, and entrapment of the brachial artery: excellent results more than 1 year after open exploration and revascularization. J Orthop Trauma. 2011;25:26–30. https://doi.org/10.1097/BOT.0b013e3181db276a.
135. Pandey K, Maravi L, Turkar R. Management of postoperative vascular compromise in supracondylar fracture of the humerus in children. Orthop J M P Chapter. 2015;21(2):70.
136. von Laer LR. Der radiale Fixateur externe zur Behandlung suprakondylarer Humerusfrakturen im Wachstumsalter. Oper Orthop Traumatol. 1997;9:265–76. https://doi.org/10.1007/s00064-006-0098-1.
137. Dormans JP, Squillante R, Sharf H. Acute neurovascular complications with supracondylar humerus fractures in children. J Hand Surg [Am]. 1995;20:1–4. https://doi.org/10.1016/S0363-5023(05)80046-2.

138. Alton TB, Werner SE, Gee AO. Classifications in brief: the Gartland classification of supracondylar humerus fractures. Clin Orthop Relat Res. 2015;473:738–41. https://doi.org/10.1007/s11999-014-4033-8.
139. Mayne AI, Perry DC, Stables G, et al. Documentation of neurovascular status in supracondylar fractures and the development of an assessment proforma. Emerg Med J. 2013;30:480–2. https://doi.org/10.1136/emermed-2012-201293.
140. Sahu RL. Percutaneous K-wire fixation in paediatric supracondylar fractures of humerus: a retrospective study. Niger Med J. 2013;54:329–34. https://doi.org/10.4103/0300-1652.122355.
141. Shaw BA, Kasser JR, Emans JB, et al. Management of vascular injuries in displaced supracondylar humerus fractures without arteriography. J Orthop Trauma. 1990;4:25–9.
142. Abbott MD, Buchler L, Loder RT, et al. Gartland type III supracondylar humerus fractures: outcome and complications as related to operative timing and pin configuration. J Child Orthop. 2014;8:473–7. https://doi.org/10.1007/s11832-014-0624-x.
143. Rasool MN, Naidoo KS. Supracondylar fractures: posterolateral type with brachialis muscle penetration and neurovascular injury. J Pediatr Orthop. 1999;19(4):518–22.
144. Mooney JF III, Hosseinzadeh P, Oetgen M, et al. AAOS appropriate use criteria: Management of pediatric supracondylar humerus fractures with vascular injury. J Am Acad Orthop Surg. 2016;24:e24–8.
145. Eren A, Güven M, Erol B, et al. Correlation between posteromedial or posterolateral displacement and cubitus varus deformity in supracondylar humerus fractures in children. J Child Orthop. 2008;2:85–9. https://doi.org/10.1007/s11832-008-0088-y.
146. Babal JC, Mehlman CT, Klein G. Nerve injuries associated with pediatric supracondylar humeral fractures: a meta-analysis. J Pediatr Orthop. 2010;30(3):253–63.
147. Wang Y-L, Chang W-N, Hsu C-J, Sun S-F, Wang J-L, Wong C-Y. The recovery of elbow range of motion after treatment of supracondylar and lateral condylar fractures of the distal humerus in children. J Orthop Trauma. 2009;23:120–5.
148. Dähnert W, Bernd W. Computer tomography determination of the torsion angle of the humerus. Z Orthop Ihre Grenzgeb. 1986;124:46–9.
149. Fuchs CC, Schmid P, Engelhardt P. Computerized tomography measurement of humerus torsion. Z Orthop Ihre Grenzgeb. 1991;129:423–5.
150. Harland U, Diepolder M, Gruber G, Knöss HP. Sonographic determination of the humerus retrotorsion angle. Z Orthop Ihre Grenzgeb. 1991;129:36–41.
151. Krahl VE. The torsion of the humerus; its localization, cause and duration in man. Am J Anat. 1947;80:275–319.
152. Kunz C, Rieder T, Viehweger R. Can ultrasonography be used to measure torsion angle of the humerus? Comparison of ultrasonographic, computerized tomographic and anthropometric methods. Z Orthop Ihre Grenzgeb. 1993;131:307–12.
153. Rogers LF, Malave S, White H, Tachdjian MO. Plastic bowing, torus and greenstick supracondylar fractures of the humerus: radiographic clues to obscure fractures of the elbow in children. Radiology. 1978;128:145–50.
154. Vocke AK, von Laer LR. Prognosis of proximal radius fractures in the growth period. Unfallchirurg. 1998;101:287–95.
155. Rockwood CA, Wikins KE. Fractures in children, vol. 3. 5th ed. Philadelphia: Lippincott Williams and Wikins; 2001.
156. Della-Giustina K, Della-Giustina DA. Emergency department evaluation and treatment of pediatric orthopedic injuries. Emerg Med Clin North Am. 1999;17:895–922.
157. Bachman D, Santora S. Orthopedic trauma. In: Fleisher GR, Ludwig S, editors. Textbook of pediatric emergency medicine. Philadelphia: Lippincott Williams and Wilkins; 2006. p. 1538–40.
158. Lyons ST, Quinn M, Stanitski CL. Neurovascular injuries in type III humeral supracondylar fractures in children. Clin Orthop Relat Res. 2000;376:62–7.

159. Griffin KJ, Walsh SR, Markar S. The pink pulseless hand: a review of the literature regarding management of vascular complications of supracondylar humeral fractures in children. Eur J Vasc Endovasc Surg. 2008;36:697–702.
160. Luria S, Sucar A, Eylon S, Pinchas-Mizrachi R, Berlatzky Y, Anner H, Liebergall M, Porat S. Vascular complications of supracondylar humeral fractures in children. J Pediatr Orthop B. 2007;16:133–43.
161. Cheng JC, Ng BK, Ying SY, Lam PK. A 10-year study of the changes in the pattern and treatment of 6,493 fractures. J Pediatr Orthop. 1999;19:344–50.
162. Landin L, Danielsson L. Elbow fractures in children. An epidemiological analysis of 589 cases. Acta Orthop Scand. 1986;57:309–12.
163. Schoenecker PL, Delgado E, Rotman M, Sicard GA, Capelli AM. Pulseless arm in association with totally displaced supracondylar fracture. J Orthop Trauma. 1996;10:410–5.
164. Copley LA, Dormans JP, Davidson RS. Vascular injuries and their sequelae in pediatric supracondylar humeral fractures: toward a goal of prevention. J Pediatr Orthop. 1996;16:99–103.
165. Endean ED, Veldenz HC, Schwarcz TH, Hyde GL. Recognition of arterial injury in elbow dislocation. J Vasc Surg. 1992;16:402–6.
166. Mitchell SL, Sullivan BT, Ho CA, Abzug JM, Raad M, Sponseller PD. Pediatric Gartland Type-IV supracondylar humeral fractures have substantial overlap with flexion-type fractures. J Bone Joint Surg Am. 2019;101(15):1351–6. PMID: 31393425; PMCID: PMC7406141
167. Wei YS, Liu WL, Bai R, et al. The use of a transolecranon pin joystick technique in the treatment of multidirectionally unstable supracondylar humeral fractures in children. J Pediatr Orthop B. 2020;29:452–7.
168. Abdelmalek A, Towner M, Clarke A. Are we staying up too late? Timing of surgery of displaced supracondylar fractures in children. Clinical audit in a paediatric tertiary UK trauma centre and literature review. Arch Orthop Trauma Surg. 2022;142:3863–7. https://doi.org/10.1007/s00402-021-04289-x.
169. Turhan E, Aksoy C, Ege A, Bayar A, Keser S, Alpaslan M. Sagittal plane analysis of the open and closed methods in children with displaced supracondylar fractures of the humerus (a radiological study). Arch Orthop Trauma Surg. 2007; https://doi.org/10.1007/s00402-007-0523-4.
170. Eckert K, Janssen N, Ackermann O, Schweiger B, Radeloff E, Liedgens P. Ultrasound diagnosis of supracondylar fractures in children. Eur J Trauma Emerg Surg. 2013; https://doi.org/10.1007/s00068-013-0306-2.
171. Sukvanich P, Samun P, Kongmalai P. Diagnostic accuracy of the shaft-condylar angle for an incomplete supracondylar fracture of elbow in children. Eur J Orthop Surg Traumatol. 2019; https://doi.org/10.1007/s00590-019-02489-1.
172. Siu C, Farrell S, Schaeffer EK, Doan Q, Dobbe A, Bone J, Reilly CW, Mulpuri K. Long-arm splinting versus above-elbow casting for type 1 supracondylar fractures of the humerus in children: a randomized controlled trial. SN Compr Clin Med. 2023; https://doi.org/10.1007/s42399-023-01417-z.
173. Kazimoglu C, Çetin M, Şener M, Aguş H, Kalanderer Ö. Operative management of type III extension supracondylar fractures in children. Int Orthop. 2008; https://doi.org/10.1007/s00264-008-0605-0.
174. Li Y, Feng Y, Chu XJ, Yuan Y, Yuan Y, Sun J. Minimally invasive techniques utilizing the "Joy Stick" method for managing irreducible flexion-type supracondylar fractures of the humerus in older children. J Orthop Surg Res. 2024; https://doi.org/10.1186/s13018-024-04922-6.
175. Zhu CM, Feng QY, Ou ZX, Zhong HB, Tang X. Minimally invasive technique combined with external fixator in the treatment of pediatric flexion-type humeral supracondylar fractures. Sci Rep. 2023; https://doi.org/10.1038/s41598-023-48158-6.

176. Sun J, Shan J, Meng L, Liu T, Wang E, Jia G. Predictive factors for open reduction of flexion-type supracondylar fracture of humerus in children. BMC Musculoskelet Disord. 2022; https://doi.org/10.1186/s12891-022-05798-5.
177. Jitprapaikulsarn S, Chantarapanich N, Apivatthakakul T, Lertvilai P, Wanchat S, Gromprasit A, Sengpanich P, Mahaisavariya C, Saramas Y, Simonet LP. Dual tension band wiring for adolescent supracondylar fractures of the humerus: mechanical assessment and a clinical series. Eur J Orthop Surg Traumatol. 2025; https://doi.org/10.1007/s00590-025-04454-7.
178. Prashant K, Lakhotia D, Bhattacharyya TD, Mahanta AK, Ravoof A. A comparative study of two percutaneous pinning techniques (lateral vs medial–lateral) for Gartland type III pediatric supracondylar fracture of the humerus. J Orthop Traumatol. 2016; https://doi.org/10.1007/s10195-016-0410-2.
179. Lin Y, Hua Z, Zhou C, Chen S, Sun X, Liu F, Meng G, Zhang S, Sun J. A new technique of intramedullary elastic reduction of the "de-sharpened" Kirschner wire for the treatment of Gartland type III posterolateral displaced supracondylar fracture of the humerus in children. Eur J Med Res. 2024; https://doi.org/10.1186/s40001-024-01671-4.
180. Maity A, Saha D, Roy DS. A prospective randomised, controlled clinical trial comparing medial and lateral entry pinning with lateral entry pinning for percutaneous fixation of displaced extension type supracondylar fractures of the humerus in children. J Orthop Surg Res. 2012; https://doi.org/10.1186/1749-799x-7-6.
181. Ersan O, Gonen E, Arik A, Dasar U, Ates Y. Treatment of supracondylar fractures of the humerus in children through an anterior approach is a safe and effective method. Int Orthop. 2008; https://doi.org/10.1007/s00264-008-0668-y.
182. Saeed MZ, Aktselis I, Mann HA, Kumar KHS, Goddard N. Reduction and stabilization of acute, displaced supracondylar fractures of distal humerus in children using the Sauvé-Kapandji technique. Eur Orthop Traumatol. 2015; https://doi.org/10.1007/s12570-015-0309-z.
183. Li J, Guo X, Wang HQ, Yue C, Chen K, Ma J, Wang J, Tang X. Locking plate versus external fixation in the treatment of displaced femoral supracondylar fracture in children. J Orthop Surg Res. 2020; https://doi.org/10.1186/s13018-020-01759-7.
184. Hussein al-Algawy AA, Aliakbar AH, Witwit IHN. Open versus closed reduction and K-wire fixation for displaced supracondylar fracture of the humerus in children. Eur J Orthop Surg Traumatol. 2018; https://doi.org/10.1007/s00590-018-2305-9.
185. Chrenko R, Hanko M, Grega M, Sýkora L', Jáger R. Peripheral nerve injuries associated with dislocated supracondylar fractures of distal humerus in children: incidence and need of surgical treatment. Childs Nerv Syst. 2024; https://doi.org/10.1007/s00381-024-06497-3.
186. Sanpera I, Salom M, Fenandez-Ansorena A, Frontera-Juan G, Pizà-Vallespir G. The fate of the malrotated elbow supracondylar fractures in children: is varus really a problem? Int Orthop. 2024; https://doi.org/10.1007/s00264-024-06153-0.
187. Latz D, Grassmann J, Schiffner E, Gehrmann S, Duran M, Windolf J, Jungbluth P. Postoperative brachial artery entrapment associated with pediatric supracondylar fracture of the humerus: a case report. J Med Case Rep. 2017; https://doi.org/10.1186/s13256-017-1240-4.
188. Hell AK, Gadomski C, Braunschweig L. Spontaneous humeral torsion deformity correction after displaced supracondylar fractures in children. BMC Musculoskelet Disord. 2021; https://doi.org/10.1186/s12891-021-04909-y.
189. Korompilias AV, Lykissas MG, Mitsionis GI, Kontogeorgakos VA, Manoudis G, Beris AE. Treatment of pink pulseless hand following supracondylar fractures of the humerus in children. Int Orthop. 2008; https://doi.org/10.1007/s00264-007-0509-4.
190. Ma H-L, Sun X-W, Liu F, Hua ZT, Sun J, Zhang S-C. Kirschner wire reconstruction of medial and lateral column periosteal hinge in the treatment of multidirectionally unstable supracondylar fracture of the humerus in children. Eur J Med Res. 2023; https://doi.org/10.1186/s40001-023-01560-2.

Lateral Condyle Fracture

5

Introduction by the Author

Lateral condyle fractures are the second most common type of surgical elbow fracture in children after supracondylar fractures. These fractures account for 12%–20% of all distal humerus fractures in children.

Due to the risk of displacement (up to 30%) and nonunion, surgical fixation is often necessary, as these complications can lead to long-term issues, such as cubitus valgus and tardy ulnar nerve palsy.

Although plain radiographs can correctly diagnose displaced fractures, some undisplaced fractures may be missed. Studies have shown that magnetic resonance imaging is particularly effective in identifying fractures with minimal displacement that are often overlooked by X-rays. Furthermore, magnetic resonance imaging allows visualization of the surrounding cartilage of the distal humerus's ossification center and helps identify fractures that would otherwise be invisible on plain radiographs.

Lateral condyle fractures can be classified into three types according to displacement: type 1 with displacement of less than 2 mm, type 2 with displacement of more than 2 mm without fragment rotation, and type 3 with complete displacement and fragment rotation.

Nondisplaced fractures are typically treated with a long arm cast. However, fractures with initial displacement tend to displace further, resulting in a high incidence of nonunion, thus requiring reduction and fixation.

While types 2 and 3 fractures are indications for surgical stabilization, there is an ongoing debate about whether type 1 fractures should be treated conservatively or surgically.

© The Author(s), under exclusive license to Springer Nature Switzerland AG 2026
F. Canavese, *Advances in Pediatric Extremity Fracture Management*,
https://doi.org/10.1007/978-3-032-33306-3_5

The optimal method of treatment is also the subject of ongoing debate: closed or open reduction. Options for stabilizing the fracture include Kirschner wires and cannulated screws. There is no consensus on the ideal fixation method, as both have distinct advantages and disadvantages. Regarding the optimal Kirschner wire configuration, finite element analysis has demonstrated that three divergent wires offer the best overall performance. However, two divergent wires at 45 or 60 degrees also provide significant stability.

Recent evidence shows that screw fixation reduces the risk of infection and elbow stiffness more effectively than Kirschner wire fixation. However, both methods have comparable union rates of over 90%. Screw fixation allows for a shorter casting period and an earlier start to range-of-motion exercises. However, screws or buried Kirschner wires require an additional procedure for removal. Regardless of the fixation method used, extensive posterior dissection should be avoided, as the lateral condyle's primary blood supply comes from the posterior region.

5.1 Machine Generated Summaries

Disclaimer: The summaries in this chapter were generated from Springer Nature publications using abstractive AI auto-summarization: An abstraction-based summarizer creates new text based on deep learning. New phrases are created to summarize the content. As the constituted sentences are machine selected, they may not fully reflect the body of the work, so we strongly advise that the original content is read and cited. The auto-generated summaries were curated by the author(s) to meet Springer Nature publication standards.

Clinical Value of MRI in Evaluating and Diagnosing of Humeral Lateral Condyle Fracture in Children [41]

This is a machine-generated summary of:

Qi, Yang; Guo, Lin; Sun, Man; Wang, Zhi Clinical value of MRI in evaluating and diagnosing of humeral lateral condyle fracture in children [41]
Published in: Journal of Orthopaedic Surgery and Research (2021)
Link to original: https://doi.org/10.1186/s13018-021-02726-6
Copyright of the summarized publication:
The Author(s) 2021
License: OpenAccess CC BY + CC0 4.0

This article is licensed under a Creative Commons Attribution 4.0 International License, which permits use, sharing, adaptation, distribution and reproduction in

any medium or format, as long as you give appropriate credit to the original author(s) and the source, provide a link to the Creative Commons licence, and indicate if changes were made. The images or other third party material in this article are included in the article's Creative Commons licence, unless indicated otherwise in a credit line to the material. If material is not included in the article's Creative Commons licence and your intended use is not permitted by statutory regulation or exceeds the permitted use, you will need to obtain permission directly from the copyright holder. To view a copy of this licence, visit http://creativecommons.org/licenses/by/4.0/. The Creative Commons Public Domain Dedication waiver (http://creativecommons.org/publicdomain/zero/1.0/) applies to the data made available in this article, unless otherwise stated in a credit line to the data.

If you want to cite the papers, please refer to the original.

For technical reasons we could not place the page where the original quote is coming from.

Research Highlights

Humeral lateral condyle fractures (HLCFs) are prevalent pediatric injuries that require timely and accurate diagnosis to prevent severe complications and joint dysfunction, which can affect the normal growth and development of children's elbow joints. Traditional radiographs are commonly used for diagnosing HLCFs, but they often fall short in evaluating articular epiphyseal cartilage damage, especially in cases without significant displacement. This poses a challenge for orthopedic pediatricians and radiologists. Now, a new study by Yang Qi and colleagues investigates the efficacy of MRI compared to radiographs in diagnosing HLCFs, assessing fracture displacement, and determining the integrity of the humeral trochlear cartilage chain.

The study involved children with acute elbow joint injuries suspected to be HLCFs. Initially, standard radiographs were used for diagnosis, followed by MRI scans after obtaining parental consent. The researchers compared the sensitivity and specificity of radiographs and MRI in diagnosing HLCFs and evaluating cartilage integrity. They also assessed the degree of fracture displacement using both methods. The study found that MRI had significantly higher sensitivity than radiographs in diagnosing HLCFs and determining cartilage chain integrity. MRI was particularly effective in identifying fractures without significant displacement, which were often underestimated by radiographs.

The findings suggest that MRI provides a more accurate assessment of fracture displacement and stability in children with HLCFs, offering valuable insights for clinical treatment decisions. Future studies could focus on larger sample sizes to further validate these results and explore long-term outcomes such as fracture nonunion or delayed union. While MRI is more expensive than radiographs, its ability to reduce complications and predict secondary fracture displacement makes it a valuable tool in managing pediatric HLCFs without significant displacement.

Comparative Study of Lateral Condyle Fracture With or Without Posteromedial Elbow Dislocation in Children [42]

This is a machine-generated summary of:

Lan, Xia; Dai, Min; Zhang, Bin; Huang, Gendong Comparative study of lateral condyle fracture with or without posteromedial elbow dislocation in children [42]
Published in: International Orthopaedics (2018)
Link to original: https://doi.org/10.1007/s00264-018-3795-0
Copyright of the summarized publication:
SICOT aisbl 2018
All rights reserved.

If you want to cite the papers, please refer to the original.

For technical reasons we could not place the page where the original quote is coming from.

Research Highlights

Lateral condyle fractures account for a significant portion of distal humeral fractures in children, with associated elbow dislocations being rare but serious injuries. These dislocations can be easily misdiagnosed due to their similarity to other types of fractures, leading to potential residual impairment if not properly treated. Now, a new study by Xia Lan and colleagues investigates the intraoperative findings and clinical outcomes in children with type II lateral condylar fractures, with or without posteromedial elbow dislocations, highlighting the differences in surgical challenges and recovery.

The study retrospectively analyzed children under 18 years old who underwent surgery for lateral humeral condylar fractures at their center between January 2010 and June 2020. Patients were divided into two groups: Group A included those with posteromedial elbow dislocation and Milch type II fractures, while Group B consisted of those with Milch type II fractures without dislocation. The surgical procedure involved open reduction and internal fixation using K-wires. The researchers found that wider exposure was necessary for Group A due to the complexity of the fracture and dislocation. Postoperative care included casting for 4 weeks followed by active rehabilitation exercises. The study assessed outcomes using the Mayo Elbow Performance Score (MEPS) and monitored complications such as bone union time and range of motion recovery.

The findings revealed that while both groups achieved satisfactory functional outcomes, Group A required a longer time to regain full range of elbow movement due to more severe soft tissue injuries. The study emphasizes the importance of recognizing this rare injury pattern early and ensuring stable fixation to achieve joint congruency and elbow stabilization. Future studies with larger sample sizes and longer follow-up periods are needed to further validate these results and explore long-term outcomes for patients with this rare injury combination.

K Wires or Cannulated Screws for Fixation of Lateral Condyle Fractures in Children: A Systematic Review of Comparative Studies [43]

This is a machine-generated summary of:

Sinha, Siddhartha; Kumar, Arvind; Meena, Sanjay; Jameel, Javed; Qureshi, Owais A.; Kumar, Sandeep K Wires or Cannulated Screws for Fixation of Lateral Condyle Fractures in Children: A Systematic Review of Comparative Studies [43]
Published in: Indian Journal of Orthopaedics (2023)
Link to original: https://doi.org/10.1007/s43465-023-00873-y
Copyright of the summarized publication:
Indian Orthopaedics Association 2023
Copyright comment: Springer Nature or its licensor (e.g. a society or other partner) holds exclusive rights to this article under a publishing agreement with the author(s) or other rightsholder(s); author self-archiving of the accepted manuscript version of this article is solely governed by the terms of such publishing agreement and applicable law.
All rights reserved.

If you want to cite the papers, please refer to the original.

For technical reasons we could not place the page where the original quote is coming from.

Research Highlights

Lateral condyle fractures are common in children, and surgical fixation is often necessary due to the risk of displacement and nonunion, which can lead to long-term complications such as cubitus valgus and tardy ulnar nerve palsy. While the need for fixation is well-established, there is ongoing debate regarding the optimal method, with options including Kirschner wires (K wires) and cannulated screws (CCS). Each method has its advantages: K wires are less damaging to the physis and easier to remove, while screws provide better compression at the fracture site, potentially leading to higher union rates. Now, a new study by Siddhartha Sinha and colleagues systematically reviews existing literature to determine whether one fixation method offers superior union rates and functional outcomes over the other.

The study involved a comprehensive search of databases such as PubMed, Medline, Cochrane, and Google Scholar for relevant articles comparing K wire and CCS fixation in pediatric lateral condyle fractures. After screening 43 articles, seven studies met the inclusion criteria for detailed analysis. The researchers extracted data on union rates, functional outcomes using the Hardacre scale, range of motion, and complications. Quality assessment was conducted using the Newcastle–Ottawa tool. The review found that while CCS showed a slightly higher union rate (94%) compared to K wires (90%), there was no significant difference in functional outcomes between the two methods. Complication rates were similar across both groups, with pin tract infections being common in K wire cases.

The study advances our understanding by highlighting that screw fixation may offer higher union rates without compromising functional outcomes or increasing complications compared to K wire fixation. However, it also underscores the need for more robust randomized clinical trials with larger sample sizes to confirm these findings. Future study could focus on differentiating between buried and unburied K wires and exploring other potential fixation methods to provide clearer guidance for clinical practice in managing pediatric lateral condyle fractures.

K-Wire Versus Screws in the Fixation of Lateral Condyle Fracture of Humerus in Pediatrics: A Systematic Review and Meta-Analysis [44]

This is a machine-generated summary of:

Cho, Yoon Joo; Kang, Se Hyun; Kang, Mu Hyun K-wire versus screws in the fixation of lateral condyle fracture of humerus in pediatrics: a systematic review and meta-analysis [44]
Published in: BMC Musculoskeletal Disorders (2023)
Link to original: https://doi.org/10.1186/s12891-023-06780-5
Copyright of the summarized publication:
The Author(s) 2023
License: OpenAccess CC BY + CC0 4.0

This article is licensed under a Creative Commons Attribution 4.0 International License, which permits use, sharing, adaptation, distribution and reproduction in any medium or format, as long as you give appropriate credit to the original author(s) and the source, provide a link to the Creative Commons licence, and indicate if changes were made. The images or other third party material in this article are included in the article's Creative Commons licence, unless indicated otherwise in a credit line to the material. If material is not included in the article's Creative Commons licence and your intended use is not permitted by statutory regulation or exceeds the permitted use, you will need to obtain permission directly from the copyright holder. To view a copy of this licence, visit http://creativecommons.org/licenses/by/4.0/. The Creative Commons Public Domain Dedication waiver (http://creativecommons.org/publicdomain/zero/1.0/) applies to the data made available in this article, unless otherwise stated in a credit line to the data.

If you want to cite the papers, please refer to the original.

For technical reasons we could not place the page where the original quote is coming from.

Research Highlights

Lateral condyle fractures of the humerus are the second most common type of elbow fracture in children, accounting for a significant portion of distal humerus fractures. While nondisplaced fractures are typically managed with casting, displaced fractures often require surgical intervention due to a high risk of further displacement and nonunion. Traditionally, open reduction and internal fixation have been the standard treatment; however, recent studies suggest that closed reduction and percutaneous pinning may yield comparable outcomes. Despite this, there remains uncertainty regarding the optimal fixation method—K-wires or screws. Now, a new study by Yoon Joo Cho and colleagues addresses this gap by conducting a meta-analysis to quantitatively compare the outcomes of K-wire versus screw fixation in pediatric patients with displaced lateral condyle fractures.

The study followed a rigorous methodology, adhering to the Preferred Reporting Items for Systematic Reviews and Meta-Analyses (PRISMA) guidelines. Researchers conducted comprehensive searches across PubMed, Embase, and Cochrane Library databases for relevant studies published before April 2023. The inclusion criteria focused on studies comparing K-wire and screw fixation in children under 18 with displaced lateral condyle fractures. Four studies met the criteria for inclusion in the meta-analysis. The primary clinical outcomes were assessed using Hardacre criteria, while complications such as infection, delayed union, nonunion, lateral overgrowth, limitation of range of motion, and avascular necrosis were also evaluated. Statistical analyses were performed using R software to determine risk ratios and assess heterogeneity.

The meta-analysis revealed that screw fixation is associated with a lower risk of superficial infection and elbow stiffness compared to K-wire fixation. Although there was no significant difference in nonunion rates between the two methods, screw fixation generally allowed for a shorter casting period and earlier initiation of range-of-motion exercises. This could contribute to reduced elbow stiffness observed in patients treated with screws. While the study provides valuable insights into the comparative effectiveness of these fixation methods, it also highlights limitations such as small sample size and short follow-up periods in included studies. Future study could benefit from larger prospective trials with longer follow-up durations to further validate these findings and explore cost implications associated with each fixation method.

Kirschner Wire vs Screw Osteosynthesis of Lateral Condyle Fractures in Paediatric Patients: A Systematic Review [45]

This is a machine-generated summary of:

Mostofi Zadeh Haghighi, D. L.; Xu, J.; Campbell, R.; Moopanar, T. R. Kirschner wire vs screw osteosynthesis of lateral condyle fractures in paediatric patients: a systematic review [45]

Published in: MUSCULOSKELETAL SURGERY (2024)
Link to original: https://doi.org/10.1007/s12306-024-00859-5
Copyright of the summarized publication:
The Author(s) 2024
License: OpenAccess CC BY 4.0

This article is licensed under a Creative Commons Attribution 4.0 International License, which permits use, sharing, adaptation, distribution and reproduction in any medium or format, as long as you give appropriate credit to the original author(s) and the source, provide a link to the Creative Commons licence, and indicate if changes were made. The images or other third party material in this article are included in the article's Creative Commons licence, unless indicated otherwise in a credit line to the material. If material is not included in the article's Creative Commons licence and your intended use is not permitted by statutory regulation or exceeds the permitted use, you will need to obtain permission directly from the copyright holder. To view a copy of this licence, visit http://creativecommons.org/licenses/by/4.0/.

Copyright comment Corrected publication 2024.

If you want to cite the papers, please refer to the original.

For technical reasons we could not place the page where the original quote is coming from.

Research Highlights

Lateral condyle fractures are the second most common type of pediatric elbow fractures, with a high risk of complications such as malunion, non-union, and angular deformities. Current literature suggests that while displaced fractures may benefit from operative management, undisplaced or minimally displaced fractures can often be managed successfully with long arm cast immobilization and close follow-up. However, there is no consensus on the ideal fixation method for surgical management, with K-wires and screw fixation each having distinct advantages and disadvantages. Now, a new study by D. L. Mostofi Zadeh Haghighi and colleagues reviews current literature to compare K-wire fixation with screw osteosynthesis for lateral condyle fractures in children, aiming to evaluate their respective outcomes and complications.

The study was conducted following the Preferred Reporting Items for Systematic Reviews and Meta-analyses guidelines. Researchers searched electronic databases such as Ovid Medline, PubMed, and Cochrane Central Register of Controlled Trials to include relevant studies up to March. The inclusion criteria focused on pediatric patients receiving K-wire or screw osteosynthesis after traumatic fracture of the lateral condyle of the humerus. Both comparative and single-arm studies were included, provided they reported at least one efficacy or safety outcome of interest. Data extraction was performed by two independent authors, focusing on primary efficacy outcomes like rates of lateral prominence, carrying angle deformities, non-union, and superficial infection. The study found that both K-wire and screw fixation methods resulted in acceptable clinical outcomes for most patients, although each method had specific complications.

The study highlights that both K-wires and cannulated screws are safe and effective methods for fixing lateral condyle fractures in children, with low complication rates and excellent clinical outcomes. However, the review also underscores the limited quality of evidence available on this topic due to heterogeneity in data reporting across studies. Future studies could benefit from using standardized outcome criteria to allow for more uniform data presentation. Prospective randomized trials could provide more definitive comparisons between K-wire and screw fixation methods to guide clinical decision-making further.

Closed Reduction and Percutaneous Pinning Versus Open Reduction and Internal Fixation for Jakob Type 3 Lateral Condyle Fractures in Children [46]

This is a machine-generated summary of:

Liu, Yanhan; Shi, Weizhe; Zhao, Hai; Li, Yiqiang; Li, Jingchun; Xun, Fuxin; Canavese, Federico; Xu, Hongwen Closed reduction and percutaneous pinning versus open reduction and internal fixation for Jakob type 3 lateral condyle fractures in children [46]
Published in: International Orthopaedics (2022)
Link to original: https://doi.org/10.1007/s00264-022-05476-0
Copyright of the summarized publication:
The Author(s) under exclusive licence to SICOT aisbl 2022
All rights reserved.

If you want to cite the papers, please refer to the original.

For technical reasons we could not place the page where the original quote is coming from.

Research Highlights

Lateral condyle fractures (LCFs) are the second most common type of elbow fracture in children that require surgical intervention, following supracondylar fractures. Traditionally, open reduction and internal fixation (ORIF) is the preferred treatment for displaced LCFs due to its ability to ensure anatomical reduction. However, closed reduction and percutaneous pinning (CRPP) has been suggested as a less invasive alternative with potential benefits such as reduced soft tissue dissection and shorter operating times. Now, a new study by Yanhan Liu and colleagues evaluates the feasibility of CRPP in treating JFC-type LCFs and compares its outcomes with ORIF.

The study was conducted at Guangzhou Women and Children's Medical Center, where 87 children with JFC-type LCFs were retrospectively reviewed. Patients were divided into two groups based on the treatment received: CRPP or ORIF, determined by the surgeon's preference on call. The researchers collected data on patient demographics, fracture characteristics, surgical details, and clinical outcomes. CRPP involved evaluating fracture displacement under fluoroscopy, using K-wires for reduction and stabilization, and converting to ORIF if necessary. The clinical outcomes were assessed using Hardacre et al.'s criteria, while complications such as avascular necrosis (AVN) and lateral spurring were monitored.

The study found that CRPP was successful in over 90% of cases with good functional outcomes comparable to ORIF. CRPP offered advantages like shorter surgical times but involved higher radiation exposure. Complications were similar between both groups, though one case of AVN occurred in the CRPP group. The authors suggest that while CRPP is a viable option for treating JFC-type LCFs in children, conversion to ORIF should be considered if satisfactory reduction is not achieved. Future studies could focus on larger sample sizes and longer follow-up periods to validate these findings further.

Finite Element Analyses of Lateral Condyle Fracture Fixation in Paediatrics Regarding Configuration of Kirschner-Wire [47]

This is a machine-generated summary of:

Jeon, Sangbin; Ahn, Wooyeol; Oh, Jongbeom; Chung, Jaiwoo; Choi, Junwon; Lee, Soonchul Finite element analyses of lateral condyle fracture fixation in paediatrics regarding configuration of Kirschner-wire [47]
Published in: BMC Musculoskeletal Disorders (2022)
Link to original: https://doi.org/10.1186/s12891-022-05897-3
Copyright of the summarized publication:
The Author(s) 2022
License: OpenAccess CC BY + CC0 4.0

This article is licensed under a Creative Commons Attribution 4.0 International License, which permits use, sharing, adaptation, distribution and reproduction in any medium or format, as long as you give appropriate credit to the original author(s) and the source, provide a link to the Creative Commons licence, and indicate if changes were made. The images or other third party material in this article are included in the article's Creative Commons licence, unless indicated otherwise in a credit line to the material. If material is not included in the article's Creative Commons licence and your intended use is not permitted by statutory regulation or exceeds the permitted use, you will need to obtain permission directly from the copyright holder. To view a copy of this licence, visit http://creativecommons.org/licenses/by/4.0/. The Creative Commons Public Domain Dedication waiver (http://creativecommons.org/publicdomain/zero/1.0/) applies to the data made available in this article, unless otherwise stated in a credit line to the data.

If you want to cite the papers, please refer to the original.

For technical reasons we could not place the page where the original quote is coming from.

Research Highlights

Lateral condyle fractures of the distal humerus are a common type of elbow fracture in children, with the Milch type II fracture being particularly unstable. Traditionally, these fractures are treated surgically using Kirschner wires (K-wires) for stabilization. Despite advancements in understanding fracture healing, complications such as nonunion and malunion remain prevalent. Now, a new study by Sangbin Jeon and colleagues explores the optimal configuration of K-wires for stabilizing lateral condyle fractures using finite element analysis (FEA), aiming to reduce these complications.

The study utilized a geometric model derived from CT images of a 7-year-old male patient to simulate a typical Milch type II fracture. The researchers employed Mimics Innovation Suite and SolidWorks software to create three-dimensional models for FEA. Various K-wire configurations were tested, including single and multiple wire setups at different angles. The simulations assessed von Mises stress distribution and stiffness under various loads, such as flexion, extension, and rotational forces. The results indicated that a single K-wire inserted at 45 degrees provided optimal stability in terms of stress distribution and stiffness. Among multiple wire configurations, three divergent K-wires demonstrated superior stability compared to two-wire setups.

The findings suggest that specific K-wire configurations can significantly enhance the stability of lateral condyle fracture fixation. A three divergent K-wire setup showed the best overall performance, while two divergent wires at 45 or 60 degrees also offered considerable stability. Future studies could focus on refining these models to include more realistic anatomical conditions and validating the results through clinical trials. Such advancements could lead to improved surgical outcomes for pediatric patients with lateral condyle fractures by minimizing complications associated with current fixation methods.

Conclusion

Fractures of the lateral condyle in children can be treated with surgery and fixed with cannulated screws or Kirschner wires. Type 1 and 2 fractures can be treated with percutaneous fixation. Severe displacement can be managed with closed reduction in select cases, though open reduction is preferred. Despite the favorable outcomes, lateral condyle fractures can still lead to complications, particularly nonunion and cubitus valgus.

Bibliography

1. Royle SG. Posterior dislocation of the elbow. Clin Orthop Relat Res. 1991;269:201.
2. Pollen AG. Fractures and dislocations in children. Edinburgh: Churchill Livingstone; 1973. p. 42–4.
3. Morrey BF. The elbow and its disorders. Philadelphia: W.B. Saunders; 1985. p. 277–88.
4. Conner AN, Smith MG. Displaced fractures of lateral humeral condyle in children. J Bone Joint Surg (Br). 1970;52:460–4.
5. Van Haaren ER, van Vugt AB, Bode PJ. Posterolateral dislocation of the elbow with concomitant fracture of the lateral humeral condyle: case report. J Trauma. 1994;36:288–90.
6. Rovinsky D, Ferguson C, Younis A, Otsuka NY. Pediatric elbow dislocation associated with a mi lch type I lateral condyle fracture of the humerus. J Orthop Trauma. 1999;13:458–60.

7. Murnaghan JM, Thompson NS, Taylor TC, Cosgrove AP, Ballard J. Fracture lateral epicondyle with associated elbow dislocation. Int J Clin Pract. 2002;56:475–7.
8. Cheng PG, Chang WN, Wang MN. Posteromedial dislocation of the elbow with lateral condyle fracture in children. J Chin Med Assoc. 2009;72(2):103–7.
9. Beaty JR, Sa JH. Lateral condylar and capitellar fractures of the distal humerus. In: Rockwood and Wilkins' fractures in children. 8th ed. Philadelphia: Wolters Kluwer Health; 2015. p. 701–25.
10. Ganeshalingam R, Donnan A, Evans O, Hoq M, Camp M, Donnan L. Lateral condylar fractures of the humerus in children: does the type of fixation matter? Bone Joint J. 2018;100(3):387–95.
11. Stein BE, Ramji AF, Hassanzadeh H, Wohlgemut JM, Ain MC, Sponseller PD. Cannulated lag screw fixation of displaced lateral humeral condyle fractures is associated with lower rates of open reduction and infection than pin fixation. J Pediatr Orthop. 2017;37(1):7–13. https://doi.org/10.1097/BPO.0000000000000579.
12. Franks D, Shatrov J, Symes M, Little D, Cheng T. Cannulated screw versus Kirschner-wire fixation for Milch II lateral condyle fractures in a paediatric sawbone model: a biomechanical comparison. J Child Orthop. 2018;12(1):29–35. https://doi.org/10.1302/1863-2548.12.170090.
13. Schlitz RS, Schwertz JM, Eberhardt AW, Gilbert SR. Biomechanical analysis of screws versus K-wires for lateral humeral condyle fractures. J Pediatr Orthop. 2015;35(8):e93–7. https://doi.org/10.1097/BPO.0000000000000450.
14. Gilbert SR, MacLennan PA, Schlitz RS, Estes AR. Screw versus pin fixation with open reduction of pediatric lateral condyle fractures. J Pediatr Orthop B. 2016;25(2):148–52. https://doi.org/10.1097/BPB.0000000000000238.
15. Page MJ, McKenzie JE, Bossuyt PM, Boutron I, Hoffmann TC, Mulrow CD, et al. The PRISMA 2020 statement: an updated guideline for reporting systematic reviews. Syst Rev. 2021;10(1):1–11.
16. Li WC, Xu RJ. Comparison of Kirschner wires and AO cannulated screw internal fixation for displaced lateral humeral condyle fracture in children. Int Orthop. 2012;36(6):1261–6. https://doi.org/10.1007/s00264-011-1452-y.
17. Singh R, Garg L, Jaiman A, Sharma V, Talwar J. Comparison of kirschner wires and cannulated screw internal fixation for displaced lateral humeral condyle fracture in skeletally immature patients. J Clin Orthop Trauma. 2015;6(1):62. https://doi.org/10.1016/j.jcot.2015.01.021.
18. Afaque SF, Singh A. Outcome of cancellous screw vs K wire fixation for management of neglected lateral condyle fracture of humerus in children. https://doi.org/10.33545/orthor.2020.v4.i4a.240
19. Eckhoff MD, Tadlock JC, Nicholson TC, Wells ME, Garcia EJ, Hennessey TA. Open reduction of pediatric lateral condyle fractures: a systematic review. Shoulder Elbow. 2022;14(3):316–24. https://doi.org/10.1177/17585732211010299.
20. Baharuddin M, Sharaf I. Screw osteosynthesis in the treatment of fracture lateral humeral condyle in children. Med J Malays. 2001;56:45–7.
21. Hasler CC, Von Laer L. Prevention of growth disturbances after fractures of the lateral humeral condyle in children. J Pediatr Orthop B. 2001;10(2):123–30.
22. Loke WP, Shukur MH, Yeap JK. Screw osteosynthesis of displaced lateral humeral condyle fractures in children: a mid-term review. Med J Malays. 2006;61:40–4.
23. Sinha S, Kumar A, Meena S, Jameel J, Qureshi OA, Kumar S. K wires or cannulated screws for fixation of lateral condyle fractures in children: a systematic review of comparative studies. Indian J Orthop. 2023;57(6):789–99.
24. Hardacre JA, Nahigian SH, Froimson AI, et al. Fracture of the lateral condyle of humerus in children. J Bone Joint Surg Am. 1971;53:1083–95.
25. Thapa P, Sapkota K, Wahegaonkar K, Ranjeet N, Onta PR, Thapa UJ. Comparison of Kirschner wires and cannulated screw internal fixation for displaced lateral humeral condyle fracture in children. Asian J Med Sci. 2019;10(6):75–9. https://doi.org/10.3126/ajms.v10i6.25727.
26. Sharma HMR, Wilson N. Lateral humeral condyle fractures in children: a comparative cohort study on screws versus K-wires. J Bone Joint Surg Br. 2006;88B:434.

27. Cummings JL, Schwabe MT, Rivera AE, Sanders J, Denning JR, Neal K, et al. K-wire versus screw fixation in displaced lateral condyle fractures of the Humerus in children: a multicenter study of 762 fractures. J Pediatr Orthop. 2023;43(4):e284–9.
28. Prusick VW, Dantzker NJ, Hysong AA, et al. Surgical technique for closed reduction and percutaneous pinning of pediatric lateral humeral condyle fractures. Tech Orthop. 2020;35(2):145–50. https://doi.org/10.1097/bto.0000000000000330.
29. Pennock AT, Salgueiro L, Upasani VV, Bastrom TP, Newton PO, Yaszay B. Closed reduction and percutaneous pinning versus open reduction and internal fixation for type II lateral condyle humerus fractures in children displaced> 2 mm. J Pediatr Orthop. 2016;36(8):780–6. https://doi.org/10.1097/BPO.0000000000000570.
30. Ikwuezunma IA, Suresh KV, Nhan DT, et al. Patient-reported outcomes after operative versus nonoperative treatment of pediatric lateral humeral condyle fractures. Medicine (Baltimore). 2021;100(41):e27440. https://doi.org/10.1097/md.0000000000027440.
31. Shirley E, Anderson M, Neal K, Mazur J. Screw fixation of lateral condyle fractures: results of treatment. J Pediatr Orthop. 2015;35(8):821–4.
32. Canavese F, Marengo L, Tiris A, Mansour M, Rousset M, Samba A, Andreacchio A, Dimeglio A. Radiological, clinical and functional evaluation using the quick disabilities of the arm, shoulder and hand questionnaire of children with medial epicondyle fractures treated surgically. Int Orthop. 2017;41:1447–52. https://doi.org/10.1007/s00264-017-3442-1.
33. Zorrilla SNJ, Prada-Cañizares A, Marti-Ciruelos R, et al. Supracondylar humeral fractures in children: current concepts for management and prognosis. Int Orthop. 2015;39:2287–96. https://doi.org/10.1007/s00264-015-2975-4.
34. Song KS, Kang CH, Min BW, Bae KC, Cho CH, Lee JH. Closed reduction and internal fixation of displaced unstable lateral condylar fractures of the humerus in children. J Bone Joint Surg Am. 2008;90(12):2673–81.
35. Song KS, Shin YW, Oh CW, et al. Closed reduction and internal fixation of completely displaced and rotated lateral condyle fractures of the humerus in children. J Orthop Trauma. 2010;24(7):434–8.
36. Xie LW, Wang J, Deng ZQ, Zhao RH, Chen W, Kang C, et al. Treatment of pediatric lateral condylar humerus fractures with closed reduction and percutaneous pinning. BMC Musculoskelet Disord. 2020;21(1):707.
37. Xie LW, Deng ZQ, Zhao RH, Wang J, Liu X, Zhou Y, Zhang H. Closed reduction and percutaneous pinning vs open reduction and internal fixation in pediatric lateral condylar humerus fractures displaced by > 4 mm: an observational cross-sectional study. BMC Muscoloskelet Disord. 2021;22(1):985. https://doi.org/10.1186/s12891-021-04880-8.
38. Milch H. Fractures and fracture dislocations of the humeral condyles. J Trauma Acute Care Surg. 1964;4(5):592–607.
39. Jakob R, Fowles JV, Rang M, Kassab MT. Observations concerning fractures of the lateral humeral condyle in children. J Bone Joint Surg Br. 1975;57(4):430–6.
40. Launay F, Leet AI, Jacopin S, Jouve JL, Bollini G, Sponseller PD. Lateral humeral condyle fractures in children: a comparison of two approaches to treatment. J Pediatr Orthop. 2004;24(4):385–91.
41. Qi Y, Guo L, Sun M, Wang Z. Clinical value of MRI in evaluating and diagnosing of humeral lateral condyle fracture in children. J Orthop Surg Res. 2021;16(1):617. https://doi.org/10.1186/s13018-021-02726-6.
42. Lan X, Dai M, Zhang B, Huang G. Comparative study of lateral condyle fracture with or without posteromedial elbow dislocation in children. Int Orthop. 2018;42(3):619–24. https://doi.org/10.1007/s00264-018-3795-0.
43. Sinha S, Kumar A, Meena S, Jameel J, Qureshi OA, Kumar S. K wires or cannulated screws for fixation of lateral condyle fractures in children: a systematic review of comparative studies. Indian J Orthop. 2023;57(6):789–99. https://doi.org/10.1007/s43465-023-00873-y.
44. Cho YJ, Kang SH, Kang MH. K-wire versus screws in the fixation of lateral condyle fracture of humerus in pediatrics: a systematic review and meta-analysis. BMC Musculoskelet Disord. 2023;24(1):649. https://doi.org/10.1186/s12891-023-06780-5.

45. Mostofi Zadeh Haghighi DL, Xu J, Campbell R, Moopanar TR. Kirschner wire vs screw osteosynthesis of lateral condyle fractures in paediatric patients: a systematic review. Musculoskelet Surg. 2024;109(1):9–15. https://doi.org/10.1007/s12306-024-00859-5.
46. Liu Y, Shi W, Zhao H, Li Y, Li J, Xun F, Canavese F, Xu H. Closed reduction and percutaneous pinning versus open reduction and internal fixation for Jakob type 3 lateral condyle fractures in children. Int Orthop. 2022;46(10):2291–7. https://doi.org/10.1007/s00264-022-05476-0.
47. Jeon S, Ahn W, Oh J, Chung J, Choi J, Lee S. Finite element analyses of lateral condyle fracture fixation in paediatrics regarding configuration of Kirschner-wire. BMC Musculoskelet Disord. 2022;23(1):940. https://doi.org/10.1186/s12891-022-05897-3.

Medial Epicondyle Fracture

6

Introduction by the Author

Fractures of the medial humeral epicondyle are a common injury in children and often require surgery. These fractures account for 11%–20% of all humerus fractures. Most occur between the ages of 11 and 12, and they are 4 times more prevalent in boys than in girls. Between 30% and 60% of medial epicondyle fractures are associated with elbow dislocation, so a medial epicondyle fracture must be ruled out in all children with a history of elbow dislocation. These fractures differ from the rarer medial condyle fractures that extend into the elbow joint.

Although plain radiographs are commonly used for diagnosis, magnetic resonance imaging is essential for accurately diagnosing unossified medial epicondylar fractures in children, which can easily be overlooked using conventional imaging techniques.

The treatment of medial epicondyle fractures in children is still a topic of debate. Undisplaced fractures can be treated conservatively. Otherwise, surgery is required to fix displaced fracture using cannulated screws or Kirschner wires. Due to the proximity of the ulnar nerve, all fractures requiring surgical treatment should undergo open reduction and internal fixation with Kirschner wires or screws. This approach yields excellent or good outcomes for most patients, resulting in stable, pain-free elbows and restored normal function in nearly all cases. Even with postoperative elbow immobilization, stiffness is rare.

Displaced fractures usually require open reduction, and avulsions with intra-articular entrapment necessitate precise anatomical reduction and fixation. Fractures involving intra-articular entrapment of the epicondyle require careful attention because they can cause joint surface damage and negatively impact functional outcomes.

© The Author(s), under exclusive license to Springer Nature Switzerland AG 2026

F. Canavese, *Advances in Pediatric Extremity Fracture Management*,
https://doi.org/10.1007/978-3-032-33306-3_6

Medial epicondyle fractures may also be complicated by avulsion from the flexor muscles and the medial collateral ligament. This often occurs alongside elbow dislocation.

Although no significant difference in functional scores is usually observed between dislocated and non-dislocated groups, limitations in flexion and extension tend to be more pronounced in the former. Children with displaced medial epicondyle fractures who undergo surgery tend to have good radiological, clinical, and functional outcomes; however, they require special attention to detect intra-articular entrapment of the broken epicondyle. Patients and their families should be warned of the potential risk of loss of elbow range of motion and poor functional outcomes in these cases, especially if treatment is delayed.

Open reduction and screw fixation are effective treatments for medial epicondyle fractures, whether or not they involve intra-articular incarceration. However, careful surgical technique is necessary to avoid complications such as hardware irritation or nerve entrapment. Despite the good overall functional and radiographic outcomes, medial epicondyle fractures may result in long-term complications, including nonunion, malunion, instability, nerve injury, growth arrest, deformity, and functional impairment.

6.1 Machine Generated Summaries

Disclaimer: The summaries in this chapter were generated from Springer Nature publications using abstractive AI auto-summarization: An abstraction-based summarizer creates new text based on deep learning. New phrases are created to summarize the content. As the constituted sentences are machine selected, they may not fully reflect the body of the work, so we strongly advise that the original content is read and cited. The auto-generated summaries were curated by the author(s) to meet Springer Nature publication standards.

Management of Medial Humeral Epicondyle Fractures in Children: A Structured Review Protocol for a Systematic Review of the Literature and Identification of a Core Outcome Set Using a Delphi Survey [34]

This is a machine-generated summary of:

Dorman, Sara L.; Shelton, James A.; Stevenson, Robert Allen; Linkman, Kenneth; Kirkham, Jamie; Perry, Daniel C. Management of medial humeral epicondyle fractures in children: a structured review protocol for a systematic review of the literature and identification of a core outcome set using a Delphi survey [34]

Published in: Trials (2018)
Link to original: https://doi.org/10.1186/s13063-018-2472-3
Copyright of the summarized publication:
The Author(s). 2018
License: OpenAccess CC BY + CC0 4.0

This article is distributed under the terms of the Creative Commons Attribution 4.0 International License (http://creativecommons.org/licenses/by/4.0/), which permits unrestricted use, distribution, and reproduction in any medium, provided you give appropriate credit to the original author(s) and the source, provide a link to the Creative Commons license, and indicate if changes were made. The Creative Commons Public Domain Dedication waiver (http://creativecommons.org/publicdomain/zero/1.0/) applies to the data made available in this article, unless otherwise stated.

If you want to cite the papers, please refer to the original.

For technical reasons we could not place the page where the original quote is coming from.

Research Highlights

Medial humeral epicondyle fractures are prevalent injuries in children, often necessitating surgical intervention. These injuries can lead to long-term complications such as non-union, mal-union, instability, nerve injury, growth arrest, deformity, and functional loss. Despite the frequency and potential severity of these fractures, there is a lack of standardized outcome measures to assess recovery in pediatric patients. This variability complicates the comparison of treatment outcomes across studies. Now, a new study by Sara L. Dorman and colleagues addresses this gap by developing a core outcome set (COS) for medial humeral epicondyle fractures in children.

The study employed a systematic review to identify outcomes previously reported in randomized controlled trials (RCTs), cohort studies, case-control studies, and case series. The researchers utilized multiple databases, including the Cochrane Central Register of Controlled Trials, SCOPUS, and MEDLINE, to ensure comprehensive coverage. Two independent reviewers screened titles and abstracts for eligibility, with disagreements resolved through discussion or consultation with a third reviewer. The study aimed to generate a list of all reported outcomes and measurement instruments. A Delphi process was then used to prioritize outcomes from the perspectives of key stakeholders: children, parents, and clinicians. This involved structured interviews with children who had experienced medial humeral epicondyle fractures and online questionnaires for parents and clinicians.

The development of this COS represents a significant advancement in pediatric orthopedics by providing a standardized framework for assessing outcomes in clinical trials and routine treatment of medial humeral epicondyle fractures in children. This standardization is expected to reduce research heterogeneity, improve data interpretation accuracy, and enhance the statistical power of meta-analyses. Future study directions may include integrating this COS into clinical trials funded by the

National Institute for Health Research (NIHR) Health Technology Assessment (HTA) program to further refine treatment strategies for these injuries in children.

Fracture of an Unossified Humeral Medial Epicondyle: Use of Magnetic Resonance Imaging for Diagnosis [35]

This is a machine-generated summary of:

Tanabe, Katsuhisa; Miyamoto, Nao Fracture of an unossified humeral medial epicondyle: use of magnetic resonance imaging for diagnosis [35]
Published in: Skeletal Radiology (2016)
Link to original: https://doi.org/10.1007/s00256-016-2434-3
Copyright of the summarized publication:
ISS 2016
All rights reserved.

If you want to cite the papers, please refer to the original.
For technical reasons we could not place the page where the original quote is coming from.

Research Highlights

Ossification of the humeral medial epicondyle apophysis typically begins at a young age, with physeal closure occurring in adolescence. Fractures of the medial epicondyle are common in children before this closure, but they are rarely detected before ossification begins due to limitations in radiographic imaging. Now, a new study by Katsuhisa Tanabe and colleagues highlights the importance of using MRI for diagnosing unossified medial epicondylar fractures, which are often undetectable with standard radiographs and CT scans.

In this study, the authors present a case of a young boy who suffered an avulsion fracture of the medial epicondylar apophysis that was not visible on initial radiographs or CT scans. Despite these imaging results, physical examination suggested a fracture, prompting the use of MRI. The MRI confirmed the presence of an avulsion fracture, allowing for appropriate surgical intervention. The patient underwent surgery involving tension band wiring to fix the displaced fracture. This approach was chosen due to concerns about potential valgus instability if left untreated. The successful surgical outcome was evidenced by the patient's full recovery and return to sports activities 2 years post-operation.

The study underscores the critical role of MRI in accurately diagnosing unossified medial epicondylar fractures in children, which can be easily overlooked with conventional imaging techniques. The authors suggest that MRI should be considered when there is clinical suspicion of such fractures despite normal radiographic findings. Future study could focus on refining diagnostic protocols and exploring less invasive imaging alternatives that provide similar diagnostic accuracy without requiring sedation in pediatric patients. This case contributes valuable insights into managing pediatric elbow injuries and highlights the need for heightened awareness among clinicians regarding potential diagnostic challenges associated with unossified fractures.

Pediatric Medial Epicondyle Fractures with Intra-Articular Elbow Incarceration [36]

This is a machine-generated summary of:

Tarallo, Luigi; Mugnai, Raffaele; Fiacchi, Francesco; Adani, Roberto; Zambianchi, Francesco; Catani, Fabio Pediatric medial epicondyle fractures with intra-articular elbow incarceration [37]
Published in: Journal of Orthopaedics and Traumatology (2014)
Link to original: https://doi.org/10.1007/s10195-014-0310-2
Copyright of the summarized publication:
The Author(s) 2014
License: OpenAccess CC BY 4.0

This article is distributed under the terms of the Creative Commons Attribution License which permits any use, distribution, and reproduction in any medium, provided the original author(s) and the source are credited.

If you want to cite the papers, please refer to the original.

For technical reasons we could not place the page where the original quote is coming from.

Research Highlights

Medial humeral epicondylar fractures are a common type of elbow fracture in children, often resulting from falls on an outstretched hand. These fractures can lead to significant complications, particularly when the fractured fragment becomes incarcerated within the elbow joint. Traditional treatment approaches have varied, with some advocating for surgical intervention and others for nonsurgical management. Now, a new study by Luigi Tarallo and colleagues investigates the outcomes of open reduction and internal fixation using screws in pediatric patients with medial epicondyle fractures complicated by intra-articular fragment incarceration.

The study involved 13 children treated at a university hospital between 2010 and 2015. All patients had closed fractures resulting from falls, with some cases involving elbow dislocation. The surgical procedure included open reduction and fixation with cannulated screws under fluoroscopic guidance, ensuring stable fixation to allow early motion. Postoperatively, patients were immobilized in a cast followed by a splint, with gradual introduction of range-of-motion exercises. Clinical evaluations were conducted at regular intervals to assess range of motion, pain levels, and functional outcomes using the Mayo Elbow Performance Score (MEPS). The study found that all patients achieved solid union and excellent functional outcomes, although some complications related to hardware prominence and nerve entrapment were noted.

The findings suggest that open reduction and screw fixation can provide excellent clinical and functional results for treating medial epicondyle fractures with intra-articular incarceration in children. However, the study highlights the importance of careful surgical technique to avoid complications such as hardware irritation or nerve entrapment. Future study could focus on refining surgical techniques to minimize these risks further or explore alternative fixation methods that might offer similar stability without the need for hardware removal. Additionally, long-term follow-up could provide insights into growth-related outcomes in pediatric patients undergoing this treatment approach.

Radiological, Clinical and Functional Evaluation Using the Quick Disabilities of the Arm, Shoulder and Hand Questionnaire of Children with Medial Epicondyle Fractures Treated Surgically [37]

This is a machine-generated summary of:

Canavese, Federico; Marengo, Lorenza; Tiris, Alexandru; Mansour, Mounira; Rousset, Marie; Samba, Antoine; Andreacchio, Antonio; Dimeglio, Alain Radiological, clinical and functional evaluation using the Quick Disabilities of the Arm, Shoulder and Hand questionnaire of children with medial epicondyle fractures treated surgically [37]

Published in: International Orthopaedics (2017)
Link to original: https://doi.org/10.1007/s00264-017-3442-1
Copyright of the summarized publication:
SICOT aisbl 2017
All rights reserved.

If you want to cite the papers, please refer to the original.

For technical reasons we could not place the page where the original quote is coming from.

Research Highlights

Medial epicondyle fractures account for a significant portion of elbow fractures in children and are distinct from the rarer medial condyle fractures that extend into the elbow joint. These injuries can be complicated by avulsion from the flexor muscles and medial collateral ligament, often occurring alongside elbow dislocation. Displaced fractures may necessitate open reduction, while avulsions with intra-articular entrapment require precise anatomical reduction and fixation. The functional outcomes of surgical management for these fractures, particularly when associated with elbow dislocation, remain uncertain. Now, a new study by Federico Canavese and colleagues retrospectively evaluates the clinical, functional, and radiographic outcomes of displaced medial epicondyle fractures in children undergoing surgical treatment, using the Quick DASH questionnaire to assess upper-extremity function.

The study involved a retrospective review of medical records for children who underwent surgical treatment for displaced medial epicondyle humeral fractures over a specified period. Patients were selected based on specific criteria, including closed displaced fractures visible on radiographs and managed surgically at a single institution. The Papavasiliou and Crawford classification system was used to categorize fracture types based on displacement. All patients underwent open reduction with fracture fixation using K-wires or screws, followed by immobilization in a long-arm cast. Functional outcomes were assessed using the Quick DASH questionnaire at follow-up visits, alongside radiographic evaluations to monitor fracture consolidation and detect complications.

The study found that children with type II, III, and IV medial epicondyle fractures who received surgical treatment generally experienced good radiological, clinical, and functional outcomes with low complication rates. However, intra-articular entrapment of the epicondyle requires careful attention due to its potential impact on joint surface damage and functional outcome. Future study could focus on optimizing surgical timing and techniques to further improve outcomes in these cases. The findings suggest that early surgical intervention can lead to similar functional results across different fracture types but highlight the importance of timely treatment to minimize risks of reduced range of motion and poor functional outcomes if delayed.

Clinical and Radiological Evaluation of Surgical Treatment of Medial Epicondyle Fractures of Humerus in Children. A Two-Centre Study [38]

This is a machine-generated summary of:

Stelmach, Wojciech; Beczkowski, Jacek; Zając, Piotr; Małecki, Krzysztof; Sibiński, Marcin; Niedzielski, Kryspin Clinical and radiological evaluation of surgical treatment of medial epicondyle fractures of humerus in children. A two-centre study [38]
Published in: Scientific Reports (2023)
Link to original: https://doi.org/10.1038/s41598-023-37063-7
Copyright of the summarized publication:
The Author(s) 2023
License: OpenAccess CC BY 4.0

This article is licensed under a Creative Commons Attribution 4.0 International License, which permits use, sharing, adaptation, distribution and reproduction in any medium or format, as long as you give appropriate credit to the original author(s) and the source, provide a link to the Creative Commons licence, and indicate if changes were made. The images or other third party material in this article are included in the article's Creative Commons licence, unless indicated otherwise in a credit line to the material. If material is not included in the article's Creative

Commons licence and your intended use is not permitted by statutory regulation or exceeds the permitted use, you will need to obtain permission directly from the copyright holder. To view a copy of this licence, visit http://creativecommons.org/licenses/by/4.0/.

If you want to cite the papers, please refer to the original.

For technical reasons we could not place the page where the original quote is coming from.

Research Highlights

Medial epicondyle fractures in the pediatric population represent a significant portion of humerus fractures, predominantly affecting boys and often associated with elbow dislocation. These fractures can result from direct trauma or more commonly from indirect mechanisms, leading to avulsion or hyperextension injuries. Diagnosis typically involves physical and radiological examinations to assess fracture displacement and nature. Now, a new study by Wojciech Stelmach and colleagues investigates the outcomes of open reduction and internal fixation (ORIF) using Kirschner wires for medial epicondyle fractures, comparing results between patients with and without elbow dislocation.

The study was conducted at two pediatric orthopedic centers, including patients who underwent surgical treatment with Kirschner wire stabilization for medial epicondyle fractures. Excluding those treated conservatively or with additional humerus or forearm fractures, the researchers performed surgeries using a medial approach with tourniquet application. Fractures were fixed with two or three Kirschner wires, followed by plaster cast immobilization. In cases of elbow dislocation, closed reduction preceded open repositioning and stabilization. Post-surgery, patients were assessed for range of motion, elbow stability, and ulnar nerve function using various clinical tests and imaging techniques. Statistical analyses were performed to evaluate treatment outcomes based on the Mayo Elbow Performance Score (MEPS).

The study found that ORIF with Kirschner wires is effective for treating medial epicondyle fractures, yielding good to excellent results in most cases. While no significant difference in MEPS scores was observed between dislocated and non-dislocated groups, flexion and extension limitations were more pronounced in the former. The study highlights the importance of fracture displacement degree in treatment decisions and suggests that future studies could explore alternative fixation methods or imaging techniques to enhance diagnostic accuracy. Additionally, addressing ulnar nerve dysfunction remains crucial in optimizing patient outcomes.

Displaced Medial Epicondyle Fractures of the Humerus: Surgical Treatment and Results. A Report of 139 Cases [39]

This is a machine-generated summary of:

Louahem, Djamel M.; Bourelle, Sophie; Buscayret, Florent; Mazeau, Philippe; Kelly, Paula; Dimeglio, Alain; Cottalorda, Jérôme Displaced medial epicondyle fractures of the humerus: surgical treatment and results. A report of 139 cases [39]

Published in: Archives of Orthopaedic and Trauma Surgery (2009)
Link to original: https://doi.org/10.1007/s00402-009-1009-3
Copyright of the summarized publication:
Springer-Verlag 2009
All rights reserved.

If you want to cite the papers, please refer to the original.
For technical reasons we could not place the page where the original quote is coming from.

Research Highlights

Medial epicondyle fractures of the humerus are a common type of elbow injury in children, often associated with elbow dislocation. While there is consensus on treating undisplaced or minimally displaced fractures with simple immobilization, the management of significantly displaced fractures remains controversial. Nonoperative treatment can lead to radiographic nonunion and potential valgus instability. Now, a new study by Djamel M. Louahem and colleagues aims to objectively assess the outcomes of operative treatment for displaced medial epicondyle fractures in a large pediatric cohort.

The study conducted a retrospective analysis at two centers, focusing on children with surgically treated displaced medial epicondyle fractures. Excluding type I fractures, the researchers categorized the injuries into four types based on displacement and instability. All patients underwent surgical exploration via a medial approach within 24 h of injury, confirming the extent of capsulomuscular damage. The medial epicondylar fragment was anatomically reduced and fixed using K-wires or compressive screws, followed by postoperative immobilization and gradual mobilization. The outcomes were evaluated using a modified Bede et al. scoring system, considering factors like residual instability, range of motion, pain, and neurological complications.

The study found that surgical intervention resulted in excellent or good outcomes for most patients, with stable and pain-free elbows and normal function restored in nearly all cases. Union was achieved in all instances, with minimal complications such as fibrous union or anatomical anomalies having little impact on function. Future study could explore long-term functional outcomes and compare operative versus nonoperative treatments more comprehensively. The findings support operative management for these fractures to ensure anatomic reduction and prevent valgus instability, highlighting the importance of addressing soft tissue damage alongside bone displacement.

Conclusion

If they are undisplaced, fractures of the medial epicondyle in children can be treated conservatively. Otherwise, surgery is required to fix the fracture with cannulated screws or Kirschner wires. Despite favorable outcomes, these fractures can lead to complications such as nonunion, malunion, instability, nerve injury, growth arrest, deformity, and functional loss.

Bibliography

1. National Institute for Health Research Health Technology Assessment Programme. NIHR HTA Commissioning Board Minutes of the 67th Meeting. 2017. https://www.nihr.ac.uk/about-us/documents/board-and-panel-documents/hta/HTA-Minutes-September-2017.pdf. Accessed 30 Jan 2018.
2. Dodd S. Classification of COS outcomes. 2017. http://www.comet-initiative.org/assets/downloads/6th-meeting/Dodd%20Classification%20of%20COS%20outcomes.pdf. Accessed 25 Apr 2017.
3. Beaty JH, Kasser JR. The elbow: physeal fractures, apophyseal injuries of the distal humerus, osteonecrosis of the trochlea, and T-condylar fractures. In: Beaty JH, Kasser JR, editors. Rockwood Wilkins' Fract. Child. 7th ed. Philadelphia: Lippincott Williams & Wilkins; 2010. p. 533–93.
4. May DA, Disler DG, Jones EA, Pearce DA. Using sonography to diagnose an unossified medial epicondyle avulsion in a child. AJR Am J Roentgenol. 2000;174:1115–7.
5. Chambers HG, Wilkins KE. Fractures involving the medial epicondylar apophysis. In: Rockwood Jr CA, Wilkins KE, Beaty JH, editors. Fractures in children. 4th ed. Philadelphia: Lippincott-Raven; 1996. p. 801–19.
6. Ireland ML, Andrews JR. Shoulder and elbow injuries in the young athlete. Clin Sports Med. 1988;7:473–94.
7. Wilkins KE. Fractures involving the medial epicondylar apophysis. In: Rockwood Jr CA, Wilkins KE, King RE, editors. Fractures in children. 3rd ed. Philadelphia: JB Lippincott; 1991. p. 509–828.
8. Papavasiliou VA, Crawford AH. Fracture-separation of the medial epicondylar epiphysis of the elbow joint. Clin Orthop Relat Res. 1982;171:172–4.
9. Patel NM, Ganley TJ. Medial epicondyle fractures of the humerus: how to evaluate and when to operate. J Pediatr Orthop. 2012;32:S10–3.
10. Morrey BF, An KN, Chao EYS. Functional evaluation of the elbow. In: Morrey BF, editor. The elbow and its disorders. 2nd ed. Philadelphia: WB Saunders; 1993. p. 86–9.
11. Carlsson AM. Assessment of chronic pain. I. Aspects of the reliability and validity of the visual analogue scale. Pain. 1983;16:87–101.
12. Lee HH, Shen HC, Chang JH, et al. Operative treatment of displaced medial epicondyle fractures in children and adolescents. J Shoulder Elb Surg. 2005;14:178–85.
13. Pimpalnerkar AL, Balasubramaniam G, Young SK, et al. Type four fracture of the medial epicondyle: a true indication for surgical intervention. Injury. 1998;29:751–6.
14. Louahem DM, Bourelle S, Buscayret F, Mazeau P, Kelly P, Dimeglio A, et al. Displaced medial epicondyle fractures of the humerus: surgical treatment and results. A report of 139 cases. Arch Orthop Trauma Surg. 2010;130:649–55.
15. Hines RF, Herndon WA, Evans JP. Operative treatment of medial epicondyle fractures in children. Clin Orthop Relat Res. 1987;223:170–4.
16. Knapik DM, Fausett CC, Gilmore A, Liu RW. Outcomes of nonoperative pediatric medial humeral epicondyle fractures with and without associated elbow dislocation. J Pediatr Orthop. 2016;37:e224–8.
17. Tarollo L, Mugnai R, Fiacchi F, Adani R, Zambianchi F, Catani F. Pediatric medial epicondyle fractures with intra-articular elbow incarceration. J Orthop Traumatol. 2015;16:117–23.
18. Beck JJ, Bowen RE, Silvia M. What's new in pediatric medial epicondyle fractures? J Pediatr Orthop. 2016;38(4):e202–6. https://doi.org/10.1097/BPO.0000000000000902.
19. Nielsen E, Andras LM, Anesi TJ, Lightdale-Miric N, Lee Pace J. Operative fixation of medial epicondyle fractures: complication rates based on mode of fixation. Medicine (Baltimore). 2020;99:e20015. https://doi.org/10.1097/MD.0000000000020015.
20. Pappas N, Lawrence JT, Donegan D, Ganley T, Flynn JM. Intraobserver and interobserver agreement in the measurement of displaced humeral medial epicondyle fractures in children. J Bone Jt Surg Am. 2010;92:322–7. https://doi.org/10.2106/JBJS.I.00493.

21. Kamath AF, Baldwin K, Horneff J, et al. Operative versus non-operative management of pediatric medial epicondyle fractures: a systematic review. J Child Orthop. 2009;3:345–57.
22. May CJ, Shore BJ. Open reduction and internal fixation of pediatric medial epicondylar humeral fractures in the prone position. JBJS Essent Surg Tech. 2021;11:e19.00069. https://doi.org/10.2106/JBJS.ST.19.00069.
23. Grahn P, Hämäläinen T, Nietosvaara Y, Ahonen M. Comparison of outcome between nonoperative and operative treatment of medial epicondyle fractures. Acta Orthop. 2021;92:114–9. https://doi.org/10.1080/17453674.2020.1832312.
24. Pezzutti D, Lin JS, Singh S, Rowan M, Balch Samora J. Pediatric medial epicondyle fracture management: a systematic review. J Pediatr Orthop. 2020;40:e697–702. https://doi.org/10.1097/BPO.0000000000001532.
25. Pathy R, Dodwell ER. Medial epicondyle fractures in children. Curr Opin Pediatr. 2015;27:58–66. https://doi.org/10.1097/MOP.0000000000000181.
26. Gottschalk HP, Eisner E, Hosalkar HS. Medial epicondyle fractures in the pediatric population. J Am Acad Orthop Surg. 2012;20:223–32.
27. Fahey JJ. Fractures of the elbow in children. AAOS Inst Course Lect. 1960;17:13–46.
28. Rang M. Children's fractures. 2nd ed. Philadelphia: JB Lippincott; 1983.
29. Lechevallier J, Lefort J. Les Fractures du coude: les fractures de l'épitrochlée. Rev Chir Orthop. 1987;73:441–7.
30. Fevre M, Roudaitis A. La réduction non sanglante des fractures de l'épitrochlée avec interposition de ce fragment dans l'interligne articulaire du coude. Rev Chir Orthop. 1933;20:300–14.
31. Woods GM, Tullos HG. Elbow instability and medial epicondyle fracture. Am J Sports Med. 1977;5:23–30.
32. Josefsson PO, Danielsson LG. Epicondylar elbow fracture in children. 35-year follow-up of 56 unreduced cases. Acta Orthop Scand. 1986;57:313–5.
33. Gilchrist AD, McKee MD. Valgus instability of the elbow due to medial epicondyle nonunion: treatment by fragment excision and ligament repair. A report of 5 cases. J Shoulder Elb Surg. 2002;11:493–7.
34. Dorman SL, Shelton JA, Stevenson RA, Linkman K, Kirkham J, Perry DC. Management of medial humeral epicondyle fractures in children: a structured review protocol for a systematic review of the literature and identification of a core outcome set using a Delphi survey. Trials. 2018; https://doi.org/10.1186/s13063-018-2472-3.
35. Tanabe K, Miyamoto N. Fracture of an unossified humeral medial epicondyle: use of magnetic resonance imaging for diagnosis. Skeletal Radiol. 2016; https://doi.org/10.1007/s00256-016-2434-3.
36. Tarallo L, Mugnai R, Fiacchi F, Adani R, Zambianchi F, Catani F. Pediatric medial epicondyle fractures with intra-articular elbow incarceration. J Orthop Traumatol. 2014; https://doi.org/10.1007/s10195-014-0310-2.
37. Canavese F, Marengo L, Tiris A, Mansour M, Rousset M, Samba A, Andreacchio A, Dimeglio A. Radiological, clinical and functional evaluation using the quick disabilities of the arm, shoulder and hand questionnaire of children with medial epicondyle fractures treated surgically. Int Orthop. 2017; https://doi.org/10.1007/s00264-017-3442-1.
38. Stelmach W, Beczkowski J, Zając P, Małecki K, Sibiński M, Niedzielski K. Clinical and radiological evaluation of surgical treatment of medial epicondyle fractures of humerus in children. A two-centre study. Sci Rep. 2023; https://doi.org/10.1038/s41598-023-37063-7.
39. Louahem DM, Bourelle S, Buscayret F, Mazeau P, Kelly P, Dimeglio A, Cottalorda J. displaced medial epicondyle fractures of the humerus: surgical treatment and results. A report of 139 cases. Arch Orthop Trauma Surg. 2009; https://doi.org/10.1007/s00402-009-1009-3.

Olecranon Fracture

7

Introduction by the Author

Olecranon fractures are uncommon in patients with skeletal immaturity, accounting for only about 5% of all elbow fractures in children. It is estimated that fewer than 2% of healthy children will sustain an olecranon fracture, though they are a more common occurrence in children with osteogenesis imperfecta. While the fracture often involves the apophysis in healthy children, apophyseal involvement is more common in patients with osteogenesis imperfecta.

Olecranon fractures in pediatric patients are often caused by high-energy trauma, such as falling on an outstretched hand. These fractures can significantly impact the articular surface of the elbow joint and the development of the ulnar bone epiphyses.

There is currently no universally accepted classification system for olecranon fractures in children.

For non-displaced or minimally displaced fractures, conservative treatment is sufficient and usually involves a long arm cast in extension or mild flexion to decrease the traction exerted by the triceps brachii muscle. However, surgical intervention is recommended for displacements of 5 mm or more, intra-articular fractures, unstable fractures, open fractures, and apophyseal involvement, as it helps prevent long-term complications, such as growth disturbances and fixed flexion deformities.

Displacements of 2–5 mm represent a gray zone. Treatment depends on the patient's age, the location and biomechanical stability of the fracture.

Olecranon fractures may occur alone or alongside other elbow injuries. In particular, transolecranon fractures associated with radial head dislocation

© The Author(s), under exclusive license to Springer Nature Switzerland AG 2026

F. Canavese, *Advances in Pediatric Extremity Fracture Management*,
https://doi.org/10.1007/978-3-032-33306-3_7

require attention because they are frequently misdiagnosed as type 1 Monteggia fractures, according to Bado. These lesions are rare and are also seen in adults. In such cases, reducing the fracture of the olecranon and restoring the normal anatomy of the humeroradial joint are necessary for a positive clinical outcome.

Due to the limited number of studies and the variety of techniques used, the optimal surgical approach for treating these fractures in skeletally immature patients is still being debated. Traditional treatments for displaced olecranon fractures include tension band wiring and suturing. However, recent evidence suggests that an isolated screw can provide similar functional and radiographic outcomes. Both methods achieve good fracture reduction and similar functional recovery, suggesting that either approach can be used effectively depending on the surgeon's preference and expertise.

7.1 Machine Generated Summaries

Disclaimer: The summaries in this chapter were generated from Springer Nature publications using abstractive AI auto-summarization: An abstraction-based summarizer creates new text based on deep learning. New phrases are created to summarize the content. As the constituted sentences are machine selected, they may not fully reflect the body of the work, so we strongly advise that the original content is read and cited. The auto-generated summaries were curated by the author(s) to meet Springer Nature publication standards.

Olecranon Fractures in Children: Treatment of a Rare Entity [57]

This is a machine-generated summary of:

Kalbitz, Miriam; Weber, Birte; Lackner, Ina; Beer, Meinrad; Pressmar, Jochen
Olecranon fractures in children: treatment of a rare entity [57]
Published in: European Journal of Trauma and Emergency Surgery (2020)
Link to original: https://doi.org/10.1007/s00068-020-01518-7
Copyright of the summarized publication:
Springer-Verlag GmbH Germany, part of Springer Nature 2020
All rights reserved.

If you want to cite the papers, please refer to the original.

For technical reasons we could not place the page where the original quote is coming from.

Research Highlights

Elbow injuries are prevalent in children, but interpreting radiographs can be challenging due to the radiolucency of cartilage and the presence of multiple ossification centers. Olecranon fractures, however, are rare in this demographic, accounting for a small percentage of elbow injuries in children. In healthy children, these fractures often involve the apophysis, whereas in those with osteogenesis imperfecta, apophyseal involvement is more common. Now, a new study by Miriam Kalbitz and colleagues investigates the classification and treatment strategies for olecranon fractures in a large cohort of pediatric patients, aiming to correlate fracture types with treatment outcomes.

The study conducted a retrospective chart review of pediatric patients under 18 years old treated for olecranon fractures at a Level I Trauma Center between 2000 and 2020. The researchers classified the fractures using the AO Pediatric Comprehensive Classification of Long Bone Fractures (AO-PCCF) and analyzed treatment strategies ranging from conservative methods like casting to surgical interventions such as tension band wiring and plate stabilization. The study included 100 patients with a mean age of 10.5 years, categorized into age groups based on developmental stages. Data analysis revealed that simple complete olecranon fractures were most common, with avulsion fractures showing significant displacement. Treatment decisions were influenced by fracture type and displacement severity.

The study highlights the need for a consistent classification system that considers both fracture morphology and displacement to guide treatment strategies effectively. Surgical intervention is recommended for displacements ≥5 mm, intra-articular fractures, unstable fracture conditions, open fractures, and apophyseal involvement. Conversely, conservative treatment suffices for non-displaced or minimally displaced fractures. Future studies could focus on long-term outcomes and refine classification systems to improve treatment precision further. This research provides valuable insights into managing olecranon fractures in children and underscores the importance of tailored treatment approaches based on comprehensive fracture assessment.

Surgical Treatment of Olecranon Fractures in Children [58]

This is a machine-generated summary of:

Arbes, Stephanie; Platzer, Patrick; Vécsei, Vilmos Surgical treatment of olecranon fractures in children [58]
Published in: European Journal of Orthopaedic Surgery & Traumatology (2011)
Link to original: https://doi.org/10.1007/s00590-011-0824-8
Copyright of the summarized publication:
Springer-Verlag 2011
All rights reserved.

If you want to cite the papers, please refer to the original.

For technical reasons we could not place the page where the original quote is coming from.

Research Highlights

Olecranon fractures in children are relatively rare, constituting a small percentage of pediatric elbow fractures. These injuries often result from falls on an outstretched hand, with associated injuries frequently observed. Treatment strategies for olecranon fractures depend on various factors, including fracture type and displacement. While conservative management is often effective for non-displaced fractures, surgical intervention is typically required for displaced fractures. Now, a new study by Stephanie Arbes and colleagues evaluates the effectiveness of different fixation techniques for displaced olecranon fractures in children, comparing clinical and radiographic outcomes across various methods.

The study involved a cohort of children treated for olecranon fractures at a single hospital over several years. Ninety patients with non-displaced or minimally displaced fractures received conservative treatment, while 12 patients with displaced fractures underwent surgical intervention. The surgical techniques assessed included open reduction with tension band wiring (TBW), absorbable tension band sutures (TBS), and other fixation methods such as screws and plates. The choice of technique was influenced by patient age and fracture characteristics. Postoperative care involved immobilization in a plaster cast, followed by clinical and radiographic evaluations using an adapted Murphey score to assess outcomes.

The study found that all fractures healed successfully within an average of 3 months, although some patients experienced complications such as incomplete reduction or secondary loss of reduction. Clinical outcomes were generally positive, with most patients achieving excellent or good results according to the Murphey score. However, radiologic outcomes were less satisfactory due to issues with reduction quality. The TBS technique showed promise by reducing hardware-related complications compared to traditional TBW methods. Future study could focus on refining surgical techniques to improve radiologic outcomes and further minimize growth disturbances associated with these injuries.

Short-Term Outcomes of Herbert Screw Fixation for Isolated Olecranon Fractures in Children: A Single-Institution Retrospective Study [59]

This is a machine-generated summary of:

Li, Yang; Wang, Kelai; Sun, Dong; Liu, Yakun; Wang, Zhe; Li, Aiwu Short-Term Outcomes of Herbert Screw Fixation for Isolated Olecranon Fractures in Children: A Single-Institution Retrospective Study [59]

Published in: Indian Journal of Orthopaedics (2022)
Link to original: https://doi.org/10.1007/s43465-022-00609-4
Copyright of the summarized publication:
Indian Orthopaedics Association 2022
All rights reserved.

If you want to cite the papers, please refer to the original.

For technical reasons we could not place the page where the original quote is coming from.

Research Highlights

Elbow fractures are common in children, but olecranon fractures are relatively rare, accounting for a small percentage of pediatric elbow injuries. These fractures often result from high-energy mechanisms and can significantly impact the elbow joint's articular surface and the development of ulnar bone epiphyses. Traditional treatments for displaced olecranon fractures include tension band wiring (TBW) and tension band suture (TBS), which, despite their effectiveness, often lead to complications such as hardware irritation and high reoperation rates. Now, a new study by Yang Li and colleagues explores the use of Herbert screws for treating isolated Mayo IIA type olecranon fractures in children, aiming to assess clinical and functional outcomes.

The study retrospectively reviewed cases of children treated with closed reduction and percutaneous Herbert screw fixation for olecranon fractures at a single institution. The inclusion criteria were displacement greater than 2 mm and ages between 5 and 15 years. The surgical procedure involved using Kirschner wires for fracture reduction followed by Herbert screw fixation, with postoperative immobilization in a functional position. Follow-ups included radiographic examinations and assessments using the QuickDASH questionnaire to evaluate elbow function. The study found that all patients achieved complete bone healing without complications such as implant migration or persistent joint pain. The Herbert screws provided stable fixation, allowing for good functional recovery with minimal soft tissue irritation.

The study suggests that Herbert screw fixation is a viable alternative to traditional methods like TBW or TBS for treating pediatric olecranon fractures, offering advantages such as reduced hardware irritation and less invasive removal procedures. Although the study's retrospective design and small sample size limit its generalizability, it provides promising evidence supporting Herbert screws as an effective treatment option. Future studies could focus on long-term outcomes and further investigate the impact on epiphyseal growth to solidify these findings.

Outcome of Isolated Olecranon Fractures in Skeletally Immature Patients: Comparison of Open Reduction and Tension Band Wiring Fixation Versus Closed Reduction and Percutaneous Screw Fixation [60]

This is a machine-generated summary of:

Corradin, Marco; Marengo, Lorenza; Andreacchio, Antonio; Paonessa, Matteo; Giacometti, Vanessa; Samba, Antoine; Rousset, Marie; Canavese, Federico Outcome of isolated olecranon fractures in skeletally immature patients: comparison of open reduction and tension band wiring fixation versus closed reduction and percutaneous screw fixation [60]

Published in: European Journal of Orthopaedic Surgery & Traumatology (2016)
Link to original: https://doi.org/10.1007/s00590-016-1774-y
Copyright of the summarized publication:
Springer-Verlag France 2016
All rights reserved.

If you want to cite the papers, please refer to the original.

For technical reasons we could not place the page where the original quote is coming from.

Research Highlights

Isolated olecranon fractures in children are relatively rare, comprising a small percentage of pediatric humeral fractures. These injuries can often be managed conservatively if minimally displaced, but surgical intervention is required for fractures with significant displacement to prevent long-term complications such as growth disturbances and fixed flexion deformities. The optimal surgical approach for treating these fractures in skeletally immature patients remains debated due to limited studies and varied techniques. Now, a new study by Marco Corradin and colleagues compares the outcomes of two surgical methods—open reduction with tension band wiring and closed reduction with percutaneous screw fixation—in treating displaced olecranon fractures in children.

The study retrospectively analyzed 22 children with isolated, displaced olecranon fractures treated at two institutions using either open reduction with tension band wiring or closed reduction with percutaneous screw fixation. Patients were selected based on specific criteria, including fracture displacement greater than 5 mm and absence of neurovascular injury. The surgical procedures were performed by experienced pediatric orthopedic teams, with postoperative care involving immobilization in a long-arm cast. Radiographic assessments were conducted to ensure proper fracture reduction, while functional outcomes were evaluated using the Quick DASH questionnaire. Statistical analyses revealed no significant differences in demographic data or clinical outcomes between the two groups.

The findings indicate that both surgical techniques provide satisfactory radiological and clinical outcomes for pediatric displaced olecranon fractures, with minimal complications. The study highlights that both methods achieve good fracture reduction and similar functional recovery, suggesting either approach can be effectively used depending on surgeon preference and expertise. Future study could focus on long-term outcomes to assess potential growth disturbances as patients reach skeletal maturity. Despite some limitations, such as the retrospective design and small sample size, this research contributes valuable insights into the management of these uncommon pediatric injuries.

Management Strategies of Pediatric Ipsilateral Olecranon with Associated Radial Neck Fractures Based on Multicenter Experience [61]

This is a machine-generated summary of:

Li, Jin; Tang, Sheng Ping; Nan, Guo Xin; Li, Ming; Chen, Shun You; Mei, Hai Bo; Shao, Jing Fan; Jiang, Fei; Lee, Rushyuan J.; Tang, Xin Management strategies of pediatric ipsilateral olecranon with associated radial neck fractures based on multicenter experience [61]
Published in: Journal of Orthopaedic Surgery and Research (2021)
Link to original: https://doi.org/10.1186/s13018-021-02373-x
Copyright of the summarized publication:
The Author(s) 2021
License: OpenAccess CC BY + CC0 4.0

This article is licensed under a Creative Commons Attribution 4.0 International License, which permits use, sharing, adaptation, distribution and reproduction in any medium or format, as long as you give appropriate credit to the original author(s) and the source, provide a link to the Creative Commons licence, and indicate if changes were made. The images or other third party material in this article are included in the article's Creative Commons licence, unless indicated otherwise in a credit line to the material. If material is not included in the article's Creative Commons licence and your intended use is not permitted by statutory regulation or exceeds the permitted use, you will need to obtain permission directly from the copyright holder. To view a copy of this licence, visit http://creativecommons.org/licenses/by/4.0/. The Creative Commons Public Domain Dedication waiver (http://creativecommons.org/publicdomain/zero/1.0/) applies to the data made available in this article, unless otherwise stated in a credit line to the data.

If you want to cite the papers, please refer to the original.

For technical reasons we could not place the page where the original quote is coming from.

Research Highlights

Monteggia fractures, characterized by a fracture of the ulna with dislocation of the radial head, have been well-documented in orthopedic literature. However, the Bado classification does not account for pediatric cases involving ipsilateral olecranon or shaft of ulna fractures with associated radial neck fractures, with or without radial head dislocation. These rare injuries have been previously described as greenstick fractures of the proximal ulnar metaphysis with concurrent radial neck fractures. Due to their rarity, there has been no established classification or recommended treatment strategy, often resulting in poor treatment outcomes. Now, a new study by Jin Li and colleagues addresses this gap by characterizing these injuries and proposing a treatment strategy based on data from multiple centers.

The study retrospectively reviewed pediatric patients with forearm fractures from seven high-volume pediatric trauma centers over a specified period. Inclusion criteria required patients to have an olecranon fracture with an associated ipsilateral radial neck fracture and complete clinical and radiological data with a minimum follow-up period. Exclusion criteria included open fractures or concomitant upper extremity fractures. The researchers collected demographic data, fracture characteristics, treatment methods, and postoperative outcomes from these centers. Fractures were classified based on anatomical and biomechanical considerations, such as fracture obliquity and displacement degree. Statistical analysis was conducted using STATA/SE software to evaluate correlations between functional outcomes and fracture subtypes or treatment choices.

The study's findings led to the development of a simplified classification system for these complex injuries, distinguishing them from classic Monteggia fractures. This new system aids in predicting mid-term treatment outcomes and guiding treatment selection. The authors propose that only type I fractures may be treated non-operatively, while types II to V require surgical intervention. Future studies could focus on prospective multicenter trials to further validate this classification system and refine treatment strategies. This research provides orthopedic surgeons with valuable insights into managing these rare injuries more effectively, potentially reducing complications and improving patient outcomes.

Trans-Olecranon Fracture–Dislocation of the Elbow in Children [62]

This is a machine-generated summary of:

Yang, Zheng; Feng, Chao; Bian, Zhen; Lu, Ming; Zhou, Dafei Trans-olecranon fracture–dislocation of the elbow in children [62]
Published in: International Orthopaedics (2021)
Link to original: https://doi.org/10.1007/s00264-021-05010-8
Copyright of the summarized publication:
SICOT aisbl 2021
All rights reserved.

If you want to cite the papers, please refer to the original.

For technical reasons we could not place the page where the original quote is coming from.

Research Highlights

Trans-olecranon fracture–dislocations in children are rare and complex injuries characterized by an anterior dislocation of the elbow with an associated fracture of the olecranon. Historically, these injuries have been underdiagnosed, often mistaken for Monteggia lesions due to a lack of understanding among surgeons. The mechanism involves an anterior force on a flexed elbow, causing the olecranon to fracture and the distal ulna to dislocate. Treatment strategies for this injury remain unclear, with various methods such as open reduction with plates, K-wires, or tension-band fixation being reported. Now, a new study by Zheng Yang and colleagues provides insights into the treatment and outcomes of trans-olecranon fracture–dislocations in children through a retrospective review at Beijing Jishuitan Hospital.

The study involved a retrospective analysis of 11 pediatric cases diagnosed with trans-olecranon fracture–dislocation. The researchers collected data on imaging techniques, treatment options, and therapeutic outcomes to provide a clearer clinical description and more accurate treatment options. All patients underwent open reduction and internal fixation through a posterior approach, followed by immobilization in a sling and supervised passive exercises postoperatively. Injuries were classified using the Tiemdjo classification system, which helped guide treatment decisions based on fracture type. The study found that early surgical intervention led to better clinical outcomes compared to delayed surgery. Statistical analysis was performed using Prism software, revealing that all cases achieved stable fracture reduction and elbow relocation at follow-up.

The study advances our understanding of trans-olecranon fracture–dislocations in children by highlighting the importance of early surgical intervention for optimal outcomes. It suggests that anatomical reduction and stable fixation are crucial for recovery, with different fixation methods recommended based on the Tiemdjo classification type. Future study could focus on developing guidelines for treating these injuries in children, as current recommendations are based on limited case series. The authors acknowledge limitations such as the small sample size and short follow-up period but emphasize that their findings could aid surgeons in identifying and treating this rare injury more effectively.

The Characteristics and Treatment Strategy for Transolecranon Fracture-Dislocation of the Elbow in Children: A Retrospective Study [63]

This is a machine-generated summary of:

Su, Fei; Sun, Chuan; Wang, Bing; Li, Min; Qu, Ji Ning; Yang, Ya Ting; Wu, Yong Tao; Jie, Qiang The characteristics and treatment strategy for transolecranon fracture-dislocation of the elbow in children: a retrospective study [63]

Published in: BMC Musculoskeletal Disorders (2022)
Link to original: https://doi.org/10.1186/s12891-022-05249-1

Copyright of the summarized publication:
The Author(s) 2022
License: OpenAccess CC BY + CC0 4.0

This article is licensed under a Creative Commons Attribution 4.0 International License, which permits use, sharing, adaptation, distribution and reproduction in any medium or format, as long as you give appropriate credit to the original author(s) and the source, provide a link to the Creative Commons licence, and indicate if changes were made. The images or other third party material in this article are included in the article's Creative Commons licence, unless indicated otherwise in a credit line to the material. If material is not included in the article's Creative Commons licence and your intended use is not permitted by statutory regulation or exceeds the permitted use, you will need to obtain permission directly from the copyright holder. To view a copy of this licence, visit http://creativecommons.org/licenses/by/4.0/. The Creative Commons Public Domain Dedication waiver (http://creativecommons.org/publicdomain/zero/1.0/) applies to the data made available in this article, unless otherwise stated in a credit line to the data.

If you want to cite the papers, please refer to the original.

For technical reasons we could not place the page where the original quote is coming from.

Research Highlights

Transolecranon fracture-dislocation of the elbow, first reported by Biga in adults, is a rare and complex injury in children, characterized by unique pathological features and treatment challenges. This condition is often misdiagnosed as other types of elbow injuries, leading to improper treatment that can result in severe complications such as forearm compartment syndrome and elbow stiffness. Now, a new study by Fei Su and colleagues from Honghui Hospital, Xi'an Jiaotong University, reviews cases of transolecranon fracture-dislocation in children to better understand its clinical characteristics and improve diagnosis and treatment strategies.

The study conducted a retrospective analysis of pediatric patients treated for transolecranon fracture-dislocation at a single institution. The researchers included children with elbow dislocations who could be followed up completely, excluding those with multiple fractures or neurovascular injuries. Treatment involved closed reduction under local anesthesia for dislocations, followed by open reduction and internal fixation for fractures if necessary. The surgical approach varied depending on the fracture type: tension-band wiring with K-wires was used for simple fractures, while comminuted fractures required additional reconstruction plates. Postoperative care included plaster immobilization and functional therapy. Outcomes were assessed using the Mayo Elbow Performance Score (MEPS), with follow-ups conducted at regular intervals to evaluate healing and joint function.

The study advances understanding of transolecranon fracture-dislocation in children by highlighting that these injuries are generally less severe than in adults due to differences in bone structure and flexibility. The findings suggest that most pediatric cases involve simple fractures that can be effectively managed with less invasive techniques compared to adults. Future study could focus on larger sample sizes and longer follow-up periods to better predict long-term outcomes and potential complications. This research underscores the importance of accurate diagnosis and tailored treatment approaches to optimize recovery in pediatric patients with this rare injury.

Outcome of Lateral Humeral Condylar Mass Fractures in Children Associated with Elbow Dislocation or Olecranon Fracture [64]

This is a machine-generated summary of:

Sharma, H.; Sibinski, M.; Sherlock, D. A. Outcome of lateral humeral condylar mass fractures in children associated with elbow dislocation or olecranon fracture [64]
Published in: International Orthopaedics (2007)
Link to original: https://doi.org/10.1007/s00264-007-0463-1
Copyright of the summarized publication:
Springer-Verlag 2007
All rights reserved.**If you want to cite the papers, please refer to the original.**

For technical reasons we could not place the page where the original quote is coming from.

Research Highlights

Lateral condylar mass (LCM) fractures of the distal humerus are a common pediatric elbow injury, second only to supracondylar fractures. While undisplaced LCM fractures can be managed conservatively, displaced fractures typically require open reduction and internal fixation. However, there is limited literature on LCM fractures occurring alongside olecranon fractures or elbow dislocations in children. Now, a new study by H. Sharma and colleagues presents the largest series of LCM fractures concurrent with olecranon fractures, aiming to elucidate management strategies, outcomes, and complication rates.

The study involved a retrospective review of elbow/humeral injuries from January to June, identifying cases with concurrent LCM and olecranon fractures. Researchers collected demographic data, injury mechanisms, diagnoses, and treatment details from medical records and radiographs. The stability of the elbow was assessed intraoperatively, with LCM fractures reduced using K-wires or screws based on surgeon preference. Undisplaced fractures were managed nonoperatively with plaster immobilization. Outcomes were evaluated using Flynn's criteria, focusing on carrying angle, range of motion, and complications. The study found that most patients achieved satisfactory outcomes; however, three patients experienced minor loss of extension.

The study advances understanding by highlighting the complexity of managing LCM fractures with associated injuries in children. It underscores the importance of thorough preoperative evaluation and appropriate management strategies to prevent complications such as nonunion or malunion. Future study could focus on refining surgical techniques and postoperative care to further improve outcomes. The authors emphasize the need for careful assessment under anesthesia for complex cases and suggest that undisplaced LCM fractures with olecranon involvement can be managed conservatively without stability testing under anesthesia. This research provides valuable insights into optimizing treatment protocols for these uncommon but challenging pediatric injuries.

Conclusion

Olecranon fractures are rare in children and can usually be treated conservatively if they are minimally displaced. However, significantly displaced fractures require surgery to prevent long-term complications, such as growth disturbances and fixed flexion deformities. Equally good results can be achieved with tension band wiring or screw fixation.

Bibliography

1. Stichhauer R, Turek J, Preis J, Zeman J, Marek O, Planka L. Verification of the necessity for the open reduction and tension band wiring of the displaced olecranon fracture in younger children. Acta Chir OrthopTraumatolCech. 2018;85(4):271–5.
2. Landin LA, Danielsson LG. Elbow fractures in children. An epidemiological analysis of 589 cases. Acta Orthop Scand. 1986;57(4):309–12.
3. Tayne S, Smith PA. Olecranon fractures in pediatric patients with osteogenesis imperfecta. J Pediatr Orthop. 2019;39(7):e558–e56262.
4. Evans MC, Graham HK. Olecranon fractures in children: part 1: a clinical review; part 2: a new classification and management algorithm. J Pediatr Orthop. 1999;19(5):559–69.
5. Gwynne-Jones DP. Displaced olecranon apophyseal fractures in children with osteogenesis imperfecta. J Pediatr Orthop. 2005;25(2):154–7.
6. Quick TJ, Gibbons P, Smith N. An olecranon chondral flap and osteochondral coronoid fracture in a spontaneously reduced elbow dislocation in a child. J Pediatr Orthop B. 2013;22(5):481–5.
7. Gicquel PH, De Billy B, Karger CS, Clavert JM. Olecranon fractures in 26 children with mean follow-up of 59 months. J Pediatr Orthop. 2001;21(2):141–7.
8. Takase K, Mizuochi J. Irreducible dislocation of the radial head with undisplaced olecranon fracture in a child: a case report. J Pediatr Orthop B. 2011;20(5):345–8.
9. Fujimori T, Kuriyama K, Yamamoto K, Moritomo H, Yoshikawa H. Occult posterolateral rotatory dislocation of the elbow with olecranon fracture in a child: a case report. J Med Case Rep. 2012;6:273.
10. Gaddy BC, Strecker WB, Schoenecker PL. Surgical treatment of displaced olecranon fractures in children. J Pediatr Orthop. 1997;17(3):321–4.
11. Gicquel P, Maximin MC, Boutemy P, Karger C, Kempf JF, Clavert JM. Biomechanical analysis of olecranon fracture fixation in children. J Pediatr Orthop. 2002;22(1):17–211.
12. Harrell RM, Tong J, Weinhold PS, Dahners LE. Comparison of the mechanical properties of different tension band materials and suture techniques. J Orthop Trauma. 2003;17(2):119–22.
13. Gortzak Y, Mercado E, Atar D, Weisel Y. Pediatric olecranon fractures: open reduction and internal fixation with removable Kirschner wires and absorbable sutures. J Pediatr Orthop. 2006;26(1):39–42.
14. Gustilo RB, Anderson JT. Prevention of infection in the treatment of one thousand and twenty-five open fractures of long bones: retrospective and prospective analyses. J Bone Joint Surg Am. 1976;58(4):453–8.
15. Gicquel P, Maximin MC, Boutemy P, Karger C, Kempf JF, Clavert JM. Biomechanical analysis of olecranon fracture fixation in children. J Pediatr Orthop. 2002;22(1):17–21.
16. Gicquel P, Giacomelli MC, Karger C, Clavert JM. Surgical technique and preliminary results of a new fixation concept for olecranon fractures in children. J Pediatr Orthop. 2003;23(3):398–401.
17. Graves SC, Canale ST. Fractures of the olecranon in children: long-term follow-up. J Pediatr Orthop. 1993;13(2):239–41.
18. Newell RL. Fractures of the olecranon in children. Injury. 1975;7(1):33–6.

19. Papavasiliou VA, Beslikas TA, Nenopoulos S. Isolated fractures of the olecranon in children. Injury. 1987;18(2):100–2.
20. Grantham SA, Kiernan HA. Displaced olecranon fractures in children. J Trauma. 1975;15(3):197–204.
21. Caterini R, Farsetti P, D'Arrigo C, Ippolito E. Fractures of the olecranon in children. Long-term follow-up of 39 cases. J Pediatr Orthop B. 2002;11(4):320–8. https://doi.org/10.1097/00009957-200210000-00010.
22. den Hamer A, Heusinkveld M, Traa W, Oomen P, Oliva F, Del Buono A, Maffulli N. Current techniques for management of transverse displaced olecranon fractures. Muscles Ligaments Tendons J. 2015;5(2):129–40.
23. Perkins CA, Busch MT, Christino MA, Axelrod J, Devito DP, Fabregas JA, et al. Olecranon fractures in children and adolescents: outcomes based on fracture fixation. J Child Orthop. 2018;12(5):497–501.
24. Macausland WR. The treatment of fractures of the olecranon by longitudinal screw or nail fixation. Ann Surg. 1942;116:293–6. https://doi.org/10.1097/00000658-194208000-00015.
25. Bosman WMPF, Emmink BL, Bhashyam AR, Houwert RM, Keizer J. Correction to: intramedullary screw fixation for simple displaced olecranon fractures. Eur J Trauma Emerg Surg. 2020;46(1):91. https://doi.org/10.1007/s00068-019-01269-0.
26. García-Elvira R, Vives-Barquiel MA, Camacho-Carrasco P. Olecranon mayo IIA fractures treated with transosseous high strength suture: a series of 29 cases. Injury. 2020;51:S94–102. https://doi.org/10.1016/j.injury.2020.02.011.
27. Claessen FM, Braun Y, Peters RM, Dyer G, Doornberg JN, Factors Ring D. Associated with reoperation after fifixation of displaced olecranon fractures. Clin Orthop Relat Res. 2016;474(1):193–200. https://doi.org/10.1007/s11999-015-4488-2.
28. Rabinovich A, Adili A, Mah J. Outcomes of intramedullary nail fixation through the olecranon apophysis in skeletally immature forearm fractures. J Pediatr Orthop. 2005;25(5):565–9. https://doi.org/10.1097/01.bpo.0000173249.04561.10.
29. Karlsson MK, Hasserius R, Karlsson C, Besjakov J, Josefsson PO. Fractures of the olecranon during growth: a 15–25-year follow-up. J Pediatr Orthop B. 2002;11:251–5.
30. Matthews JG. Fractures of the olecranon in children. Injury. 1980;12(3):207–12.
31. Wright PR. Greenstick fracture of the upper end of the ulna with dislocation of the radio-humeral joint or displacement of the superior radial epiphysis. J Bone Joint Surg Br. 1963;45:727–31.
32. Ruchelsman DE, Christoforou D, Jupiter JB. Fractures of the radial head and neck. J Bone Joint Surg Am. 2013;95(5):469–78. https://doi.org/10.2106/JBJS.J.01989.
33. Sur YJ, Park JB, Song SW. Pediatric posterior monteggia lesion: a greenstick fracture of the proximal ulnar metaphysis with radial neck fracture. A case report. J Orthop Trauma. 2010 Feb;24(2):e12–6. https://doi.org/10.1097/BOT.0b013e3181a5e441.
34. Foruria AM, Augustin S, Morrey BF, Sanchez-Sotelo J. Heterotopic ossification after surgery for fractures and fracture-dislocations involving the proximal aspect of the radius or ulna. J Bone Joint Surg Am. 2013;95(10):e66.
35. Giannicola G, Scacchi M, Sacchetti FM, Cinotti G. Clinical usefulness of proximal ulnar and radial fracture-dislocation comprehensive classification system (PURCCS): prospective study of 39 cases. J Shoulder Elb Surg. 2013;22(12):1729–36.
36. Arain AR, Haddad S, Anderson M, Murtaza H, Rosenbaum A. Isolated pediatric transolecranon fracture-dislocation of the elbow managed nonoperatively: a case report and review of literature. Clin Case Reports. 2019;7(7):1435–8.
37. Bouaziz W, Guidara AR, Trabelsi A, Bardaa T, Hammami M, Ellouz Z, Keskes H. Anterior transolecranon dislocation of the elbow in a child: a case report and review of literature. World J Orthop. 2018;9(7):100–4.
38. Butler MA, Martus JE, Schoenecker JG. Pediatric variants of the transolecranon fracture dislocation: recognition and tension band fixation: report of 3 cases. J Hand Surg [Am]. 2012;37(5):999–1002.

39. Guitton TG, Albers RG, Ring D. Anterior olecranon fracture-dislocations of the elbow in children. A report of four cases. J Bone Joint Surg Am. 2009;91(6):1487–90.
40. Tiemdjo H, Kinkpe C, Coulibaly NF, Sane A, Ndiaye A, Seye SI. Anterior transolecranon fracture-dislocations of the elbow in children: a case report and review of the literature. Arch Pediatr. 2015;22(7):737–40.
41. Wilkerson RD. Anterior elbow dislocation associated with olecranon fractures–review of the literature and case report. Iowa Orthop J. 1993;13:223–5.
42. Rasool MN. Dislocations of the elbow in children. J Bone Joint Surg (Br). 2004;86:1050–8. https://doi.org/10.1302/0301-620X.86B7.14505.
43. Ring D, Jupiter JB, Sanders RW, Mast J, Simpson NS. Transolecranon fracture-dislocation of the elbow. J Orthop Trauma. 1997;11(8):545–50.
44. Mouhsine E, Akiki A, Castagna A, Cikes A, Wettstein M, Borens O, Garofalo R. Transolecranon anterior fracture dislocation. J Shoulder Elb Surg. 2007;16(3):352–7.
45. Valisena S, Hamitaga F, Gonzalez JG, Voumard NM, Ciritsis BD, De Rosa V, Mendoza Sagaon M. Osteochondral flap fracture of the coronoid in pediatric elbow dislocation: a case report and literature review. Eur J Orthop Surg Traumatol. 2019;29(1):213–20.
46. Biga N, Thomine JM. La luxation trans-olécranienne du coude [Trans-olecranal dislocations of the elbow]. Rev Chir Orthop Reparatrice Appar Mot. 1974;60(7):557–67. French.
47. Suzuki T, Yoshida H, Matsumura N, Iwamoto T, Ochi K, Sato K. Anterior transverse divergent dislocation of the elbow in a child: a case report. JBJS Case Connect. 2015;5(3):e75.
48. Hardacre JA, Nahigian SH, Froimson AI, Brown JE. Fractures of the lateral condyle of the humerus in children. J Bone Jt Surg [Am]. 1971;53:1083–95.
49. Jakob R, Fowles JV, Rank M, Kassab MT. Observations concerning fractures of the lateral humeral condyle in children. J Bone Joint Surg (Br). 1975;57:430–6.
50. Milch H. Fractures and fracture dislocations of the humeral condyles. J Trauma Acute Care Surg. 1964;4(5):592–607.
51. Sharma H, Ayer R, Taylor GR. Complex pediatric elbow trauma: an uncommon case. BMC Musculoskelet Disord. 2005;6:13.
52. Kirkos JM, Beslikas TA, Papavasiliou VA. Posteromedial dislocation of the elbow with lateral condyle fracture in children. Clin Orthop Relat Res. 2003;1:232–6.
53. Van Haaren ER, van Vugt AB, Bode PJ. Posterolateral dislocation of the elbow with concomitant fracture of the lateral humeral condyle: case report. J Trauma. 1994;36:288–90.
54. Pace A, Gibson A, Al-Mousawi A, Matthews SJ. Distal humerus lateral condyle mass fracture and olecranon fracture in a 4-year-old female-review of literature. Injury. 2005;36:368–72.
55. Murnaghan JM, Thompson NS, Taylor TC, Cosgrove A, Ballard J. Fractured lateral epicondyle with associated elbow dislocation. Int J Clin Pract. 2002;56:475–7.
56. Rovinsky D, Ferguson C, Younis A, Otsuka NY. Pediatric elbow dislocation associated with a mi lch type I lateral condyle fracture of the humerus. J Orthop Trauma. 1999;13:458–60.
57. Kalbitz M, Weber B, Lackner I, Beer M, Pressmar J. Olecranon fractures in children: treatment of a rare entity. Eur J Trauma Emerg Surg. 2020; https://doi.org/10.1007/s00068-020-01518-7.
58. Arbes S, Platzer P, Vécsei V. surgical treatment of olecranon fractures in children. Eur J Orthop Surg Traumatol. 2011; https://doi.org/10.1007/s00590-011-0824-8.
59. Li Y, Wang K, Sun D, Liu Y, Wang Z, Li A. Short-term outcomes of Herbert screw fixation for isolated olecranon fractures in children: a single-institution retrospective study. Indian J Orthop. 2022; https://doi.org/10.1007/s43465-022-00609-4.
60. Corradin M, Marengo L, Andreacchio A, Paonessa M, Giacometti V, Samba A, Rousset M, Canavese F. Outcome of isolated olecranon fractures in skeletally immature patients: comparison of open reduction and tension band wiring fixation versus closed reduction and percutaneous screw fixation. Eur J Orthop Surg Traumatol. 2016; https://doi.org/10.1007/s00590-016-1774-y.
61. Li J, Tang SP, Nan GX, Li M, Chen SY, Mei HB, Shao JF, Jiang F, Lee RJ, Tang X. Management strategies of pediatric ipsilateral olecranon with associated radial neck fractures based on multicenter experience. J Orthop Surg Res. 2021; https://doi.org/10.1186/s13018-021-02373-x.

62. Yang Z, Feng C, Bian Z, Lu M, Zhou D. trans-olecranon fracture–dislocation of the elbow in children. Int Orthop. 2021; https://doi.org/10.1007/s00264-021-05010-8.
63. Su F, Sun C, Wang B, Li M, Qu JN, Yang YT, Wu YT, Jie Q. The characteristics and treatment strategy for transolecranon fracture-dislocation of the elbow in children: a retrospective study. BMC Musculoskelet Disord. 2022; https://doi.org/10.1186/s12891-022-05249-1.
64. Sharma H, Sibinski M, Sherlock DA. Outcome of lateral humeral condylar mass fractures in children associated with elbow dislocation or olecranon fracture. Int Orthop. 2007; https://doi.org/10.1007/s00264-007-0463-1.

Radial Head and Neck Fractures

8

Introduction by the Author

Radial neck fractures are relatively uncommon in children, accounting for only a small percentage of all fractures (5% to 10% of elbow fractures and 1% of all fractures). These injuries often result from falling on an outstretched arm and frequently occur alongside other elbow injuries. If these fractures are not properly managed, they can lead to significant complications and impaired elbow function.

The cartilaginous nature of the radial head in young children makes visualization via radiography difficult, often necessitating increased exposure to ionizing radiation during surgery. Ultrasound can facilitate diagnosis and guide closed reduction.

Treatment strategies for these injuries, especially those involving varying degrees of displacement, are still controversial. These fractures are classified using the Judet system, which guides treatment decisions based on the degree of angulation and displacement. Less severe fractures (Judet types I and II with less than 30 degrees of angulation) typically require only cast immobilization, while more severe cases (Judet types III and IV with more than 30 degrees of angulation) usually necessitate surgery.

A combination of closed reduction techniques and elastic intramedullary nail fixation or Kirchner wires offers favorable outcomes while minimizing complications. Although both methods result in favorable clinical outcomes for most patients, the use of elastic stable intramedullary nailing has become the primary treatment method for head and radial neck fractures in children. However, elastic stable intramedullary nailing is more expensive than Kirschner wires. It is also associated with higher hospitalization costs due to the need for a second surgery to remove the nail.

© The Author(s), under exclusive license to Springer Nature Switzerland AG 2026

F. Canavese, *Advances in Pediatric Extremity Fracture Management*,
https://doi.org/10.1007/978-3-032-33306-3_8

Some authors have reported that elastic stable intramedullary nailing leads to faster bone healing and fewer complications than Kirschner wire fixation. While both methods ultimately result in good long-term outcomes, early stabilization is more common with elastic stable intramedullary nailing. Recent studies have shown that age, length of hospitalization, and preoperative angulation are independent risk factors for postoperative complications.

Open reduction should be avoided when treating displaced fractures because it often results in poor outcomes, such as radial head necrosis or iatrogenic radio-ulnar synostosis. To avoid open reduction, a Kirschner wire can be percutaneously inserted at the fracture site to act as a lever for reduction and subsequent elastic intramedullary nailing fixation. Reduction can be assessed with ultrasound or fluoroscopy, both of which have a similar success rate. Transcapitellar pinning carries risks of pin breakage, damage to articular cartilage, and nerve injury.

8.1 Machine Generated Summaries

Disclaimer: The summaries in this chapter were generated from Springer Nature publications using abstractive AI auto-summarization: An abstraction-based summarizer creates new text based on deep learning. New phrases are created to summarize the content. As the constituted sentences are machine selected, they may not fully reflect the body of the work, so we strongly advise that the original content is read and cited. The auto-generated summaries were curated by the author(s) to meet Springer Nature publication standards.

Effect Analysis of Different Methods on Radial Neck Fracture in Children [72]

This is a machine-generated summary of:

Meng, Hailiang; Li, Min; Jie, Qiang; Wu, Yongtao Effect analysis of different methods on radial neck fracture in children [72]
Published in: Scientific Reports (2023)
Link to original: https://doi.org/10.1038/s41598-023-28294-9
Copyright of the summarized publication:
The Author(s) 2023
License: OpenAccess CC BY 4.0

This article is licensed under a Creative Commons Attribution 4.0 International License, which permits use, sharing, adaptation, distribution and reproduction in any medium or format, as long as you give appropriate credit to the original author(s)

and the source, provide a link to the Creative Commons licence, and indicate if changes were made. The images or other third party material in this article are included in the article's Creative Commons licence, unless indicated otherwise in a credit line to the material. If material is not included in the article's Creative Commons licence and your intended use is not permitted by statutory regulation or exceeds the permitted use, you will need to obtain permission directly from the copyright holder. To view a copy of this licence, visit http://creativecommons.org/licenses/by/4.0/.

Copyright comment: corrected publication 2023.

If you want to cite the papers, please refer to the original.

For technical reasons we could not place the page where the original quote is coming from.

Research Highlights

Pediatric radial neck fractures (RNFs) are relatively rare, comprising a small percentage of elbow fracture injuries in children. Improper management of these fractures can lead to significant complications and impaired elbow function. The treatment strategies for RNFs, particularly those with varying degrees of displacement, remain controversial. Children with non-displaced or minimally displaced RNFs can often be treated conservatively, while more severe cases may require surgical intervention. Now, a new study by Hailiang Meng and colleagues retrospectively analyzes RNF cases treated at Honghui Hospital, Xi'an Jiaotong University, to identify prognostic factors associated with these injuries.

The study involved a retrospective analysis of pediatric patients with RNFs treated over a one-year period. Clinical data were collected, including patient demographics, injury causes, treatment methods, and follow-up outcomes. Patients were classified using the O'Brien classification criteria and divided into groups based on treatment methods: plaster fixation, closed reduction, percutaneous Kirschner wire fixation, and open reduction. The study evaluated outcomes such as elbow movement, pain levels, and complications over an average follow-up period of 18 months. Statistical analyses were conducted to assess the impact of age, fracture classification, and treatment method on prognosis. The results indicated that age and treatment method significantly influenced outcomes, with closed reduction showing higher success rates compared to open reduction.

The study advances our understanding of pediatric RNF management by highlighting the importance of tailored treatment strategies based on fracture type and patient age. It suggests that closed reduction techniques combined with elastic intramedullary nail fixation offer favorable outcomes while minimizing complications. Future studies could focus on larger sample sizes and include additional factors such as rehabilitation exercises to further refine treatment protocols. The findings underscore the need for individualized approaches in managing pediatric RNFs to optimize functional recovery and reduce the risk of long-term complications.

Closed Reduction of Severely Displaced Radial Neck Fractures in Children [59]

This is a machine-generated summary of:

Qiao, Fei; Jiang, Fei Closed reduction of severely displaced radial neck fractures in children [59]
Published in: BMC Musculoskeletal Disorders (2019)
Link to original: https://doi.org/10.1186/s12891-019-2947-8
Copyright of the summarized publication:
The Author(s). 2019
License: OpenAccess CC BY + CC0 4.0

This article is distributed under the terms of the Creative Commons Attribution 4.0 International License (http://creativecommons.org/licenses/by/4.0/), which permits unrestricted use, distribution, and reproduction in any medium, provided you give appropriate credit to the original author(s) and the source, provide a link to the Creative Commons license, and indicate if changes were made. The Creative Commons Public Domain Dedication waiver (http://creativecommons.org/publicdomain/zero/1.0/) applies to the data made available in this article, unless otherwise stated.

If you want to cite the papers, please refer to the original.

For technical reasons we could not place the page where the original quote is coming from.

Management of Displaced Radial Neck Fractures in Children: Percutaneous Pinning vs. Elastic Stable Intramedullary Nailing [58]

This is a machine-generated summary of:

Tarallo, Luigi; Mugnai, Raffaele; Fiacchi, Francesco; Capra, Francesco; Catani, Fabio Management of displaced radial neck fractures in children: percutaneous pinning vs. elastic stable intramedullary nailing [58]
Published in: Journal of Orthopaedics and Traumatology (2013)
Link to original: https://doi.org/10.1007/s10195-013-0252-0
Copyright of the summarized publication:
The Author(s) 2013
License: OpenAccess CC BY 2.0

This article is distributed under the terms of the Creative Commons Attribution License which permits any use, distribution, and reproduction in any medium, provided the original author(s) and the source are credited.

If you want to cite the papers, please refer to the original.

For technical reasons we could not place the page where the original quote is coming from.

Research Highlights

Radial neck fractures in children are typically treated based on the degree of displacement, angulation, and skeletal maturity. While most fractures can be managed with closed reduction and casting, displaced fractures with significant angulation often require surgical intervention. Various surgical techniques exist, including percutaneous pinning and open reduction, though the latter is associated with higher complication rates such as avascular necrosis. Now, a new study by Luigi Tarallo and colleagues investigates the clinical and radiographical outcomes of intramedullary versus percutaneous pinning in children with displaced radial neck fractures.

The study retrospectively analyzed a cohort of children treated at a university hospital for displaced radial neck fractures with angulation greater than 30 degrees. The researchers compared two minimally invasive techniques: elastic stable intramedullary nailing (ESIN) and percutaneous pinning. Twenty patients were included, with the choice of technique depending on the surgeon's preference. The procedures involved closed reduction under general anesthesia, followed by either intramedullary fixation using a contoured K-wire or percutaneous pinning to stabilize the fracture. Postoperative care included casting and regular follow-up assessments to evaluate healing and function. Clinical outcomes were measured using the Mayo Elbow Performance Score (MEPS), while radiological assessments determined fracture alignment.

The study found that both ESIN and percutaneous pinning resulted in excellent clinical and radiological outcomes, with no major complications such as nonunion or avascular necrosis observed. However, patients treated with ESIN demonstrated superior range of motion in flexion, extension, and pronation compared to those who underwent percutaneous pinning. Additionally, minor complications like asymptomatic radial head enlargement were noted only in the percutaneous group. This research suggests that while both techniques are effective, ESIN may offer advantages in terms of range of motion and lower complication rates. Future studies could focus on larger sample sizes and randomized trials to further validate these findings and refine treatment protocols for pediatric radial neck fractures.

Percutaneous Reduction and Leverage Fixation Using K-Wires in Paediatric Angulated Radial Neck Fractures [111]

This is a machine-generated summary of:

Cha, Soo Min; Shin, Hyun Dae; Kim, Kyung Cheon; Han, Sun Cheol Percutaneous reduction and leverage fixation using K-wires in paediatric angulated radial neck fractures [111]
Published in: International Orthopaedics (2011)
Link to original: https://doi.org/10.1007/s00264-011-1387-3
Copyright of the summarized publication:
Springer-Verlag 2011
All rights reserved.

If you want to cite the papers, please refer to the original.

For technical reasons we could not place the page where the original quote is coming from.

Research Highlights

Radial neck fractures in children, though relatively rare, present a significant treatment challenge due to the protective nature of surrounding soft tissues and the potential for complications such as dislocation of the radial head. These injuries typically occur from falls onto an outstretched arm, leading to debates over the best treatment approach, especially for fractures with severe angulation. While conservative management is often preferred for slight angulations, more severe cases may require surgical intervention. Now, a new study by Soo Min Cha and colleagues explores a modified percutaneous reduction and temporary leverage fixation method using K-wires, reporting excellent outcomes after a follow-up period of at least 2 years.

The study evaluated pediatric patients with radial neck fractures treated between 2010 and 2015 using percutaneous reduction and leverage fixation with K-wires. The researchers focused on cases with more than 30° angulation seen within 24 hours of injury, excluding those requiring invasive operations for associated fractures. The average patient age was 9.3 years, with a follow-up period averaging 3.2 years. Under general anesthesia, radiographs were used to assess fracture angulation and translation. The surgical technique involved inserting a K-wire percutaneously at the fracture site to act as a lever for reduction, avoiding penetration into the fracture line to prevent epiphyseal injury. Postoperative evaluations showed significant improvements in angulation and minimal complications such as nonunion or nerve injury.

The study's findings suggest that this modified technique offers a promising alternative for treating severely displaced radial neck fractures in children, minimizing risks associated with open reduction methods. Future study could focus on refining this technique further or exploring its applicability to other types of pediatric fractures. The authors emphasize the importance of careful surgical technique to avoid additional damage to the physis and highlight the potential for this method to improve clinical outcomes while reducing complications traditionally associated with more invasive procedures.

Close Reduction Technique for Severely Displaced Radial Neck Fractures in Children [95]

This is a machine-generated summary of:

Shah, Maulin M.; Gupta, Gaurav; Rabbi, Qaisur; Bohra, Vikas; Wang, Kemble K. Close Reduction Technique for Severely Displaced Radial Neck Fractures in Children [95]
Published in: Indian Journal of Orthopaedics (2020)
Link to original: https://doi.org/10.1007/s43465-020-00168-6
Copyright of the summarized publication:
Indian Orthopaedics Association 2020
All rights reserved.

If you want to cite the papers, please refer to the original.

For technical reasons we could not place the page where the original quote is coming from.

Research Highlights

Radial neck fractures represent a significant portion of pediatric elbow trauma, often resulting from falls on an outstretched hand. These injuries can be challenging to manage, particularly when the fracture is severely displaced, as traditional closed reduction techniques may not suffice. Surgical intervention, while effective, carries risks such as nerve injury and avascular necrosis. Now, a new study by Maulin M. Shah and colleagues introduces a modified closed reduction technique that successfully achieves anatomical reduction in severely displaced pediatric radial neck fractures without the need for surgical fixation.

The study involved ten consecutive patients with completely displaced radial neck fractures classified as type IVa or IVb according to the Judet classification. The researchers employed a novel combination of maneuvers under general anesthesia and fluoroscopic guidance. The technique involved positioning the affected limb in elbow extension and full supination, applying longitudinal traction with varus stress at the elbow joint, and using thumb pressure on the displaced radial head fragment. This was followed by pronation and flexion of the elbow to achieve complete reduction. The fractures were immobilized in a mid-prone position with 90° elbow flexion for 3 weeks before initiating gradual active exercises. All patients achieved full range of motion at an average follow-up of 6 months, with no evidence of complications such as avascular necrosis or heterotopic ossification.

This study presents a significant advancement in the non-surgical management of severely displaced radial neck fractures in children. The described technique consistently achieved anatomical reduction without requiring k-wire or nail fixation, potentially reducing the risks associated with surgical intervention. Future studies could focus on increasing the sample size to validate these findings further and explore long-term outcomes to assess any potential for premature epiphyseal fusion. This approach may offer a promising alternative for treating complex pediatric elbow injuries while minimizing complications associated with more invasive procedures.

Pediatric Displaced Radial Neck Fractures: Retrospective Results of a Modified Metaizeau Technique [112]

This is a machine-generated summary of:

Bither, Nitin; Gupta, Parmanand; Jindal, Nipun Pediatric displaced radial neck fractures: retrospective results of a modified Metaizeau technique [112]
Published in: European Journal of Orthopaedic Surgery & Traumatology (2014)
Link to original: https://doi.org/10.1007/s00590-014-1452-x
Copyright of the summarized publication:
Springer-Verlag France 2014
All rights reserved.

If you want to cite the papers, please refer to the original.
For technical reasons we could not place the page where the original quote is coming from.

Research Highlights

Radial neck fractures in children, particularly those that are severely displaced or occur in older children, pose a significant challenge in orthopedic treatment. Traditional methods such as open reduction often result in fair to poor outcomes, while transcapitellar pinning carries risks of pin breakage and nerve injury. Now, a new study by Nitin Bither and colleagues explores the efficacy of a modified Metaizeau technique for intramedullary pinning in treating severely displaced radial neck fractures in children.

The study retrospectively analyzed 14 pediatric patients with Judet type IV radial neck fractures treated at their institute. The researchers employed a modified version of the Metaizeau technique, which involved using a bent K-wire introduced through a drill hole proximal to the distal physis. This modification aimed to prevent iatrogenic nerve injury and improve fracture reduction precision. The procedure included percutaneous K-wire assistance for reduction, with open reduction reserved for cases where closed reduction was unsuccessful. Postoperative care involved immobilization and subsequent K-wire removal after fracture consolidation. The outcomes were assessed using the Mayo elbow performance score and radiographic evaluations.

The study found that all patients achieved excellent clinical outcomes, with no cases of avascular necrosis or growth arrest at final follow-up. The modifications to the Metaizeau technique appeared to offer significant advantages, such as reducing the risk of nerve injury and improving reduction accuracy. Future study could focus on evaluating the role of the periosteal hinge as a predictor of successful closed reduction in a larger cohort. These findings suggest that the modified Metaizeau technique could be a valuable approach for managing complex radial neck fractures in pediatric patients, potentially improving both functional and radiological outcomes.

Percutaneous k-Wire Leverage Reduction and Retrograde Transphyseal k-Wire Fixation of Angulated Radial Neck Fractures in Children [113]

This is a machine-generated summary of:

Massetti, Daniele; Marinelli, Mario; Facco, Giulia; Falcioni, Danya; Giampaolini, Nicola; Specchia, Nicola; Gigante, Antonio Pompilio Percutaneous k-wire leverage reduction and retrograde transphyseal k-wire fixation of angulated radial neck fractures in children [113]

Published in: European Journal of Orthopaedic Surgery & Traumatology (2020)
Link to original: https://doi.org/10.1007/s00590-020-02654-x
Copyright of the summarized publication:
Springer-Verlag France SAS, part of Springer Nature 2020
All rights reserved.

If you want to cite the papers, please refer to the original.

For technical reasons we could not place the page where the original quote is coming from.

Research Highlights

The radial head is the second ossification center to appear in children and fuses with the radial neck during adolescence. Isolated radial neck fractures account for a small percentage of elbow fractures in children, often resulting from falls with the elbow extended and forearm supinated. These fractures can be complicated by other injuries, such as elbow dislocation or proximal ulnar fracture. While most fractures are undisplaced and treatable with closed reduction and casting, angulated radial neck fractures with more than 30° angulation typically require surgical intervention. Now, a new study by Daniele Massetti and colleagues explores the clinical and radiographic outcomes of treating angulated radial neck fractures Judet type III and IV using a combined technique of percutaneous k-wire leverage reduction and retrograde transphyseal k-wire fixation.

The study was conducted at Salesi Children's Hospital, where records of patients with angulated radial neck fractures from November 2015 to March 2020 were reviewed. The inclusion criteria focused on fractures with more than 30° angulation treated surgically using the specified technique. A total of 20 children participated, with a mean age of 9.3 years. The surgical procedure involved placing patients in a supine position under sedation, followed by percutaneous k-wire leverage reduction and retrograde transphyseal k-wire fixation under fluoroscopic guidance. Postoperative care included immobilization in an above-elbow cast for 3 weeks, followed by gradual return to daily activities. Clinical outcomes were assessed using the Mayo Elbow Performance Score (MEPS) and radiographic evaluations were performed to assess fracture healing.

The study demonstrated that this combined surgical technique is effective for treating angulated radial neck fractures in children, showing excellent or good outcomes in all patients according to MEPS and Tibone and Stoltz scores. The technique was associated with low complication rates, no nerve injuries or infections, and satisfactory radiographic healing in all cases. Future study could explore long-term outcomes beyond the average follow-up period of 12 months or compare this method directly with other minimally invasive techniques to further validate its efficacy and safety profile.

Management of Severely Displaced Radial Neck Fractures in Children: A Systematic Review and Meta-Analysis of Outcomes [96]

This is a machine-generated summary of:

Narang, Ashish M.; Pandey, Anuja A.; Bhat, Murlidhar Management of Severely Displaced Radial Neck Fractures in Children: A Systematic Review and Meta-analysis of Outcomes [96]
Published in: Indian Journal of Orthopaedics (2020)
Link to original: https://doi.org/10.1007/s43465-019-00032-2
Copyright of the summarized publication:
Indian Orthopaedics Association 2020
All rights reserved.

If you want to cite the papers, please refer to the original.

For technical reasons we could not place the page where the original quote is coming from.

Research Highlights

Radial neck fractures in children, accounting for a small percentage of pediatric fractures, present a complex treatment challenge, particularly when the displacement exceeds 30 degrees. These injuries often result from falls on an outstretched arm and can be associated with other elbow injuries. The management of these fractures is complicated by factors such as patient age and fracture characteristics, with various surgical techniques available. However, the evidence base for treating severely displaced radial neck fractures is limited, with previous studies often including all types of radial neck fractures without focusing on the severely displaced subgroup. Now, a new study by Ashish M. Narang and colleagues provides a systematic review and meta-analysis of the literature specifically addressing the surgical management of severely displaced radial neck fractures in skeletally immature patients.

The study conducted a comprehensive search across MEDLINE, EMBASE, and CINAHL PLUS databases to identify relevant articles published within a specified timeframe. A total of 14 studies involving patients with radial neck fractures displaced more than 30 degrees were included in the final review. The researchers employed a rigorous methodology, including independent data extraction and quality assessment using the NHLBI Quality Assessment Tool. The analysis focused on outcomes reported using standard scoring systems such as the Metaizeau outcome classification and Mayo Elbow Performance Score. The study found that closed reduction techniques had a higher success rate (87%) compared to open reduction techniques (70%). Subgroup analyses were performed to compare different surgical approaches, highlighting that meticulous surgical techniques can lead to excellent or good outcomes in most cases.

The findings from this systematic review underscore the effectiveness of surgical management for severely displaced radial neck fractures in children, with closed reduction methods showing particularly promising results. The study highlights the need for future research to address existing evidence gaps through long-term, prospective multicenter studies with standardized outcome measures. Such research could provide more definitive guidance on optimal treatment strategies for these complex injuries and improve prognostic discussions between surgeons and patients' families.

Modified Kirschner Wire Percutaneous Rotation Prying Reduction Combined with Elastic Stable Intramedullary Nailing in Children with Judet IV Radial Neck Fracture [114]

This is a machine-generated summary of:

Fan, YongFei; Xu, WenQiang; Liu, QiXin; Liu, ChaoYu; Wang, Wei Modified Kirschner wire percutaneous rotation prying reduction combined with elastic stable intramedullary nailing in children with Judet IV radial neck fracture [114]
Published in: BMC Musculoskeletal Disorders (2023)
Link to original: https://doi.org/10.1186/s12891-023-07008-2
Copyright of the summarized publication:
The Author(s) 2023
License: OpenAccess CC BY + CC0 4.0

This article is licensed under a Creative Commons Attribution 4.0 International License, which permits use, sharing, adaptation, distribution and reproduction in any medium or format, as long as you give appropriate credit to the original author(s) and the source, provide a link to the Creative Commons licence, and indicate if changes were made. The images or other third party material in this article are included in the article's Creative Commons licence, unless indicated otherwise in a credit line to the material. If material is not included in the article's Creative Commons licence and your intended use is not permitted by statutory regulation or exceeds the permitted use, you will need to obtain permission directly from the copyright holder. To view a copy of this licence, visit http://creativecommons.org/licenses/by/4.0/. The Creative Commons Public Domain Dedication waiver (http://creativecommons.org/publicdomain/zero/1.0/) applies to the data made available in this article, unless otherwise stated in a credit line to the data.

If you want to cite the papers, please refer to the original.

For technical reasons we could not place the page where the original quote is coming from.

Research Highlights

Radial neck fractures are a common type of pediatric elbow fracture, often requiring surgical intervention due to the vulnerability of the developing bone structure. The Judet classification system indicates that type III and IV fractures typically necessitate surgical treatment, with Metaizeau's percutaneous ESIN fixation being a common approach. However, achieving satisfactory reduction in severe cases, particularly Judet type IV fractures, can be challenging with ESIN alone. Now, a new study by YongFei Fan and colleagues explores a modified technique combining K-wire percutaneous rotation prying reduction with ESIN to improve outcomes for children with these complex fractures.

The study retrospectively reviewed patient records from April to November, focusing on children with Judet type IV closed radial neck fractures. Excluding open fractures, the study included patients who underwent surgery within an average of 3.5 days post-injury. The surgical procedure involved using a pre-bent K-wire for prying reduction under fluoroscopic guidance, followed by ESIN insertion for stabilization. This method aimed to enhance reduction quality while minimizing complications such as iatrogenic injury and excessive radiation exposure. Post-surgery, patients were immobilized in a long-arm cast and monitored through follow-up visits to assess healing and functional recovery.

The modified technique demonstrated promising results, achieving excellent or good reduction quality in all cases according to Metaizeau radiographic criteria. The study reported no significant complications like premature epiphyseal closure or nerve injury, and functional outcomes were comparable to the unaffected side at final follow-up. While the findings suggest that this approach can effectively manage severe radial neck fractures in children, the authors note the need for further research with larger sample sizes and control groups to validate these results comprehensively. Future study could focus on long-term outcomes and comparisons with other treatment modalities to refine pediatric fracture management strategies further.

Faster Healing of Radial Neck Fractures in Children Treated with the Metaizeau Technique Compared with Percutaneous Kirschner Wire Fixation: A Population-Based Study [115]

This is a machine-generated summary of:

Stöckell, Markus; Lampio, Emmi; Sagstetter, Felicitas; Sinikumpu, Jaakko Faster healing of radial neck fractures in children treated with the Metaizeau technique compared with percutaneous Kirschner wire fixation: a population-based study [115]

Published in: BMC Musculoskeletal Disorders (2025)
Link to original: https://doi.org/10.1186/s12891-025-08830-6
Copyright of the summarized publication:
The Author(s) 2025
License: OpenAccess CC BY 4.0

This article is licensed under a Creative Commons Attribution 4.0 International License, which permits use, sharing, adaptation, distribution and reproduction in any medium or format, as long as you give appropriate credit to the original author(s) and the source, provide a link to the Creative Commons licence, and indicate if changes were made. The images or other third party material in this article are included in the article's Creative Commons licence, unless indicated otherwise in a credit line to the material. If material is not included in the article's Creative Commons licence and your intended use is not permitted by statutory regulation or exceeds the permitted use, you will need to obtain permission directly from the copyright holder. To view a copy of this licence, visit http://creativecommons.org/licenses/by/4.0/.

If you want to cite the papers, please refer to the original.

For technical reasons we could not place the page where the original quote is coming from.

Research Highlights

Proximal radius fractures, accounting for a significant portion of elbow fractures, often result from falls on an outstretched arm. These injuries can be classified into metaphyseal fractures of the radial neck and epiphyseal fractures of the radial head, with the former being more prevalent. Complications such as nonunion and stiffness in movement are common due to the fragile vascular supply to the proximal radius. Now, a new study by Markus Stöckell and colleagues investigates the efficacy of two surgical techniques—Metaizeau technique using elastic stable intramedullary nails (ESIN) and K-wire fixation—in treating radial neck fractures in children.

The study included all children with radial neck fractures treated at Oulu University Hospital over a specified period. Researchers compared fracture healing outcomes between those treated with the Metaizeau technique and those with K-wire fixation. The primary outcome was radiographic bone healing at a six-month follow-up, assessed using the Lane–Sandhu score. Data were collected from hospital records, including patient characteristics, type of injury, treatment details, and follow-up outcomes. Statistical analyses were conducted to compare categorical and continuous variables between the two groups, ensuring robust results despite the retrospective nature of the study.

The findings suggest that the Metaizeau technique leads to faster bone healing and fewer complications compared to K-wire fixation. While both methods ultimately resulted in good long-term outcomes, early stabilization was more common with ESIN. This supports its use as a primary treatment method for radial neck fractures in children. Future studies could focus on larger sample sizes and randomized trials to further validate these findings and explore subgroup analyses based on reduction methods combined with surgical techniques. The study highlights the importance of surgical expertise in choosing appropriate treatment methods for optimal patient outcomes.

Open Reduction of Displaced Radial Neck Fractures in Children by Internal Fixation Techniques: Comparison of Percutaneous Kirschner Wiring and Elastic Stable Intramedullary Nailing [116]

This is a machine-generated summary of:

Liu, Yao; Zhu, Lun-Qing; Zhang, Fu-Yong; Liu, Ya; Zhen, Yun-Fang; Zhao, Tan-Tan
Open Reduction of Displaced Radial Neck Fractures in Children by Internal Fixation Techniques: Comparison of Percutaneous Kirschner Wiring and Elastic Stable Intramedullary Nailing [116]
Published in: Indian Journal of Orthopaedics (2022)
Link to original: https://doi.org/10.1007/s43465-022-00631-6
Copyright of the summarized publication:
Indian Orthopaedics Association 2022
All rights reserved.

If you want to cite the papers, please refer to the original.

For technical reasons we could not place the page where the original quote is coming from.

Research Highlights

Radial neck fractures are common injuries in children, often resulting from falls on an outstretched hand. These fractures are classified using the Judet system, which guides treatment decisions based on the degree of angulation and displacement. While less severe fractures (Judet type I and II) typically require only cast immobilization, more severe cases (type III and IV) may necessitate reduction techniques, with open reduction considered a last resort. However, there is no consensus on the optimal internal fixation method following open reduction. Now, a new study by Yao Liu and colleagues investigates the comparative effectiveness of Kirschner wire (KW) fixation versus elastic stable intramedullary nailing (ESIN) in the open reduction of displaced radial neck fractures in children.

The study reviewed records of 24 children with displaced radial neck fractures treated at a hospital over a five-year period. Patients were included if they underwent open reduction with either ESIN or KW fixation and had at least 1 year of follow-up. The surgical procedures involved initial attempts at manual reduction, followed by closed or percutaneous techniques if necessary, with open reduction performed after failed attempts. In the ESIN group, nails were inserted intramedullarily after percutaneous reduction, while in the KW group, wires were inserted percutaneously across the fracture site. Clinical outcomes were assessed using radiological criteria and the Steele and Graham classification system during follow-up visits.

The study found that both KW and ESIN fixation methods resulted in good clinical outcomes for most patients, although ESIN was associated with higher hospitalization costs due to secondary surgery for nail removal. Complications such as nail migration were observed in the ESIN group but not in the KW group. The authors suggest that while both methods are effective, KW fixation may be preferable due to lower costs and fewer complications. Future studies could focus on larger sample sizes and longer follow-up periods to further validate these findings and explore additional predictors for successful outcomes in pediatric radial neck fracture treatments.

Comparison of Different Treatments for Children with Radial Neck Fracture and Analysis of Prognostic Factors [117]

This is a machine-generated summary of:

Xia, Anning; You, Chao; Han, Jingming; Wu, Dechao; Xia, Yongjie; Wang, Jiangsheng Comparison of different treatments for children with radial neck fracture and analysis of prognostic factors [117]
Published in: Archives of Orthopaedic and Trauma Surgery (2021)
Link to original: https://doi.org/10.1007/s00402-021-04178-3
Copyright of the summarized publication:
The Author(s) 2021
License: OpenAccess CC BY 4.0

This article is licensed under a Creative Commons Attribution 4.0 International License, which permits use, sharing, adaptation, distribution and reproduction in any medium or format, as long as you give appropriate credit to the original author(s) and the source, provide a link to the Creative Commons licence, and indicate if changes were made. The images or other third party material in this article are included in the article's Creative Commons licence, unless indicated otherwise in a credit line to the material. If material is not included in the article's Creative Commons licence and your intended use is not permitted by statutory regulation or exceeds the permitted use, you will need to obtain permission directly from the copyright holder. To view a copy of this licence, visit http://creativecommons.org/licenses/by/4.0/.

If you want to cite the papers, please refer to the original.

For technical reasons we could not place the page where the original quote is coming from.

Research Highlights

Radial neck fractures in children are relatively rare, comprising a small percentage of all body and elbow fractures. The complexity of treatment options and varying efficacy evaluations make it challenging for physicians to choose the best approach, with adverse outcomes affecting a significant number of cases. Now, a new study by Anning Xia and colleagues retrospectively analyzes clinical data from children with radial neck fractures treated at their hospital over several years. The study explores differences in clinical characteristics and treatment efficacy across various surgical regimens, aiming to identify factors influencing outcomes and provide guidance for clinical practice.

The study involved a retrospective review of patient records from January to December, excluding cases with nontraumatic fractures or other medical conditions requiring special treatment. Patients were divided into six groups based on surgical methods and materials used for internal fixation, such as Kirschner wires (K-wires) and elastic stable intramedullary nails (ESINs). The researchers assessed preoperative fracture angulation using the Judet classification and evaluated postoperative complications like bony deformities, neurovascular injuries, and infections. Functional outcomes were measured using the Tibone elbow outcome scoring system. Statistical analyses were conducted to compare treatment groups, revealing significant differences in factors such as age, hospitalization duration, preoperative angulation, and functional scores. Group B (manipulative reduction with ESINs) showed the most favorable outcomes.

The study highlights that age, hospitalization duration, and preoperative angulation are independent risk factors for postoperative complications. While ESINs were preferred for older patients due to their elasticity and effectiveness in fracture reduction, they also incurred higher costs and longer indwelling times compared to K-wires. The findings suggest that manual reduction combined with ESIN fixation may be optimal for achieving good functional recovery with minimal complications. However, open reduction remains necessary for severe cases with large preoperative angulation degrees. Future studies could further explore these findings to refine treatment strategies for pediatric radial neck fractures.

Ultrasound-Guided vs. Fluoroscopy-Guided Percutaneous Leverage Reduction for Severely Displaced Radial Neck Fractures in Children: A Comparative Analysis of Clinical and Radiological Outcomes [118]

This is a machine-generated summary of:

Wu, Xing; Xia, Jingdong; Li, Xiongtao; Chen, Xiaoliang; Wang, Si; Shen, Xiantao
Ultrasound-guided vs. fluoroscopy-guided percutaneous leverage reduction for severely displaced radial neck fractures in children: a comparative analysis of clinical and radiological outcomes [118]
Published in: BMC Musculoskeletal Disorders (2025)
Link to original: https://doi.org/10.1186/s12891-025-08312-9
Copyright of the summarized publication:
The Author(s) 2025
License: OpenAccess CC BY-NC-ND 4.0

This article is licensed under a Creative Commons Attribution-NonCommercial-NoDerivatives 4.0 International License, which permits any non-commercial use, sharing, distribution and reproduction in any medium or format, as long as you give appropriate credit to the original author(s) and the source, provide a link to the

Creative Commons licence, and indicate if you modified the licensed material. You do not have permission under this licence to share adapted material derived from this article or parts of it. The images or other third party material in this article are included in the article's Creative Commons licence, unless indicated otherwise in a credit line to the material. If material is not included in the article's Creative Commons licence and your intended use is not permitted by statutory regulation or exceeds the permitted use, you will need to obtain permission directly from the copyright holder. To view a copy of this licence, visit http://creativecommons.org/licenses/by-nc-nd/4.0/.

If you want to cite the papers, please refer to the original.

For technical reasons we could not place the page where the original quote is coming from.

Research Highlights

Radial neck fractures are a common type of elbow injury in children, accounting for a significant percentage of such cases. Various surgical techniques have been developed to manage these fractures, with closed reduction being preferred over open reduction due to its less invasive nature. However, the optimal treatment approach remains controversial, particularly concerning the guidance method used during percutaneous pin leverage reduction. Currently, fluoroscopic (FL) guidance is widely used but poses challenges such as ionizing radiation exposure and difficulty visualizing the ossifying radial head. Now, a new study by Xing Wu and colleagues explores the use of ultrasound (US) as an alternative guidance method, hypothesizing that it can effectively replace FL guidance while reducing radiation exposure and operative time.

The study was conducted as a retrospective analysis approved by the institution's internal review board. It included children with closed, displaced radial neck fractures with angulation greater than a specified degree. Patients were divided into two groups based on the guidance technique used: US-guided and FL-guided percutaneous pin leverage reduction. The US-guided procedure involved positioning patients supine with the elbow in semiflexion and using a GE LOGIQ e ultrasound system for real-time visualization during surgery. A Kirschner wire was inserted under US guidance to achieve fracture reduction, with final assessments confirmed via FL. The study measured operative times, radiation exposure, and clinical outcomes using established classification systems.

The findings suggest that US-guided percutaneous pinning is an effective alternative to FL-guided methods for treating displaced radial neck fractures in children. The US group demonstrated significantly shorter operative times and reduced radiation exposure compared to the FL group, with comparable success rates in fracture reduction and clinical outcomes. While both techniques achieved similar functional results, US offers advantages such as real-time visualization and enhanced convenience without compromising efficacy. Future studies could focus on larger, multicenter trials to validate these findings further and explore long-term outcomes of US-guided techniques in pediatric orthopedic surgery.

Treatment of Displaced Radial Neck Fractures Under Ultrasonographic Guidance in Children [93]

This is a machine-generated summary of:

Su, Yuxi; Jin, Chen; Duan, Xiaokun; Wang, Jing; Li, Kuang Treatment of displaced radial neck fractures under ultrasonographic guidance in children [93]
Published in: International Orthopaedics (2020)
Link to original: https://doi.org/10.1007/s00264-020-04630-w
Copyright of the summarized publication:
SICOT aisbl 2020
All rights reserved.

If you want to cite the papers, please refer to the original.

For technical reasons we could not place the page where the original quote is coming from.

Research Highlights

Radial neck fractures (RNFs) in children, often resulting from falls, account for a small percentage of pediatric fractures. Traditionally, these fractures are treated conservatively if the displacement and angulation are minimal, with the Métaizeau technique being favored for its positive outcomes. However, challenges remain in reducing severely displaced RNFs, particularly Judet type IV, and current methods expose patients and medical staff to harmful radiation. Now, a new study by Yuxi Su and colleagues explores the use of ultrasonography (US) as a radiation-free alternative to guide the reduction and fixation of RNFs using Kirschner wires and elastic stable intramedullary nails.

The study retrospectively reviewed patient records from September to November at a single clinical center. Fifty patients with specific types of RNFs were included based on defined criteria. The surgical procedure involved using US to locate nerves and the fracture site, followed by the insertion of a K-wire for fracture reduction and fixation with an intramedullary nail. The surgeries were performed under general anesthesia with US guidance provided by a trained clinician. Post-operative evaluations included radiological assessments and functional outcomes measured by the Mayo Elbow Performance Index (MEPI). Statistical analyses showed that US guidance significantly reduced radiation exposure and operation time compared to traditional methods.

The study demonstrates that US can effectively guide RNF reduction while minimizing radiation exposure and reducing the risk of iatrogenic injury to the posterior interosseous nerve (PIN). Although mastering US technology requires training, its advantages make it a promising tool for pediatric orthopedic surgery. Future studies could focus on larger sample sizes and further explore the learning curve associated with US-guided fracture reduction. The findings suggest that US could become a standard practice in treating RNFs, offering a safer alternative to traditional radiographic methods.

Ultrasonography-Guided Reduction of Pediatric Radial Neck Fractures [119]

This is a machine-generated summary of:

Lee, Jung Eun; Kim, Jung Bong; Choi, Eun Seok Ultrasonography-guided reduction of pediatric radial neck fractures [119]
Published in: BMC Musculoskeletal Disorders (2017)
Link to original: https://doi.org/10.1186/s12891-017-1891-8
Copyright of the summarized publication:
The Author(s). 2017
License: OpenAccess CC BY + CC0 4.0

This article is distributed under the terms of the Creative Commons Attribution 4.0 International License (http://creativecommons.org/licenses/by/4.0/), which permits unrestricted use, distribution, and reproduction in any medium, provided you give appropriate credit to the original author(s) and the source, provide a link to the Creative Commons license, and indicate if changes were made. The Creative Commons Public Domain Dedication waiver (http://creativecommons.org/publicdomain/zero/1.0/) applies to the data made available in this article, unless otherwise stated.

If you want to cite the papers, please refer to the original.

For technical reasons we could not place the page where the original quote is coming from.

Research Highlights

Radial neck fractures in children, though relatively uncommon, present significant challenges in treatment, particularly when the fractures are displaced and angulated. Traditional surgical techniques, such as closed reduction with percutaneous pinning or intramedullary elastic nails, carry risks of inadequate reduction and potential nerve injury. Additionally, the cartilaginous nature of the radial head in young children complicates radiographic visualization, often necessitating increased exposure to ionizing radiation during surgery. Now a new study by Jung Eun Lee and colleagues explores the use of intraoperative ultrasonography (US) as a novel approach to guide the reduction and fixation of radial neck fractures in pediatric patients.

The study retrospectively reviewed medical records of 12 children with severely angulated radial neck fractures classified as type III or IV according to the Judet classification. These patients underwent US-guided reduction and fixation using Kirschner wires at a single institution. Under general anesthesia, the fractured elbow was extended and supinated while a mobile image intensifier and US were used simultaneously. A Steinmann pin was inserted under US guidance to monitor fracture reduction continuously. Once satisfactory reduction was confirmed via US, fluoroscopy was employed for in situ fixation with a second K-wire. Postoperative care involved immobilization with a long arm cast followed by a hinged brace. The study evaluated clinical outcomes using the Metaizeau criteria and assessed radiation exposure through dose area product measurements.

The findings suggest that US-guided reduction is a safe and effective method for treating displaced radial neck fractures in children, offering reduced radiation exposure compared to traditional methods. The study reported no nerve injuries or long-term complications such as avascular necrosis or synostosis during follow-up. While promising, the authors acknowledge limitations due to the small sample size and retrospective design. Future studies could focus on larger cohorts and randomized trials to further validate these findings and explore the broader application of US guidance in pediatric orthopedic surgeries.

Conclusion

Undisplaced fractures of the radial head and neck can be treated conservatively. Depending on the quality of the reduction, displaced fractures should undergo closed reduction with or without fixation. If displacement persists by more than 30 degrees, reduction should be completed using elastic nailing or Kirschner wires.

Bibliography

1. Beaty JH, et al. Rockwood and Wilkins' fractures in children (8th edition) [M]. People's military Medical Publishing House; 2018. p. 387–9.
2. Du X, et al. Percutaneous leverage reduction with two Kirschner wires combined with the Métaizeau technique versus open reduction plus internal fixation with a single Kirschner-wire for treating Judet IV radial neck fractures in children. J Int Med Res. 2019;47:5497–507.
3. Karthick SR, Gopinathan NR, Vashisht S. Arthrogram assisted reduction of radial neck fracture in a child with unossified radial head—a case report and review of literature. J Clin Orthop Trauma. 2020;11:324–7.
4. Metaizeau JP. Reduction and osteosynthesis of radial neck fractures in children by centromedullary pinning. Injury. 2005;36(1):75–7.
5. Kaiser M, et al. Judet type-IV radial neck fractures in children: comparison of the outcome of fractures with and without bony contact. Acta Orthop. 2016;87(5):529–32.
6. Metaizeau JP, Lascombes P, Lemelle JL, Finlayson D, Prevot J. Reduction and fixation of displaced radial neck fractures by closed intramedullary pinning. J Pediatr Orthop MayeJun. 1993;13(3):355–60.
7. Gutiérrez-de la Iglesia D, Pérez-López LM, Cabrera-González M, Knorr-Gimenez J. Surgical rechniques for displaced radial neck fractures: predictive factors of functional results. J Pediatr Orthop. 2017;37(3):159–65. https://doi.org/10.1097/BPO.0000000000000617.
8. Ma YP, et al. Treatment of pediatric radial neck fractures by kirschner wire assisted reduction and intramedullary nail fixation. Chin J Hand Surg. 2016;32(2):96–7.
9. Gagliardi Ida C, et al. Evaluation of children with radial neck fractures treated with flexible intramedullary nail. Acta Ortop Bras. 2016;24(2):81–4.
10. Kaufman B, Rinott MG, Tanzman M. Closed reduction of fractures of the proximal radius in children. J Bone Joint Surg Br. 1989;71(1):66–7.
11. Ugutmen E, Ozkan K, Ozkan FU, Eceviz E, Altintas F, Unay K. Reduction and fixation of radius neck fractures in children with intramedullary pin. J Pediatr Orthop B. 2010;19(4):289–93.

12. Pesudo JV, Aracil J, Barcelo M. Leverage method in displaced fractures of the radial neck in children. Clin Orthop Relat Res. 1982;169:215–8.
13. Klitscher D, Richter S, Bodenschatz K, Huckstadt T, Weltzien A, Muller LP, Schier F, Rommens PM. Evaluation of severely displaced radial neck fractures in children treated with elastic stable intramedullary nailing. J Pediatr Orthop. 2009;29(7):698–703.
14. Metaizeau JP, Prevot J, Schmitt M. Reduction and fixation of fractures of the neck of the radious be centro-medullary pinning. Original technic. Rev Chir Orthop Reparatrice Appar Mot. 1980;66(1):47–9.
15. Wood SK. Reversal of the radial head during reduction of fracture of the neck of the radius in children. J Bone Joint Surg Br. 1969;51(4):707–10.
16. Steele JA, Graham HK. Angulated radial neck fractures in children. A prospective study of percutaneous reduction. J Bone Joint Surg Br. 1992;74(5):760–4 Erratum in: J Bone Joint Surg Br 1993 Jan;75(1):169.
17. Judet J, Judet R, Lefrance J. Fracture of the radial head in the child. Ann Chir. 1962;16:1377–85.
18. Steinberg EL, Golomb D, Salama R, Wientroub S. Radial head and neck fractures in children. J Pediatr Orthop. 1988;8(1):35–40.
19. Steele JA, Graham HK. Angulated radial neck fractures in children. A prospective study of percutaneous reduction. J Bone Joint Surg Br. 1992;74:760–4.
20. Prathapkumar KR, Garg NK, Bruce CE. Elastic stable intramedullary nail fixation for severely displaced fractures of the neck of the radius in children. J Bone Joint Surg Br. 2006;88(3):358–61.
21. D'souza S, Vaishya R, Klenerman L. Management of radial neck fractures in children: a retrospective analysis of one hundred patients. J Pediatr Orthop. 1993;13:232–8.
22. Chotel F, Vallese P, Parot R, Laville JM, Hodgkinson I, Muller C, Berard J. Complete dislocation of the radial head following fracture of the radial neck in children: the Jeffery type II lesion. J Pediatr Orthop B. 2004;13(4):268–74.
23. Radomisli TE, Rosen AL. Controversies regarding radial neck fractures in children. Clin Orthop. 1998;353:30–9.
24. O'Brien PI. Injuries involving the proximal radial epiphysis. Clin Orthop. 1965;41:51–8.
25. Biyani A, Mehara A, Bhan S. Percutaneous pinning for radial neck fractures. Injury. 1994;25(3):169–71.
26. Futami T, Tsukamot Y, Itoman M. Percutaneous reduction of displaced radial neck fractures. J Shoulder Elb Surg. 1995;4:162–7.
27. Bohler J. Conservative treatment of fractures of the radial neck. Chirurg. 1950;21(12):687–8.
28. Kapandji A. Intra-focal pinning of fractures of the distal end of the radius 10 years later. Ann Chir Main. 1987;6:57–63.
29. Fowles JV, Kassab MT. Observations concerning radial neck fractures in children. J Pediatr Orthop. 1986;6(1):51–7.
30. Ursei M, Sales de Gauzy J, Knorr J, Abid A, Darodes P, Cahuzac JP. Surgical treatment of radial neck fractures in children by intramedullary pinning. Acta Orthop Belg. 2006;72(2):131–7.
31. Al-Aubaidi Z, Pedersen NW, Nielsen KD. Radial neck fractures in children treated with the centromedullary Métaizeau technique. Injury. 2012;43(3):301–5.
32. Brandão GF, Soares CB, Teixeira LE, Boechat Lde C. Displaced radial neck fractures in children: association of the Metaizeau and Böhler surgical techniques. J Pediatr Orthop. 2010;30(2):110–4.
33. Eberl R, Singer G, Fruhmann J, Saxena A, Hoellwarth ME. Intramedullary nailing for the treatment of dislocated pediatric radial neck fractures. Eur J Pediatr Surg. 2010;20(4):250–2.
34. Vocke AK, Von Laer L. Displaced fractures of the radial neck in children: long-term results and prognosis of conservative treatment. J Pediatr Orthop B. 1998;7(3):217–22.
35. Green NE. Fractures and dislocations about the elbow. In: Green NE, Swiontkowski MF, editors. Skeletal trauma in children. Philadelphia: WB Saunders; 1994. p. 213–56.
36. Metaizeau JP, Prevot J, Schmitt M. Reduction and fixation of fractures of the neck of the radius by centro-medullary pinning. Original technique. Rev Chir Orthop. 1980;66:47–9.

37. Steele JA, Graham HK. Angulated radial neck fractures in children. A prospective study of percutaneous reduction. J Bone Joint Surg. 1992;74B:760–4.
38. Jones ERL, Esah M. Displaced fractures of the neck of the radius in children. J Bone Joint Surg. 1971;53B:429–39.
39. Judet J, Judet R, Lefranc J. Fracture of the radial head in the child. Ann Chir. 1962;16:1377–85.
40. Landin L. Fracture patterns in children. Acta Orthop Scand. 1983;202:1–109.
41. Neher CG, Torch MA. New reduction technique for severely displaced pediatric radial neck fractures. J Pediatr Orthop. 2003;23:626–8.
42. Sessa S, Lascombes P, Prevot J, et al. Fractures of the radial head and associated elbow injuries in children. J Pediatr Orthop B. 1996;5:200.
43. Patterson RF. Treatment of displaced transverse fractures of the neck of the radius in children. J Bone Joint Surg. 1934;16:696–8.
44. Monson R, Black B, Reed M. A new closed reduction technique for the treatment of radial neck fractures in children. J Pediatr Orthop. 2009;29:243–7.
45. Augustithis GA, Huntley JS. Closed reduction of paediatric radial neck fractures. Ann R Coll Surg Engl. 2015;97:315–20.
46. Chambers HG, Wilkins K. Fractures of the neck and head of the radius. In: Rockwood Jr CA, Wilkins K, Beaty J, editors. Fractures in children. 3rd ed. Philadelphia: Lippincott-Raven; 1996. p. 586.
47. Kiefer GN. Fractures of the radial head and neck. In: Letts M, editor. Management of pediatric fractures. New York: Churchill Livingstone; 1994. p. 376.
48. Chambers H. Fractures of the proximal radius and ulna. In: Kasser J, Beaty J, editors. Rockwood and Wilkins fractures in children. 5th ed. Philadelphia: Lippincott William and Wilkins; 2001. p. 483–528.
49. Wedge JH, Robertson DE. Displaced fractures of the neck of the radius. J Bone Joint Surg Br. 1982;64:256.
50. Jeffrey CC. Fractures of the head of the radius in children. J Bone Joint Surg Br. 1950;32:314–24.
51. Safran MR, Baillargeon D. Soft-tissue stabilizers of the elbow closed meeting of the american-shoulder-and-elbow-surgeons. St. Louis: Mosby-Elsevier; 2005. p. 179S–85S.
52. Tibone JE, Stoltz M. Fractures of the radial head and neck in children. J Bone Joint Surg Am. 1981;63(1):100–6.
53. Waters PM, Stewart SL. Radial neck fracture nonunion in children. J Pediatr Orthop. 2001;21:570–6.
54. Wood SK. Reversal of the radial head during reduction of fracture of the neck of the radius in children. J Bone Joint Surg (Br). 1969;51:707–10.
55. Steele JA, Graham HK. Angulated radial neck fractures in children. A prospective study of percutaneous reduction. J Bone Joint Surg (Br). 1992;74-B:760–4.
56. Biyani A, Mehara A, Bhan S. Percutaneous pinning for radial neck fractures. Injury. 1994;25(169):71.
57. Zhang FY, Wang XD, Zhen YF, Guo ZX, Dai J, Zhu LQ. Treatment of severely displaced radial neck fractures in children with percutaneous K-wire leverage and closed intramedullary pinning. Medicine (Baltimore). 2016;95(1):e2346.
58. Tarallo L, Mugnai R, Fiacchi F, Capra F, Catani F. Management of displaced radial neck fractures in children: percutaneous pinning vs. elastic stable intramedullary nailing. J Orthop Traumatol. 2013;14(4):291–7.
59. Qiao F, Jiang F. Closed reduction of severely displaced radial neck fractures in children. BMC Musculoskelet Disord. 2019;20:567. https://doi.org/10.1186/s12891-019-2947-8.
60. Giannini S, Faldini C, Vannini F, Digennaro V, Bevoni R, Luciani D. The minimally invasive osteotomy. Foot Ankle Int. 2008;29(3):282–6. https://doi.org/10.3113/fai.2008.0282.
61. Zwingmann J, Welzel M, Dovi-Akue D, Schmal H, Südkamp NP, Strohm PC. Clinical results after different operative treatment methods of radial head and neck fractures: a systematic review and meta-analysis of clinical outcome. Injury. 2013;44(11):1540–50.

62. Morrey B, An K, Chao E. Functional evaluation of the elbow. In: Morrey B, editor. The elbow and its disorders. Philadelphia: W.B. Saunders Company; 1993. p. 86–97.
63. Tibone JE, Stoltz M. Fractures of the radial head and neck in children. J Bone Joint Surg Am. 1981;63(1):100–6. https://doi.org/10.2106/00004623-198163010-00013.
64. Linscheid RL, Wheeler DK. Elbow dislocations. JAMA. 1965;194(11):1171–6. *(PubMed PMID: 4284719)*
65. Schmittenbecher PP, Haevernick B, Herold A, Knorr P, Schmid E. Treatment decision, method of osteosynthesis, and outcome in radial neck fractures in children: a multicenter study. J Pediatr Orthop. 2005;25(1):45–50.
66. Okçu G, Aktuğlu K. Surgical treatment of displaced radial neck fractures in children with Metaizeau technique. Ulus Travma Acil Cerrahi Derg. 2007;13(2):122–7.
67. Cossio A, Cazzaniga C, Gridavilla G, Gallone D, Zatti G. Paediatric radial neck fractures: one-step percutaneous reduction and fixation. Injury. 2014;45(Suppl 6):S80–4.
68. Bither N, Gupta P, Jindal N. Pediatric displaced radial neck fractures: retrospective results of a modified Metaizeau technique. Eur J Orthop Surg Traumatol. 2015;25(1):99–103.
69. Sandra E, Thomas W, Oliver E, Francisco F. The treatment of radial neck fractures in children according to Métaizeau[J]. J Pediatr Orthop B. 2010;19(3):246.
70. Zimmerman RM, Kalish LA, Hresko MT, Waters PM, Bae DS. Surgical management of pediatric radial neck fractures. J Bone Joint Surg Am. 2013;95(20):1825–32.
71. Stiefel D, Meuli M, Altermatt S. Fractures of the neck of the radius in children. J Bone Joint Surg. 2001;83(4):536–41.
72. Meng H, Li M, Jie Q, Wu Y. Effect analysis of different methods on radial neck fracture in children. Sci Rep. 2023;13:1181. https://doi.org/10.1038/s41598-023-28294-9.
73. Cevik N, Cansabuncu G, Akalin Y, Otuzbir A, Ozturk A, Ozkan Y. Functional and radiological results of percutaneous K-wire aided Metaizeau technique in the treatment of displaced radial neck fractures in children. Acta Orthop Traumatol Turc. 2018;52:428–34. https://doi.org/10.1016/j.aott.2018.07.007.
74. Dietzel M, Scherer S, Esser M, et al. Fractures of the proximal radius in children: management and results of 100 consecutive cases. Arch Orthop Trauma Surg. 2022;142:1903–10. https://doi.org/10.1007/s00402-021-03917-w.
75. Lascombes P, Haumont T, Journeau P. Use and abuse of flexible intramedullary nailing in children and adolescents. J Pediatr Orthop. 2006;26:827–34.
76. Lin HM, Ma YP, Hu CT, et al. Modified metaizeau's technique for the treatment of radial neck fractures of Judet III or IV in children. Zhongguo Gu Shang. 2018;31:790–3. https://doi.org/10.3969/j.issn.1003-0034.2018.09.002.
77. Nicholson LT, Skaggs DL. Proximal radius fractures in children. J Am Acad Orthop Surg. 2019;27:E876–86. https://doi.org/10.5435/JAAOS-D-18-00204.
78. Schmittenbecher PP, Haevernick B, Herold A, et al. Treatment decision, method of osteosynthesis, and outcome in radial neck fractures in children a multicenter study. J Pediatr Orthop. 2005;25:45–50.
79. Degnan AJ, Ho-Fung VM, Nguyen JC, et al. Proximal radius fractures in children: evaluation of associated elbow fractures. Pediatr Radiol. 2019;49:1177–84. https://doi.org/10.1007/s00247-019-04445-x.
80. Su Y, Xie Y, Qin J, et al. Internal fixation with absorbable rods for the treatment of displaced radial neck fractures in children. J Pediatr Orthop. 2016;36:797–802. https://doi.org/10.1097/BPO.0000000000000572.
81. Tian K, Cao J, Pei X, et al. Comparison of elastic stable intramedullary nailing versus Kirschner wires in treatment of pediatric radial neck fractures. J Child Orthop. 2024; https://doi.org/10.1177/18632521241233444.
82. Kumar SMA, Odak S, Dwyer J. Treatment principles, prognostic factors and controversies in radial neck fractures in children: a systematic review. J Clin Orthop Trauma. 2020;11(Suppl 4):456–S463. https://doi.org/10.1016/j.jcot.2020.04.022.

83. Kalem M, Sahin E, Kocaoglu H, Basarir K, Kinik H. Comparison of two closed surgical techniques at isolated pediatric radial neck fractures. Injury. 2018;49:618–23. https://doi.org/10.1016/j.injury.2018.01.012.
84. Basmajian HG, Choi PD, Huh K, Sankar WN, Wells L, Arkader A. Radial neck fractures in children: experience from two level-1 trauma centers. J Pediatr Orthop. 2014;23(4):369.
85. Gutiérrez-de la Iglesia D, Pérez-López LM, Cabrera-González M, Knörr-Giménez J. Surgical techniques for displaced radial neck fractures: predictive factors of functional results. J Pediatr Orthop. 2017;37(3):159–65.
86. Fuller CB, Guillen PT, Wongworawat MD, Riedel BB. Bioabsorbable pin fixation in late presenting pediatric radial neck fractures. J Pediatr Orthop. 2016;36:793–6. https://doi.org/10.1097/BPO.0000000000000576.
87. Pring ME. Pediatric radial neck fractures: when and how to fix. J Pediatr Orthop. 2012;32(Suppl 1):S14–21.
88. Basmajian HG, Choi PD, Huh K, et al. Radial neck fractures in children experience from two level-1 trauma centers. J Pediatr Orthop B. 2014;23:369–74. https://doi.org/10.1097/BPB.0000000000000057.
89. Newman JH. Displaced radial neck fractures in children. Injury. 1977;9(2):114–21.
90. Lee JE, Kim JB, Choi ES. Ultrasonograhy-guided reduction of pediatric radial neck fracture[J]. BMC Musculoskelet Disord. 2017;18(1):516.
91. Shen XT, Chen XL, Li XT, Wu X, Li J, Zhang P, Sun J, Zhao YP. Ultrasound guided percutaneous Kirschner-Wire leverage and reduction for radial neck fracture in children. Chin J Pediatr Surg. 2015;36(5):363–7.
92. Baghdadi S, Shah AS, Lawrence JTR. Open reduction of radial neck fractures in children: injury severity predicts the radiographic and clinical outcomes. J Shoulder Elb Surg. 2021;30(10):2418–27.
93. Su Y, Jin C, Duan X, Wang J, Li K. Treatment of displaced radial neck fractures under ultrasonographic guidance in children. Int Orthop. 2020;44:2337–42. https://doi.org/10.1007/s00264-020-04630-w.
94. Yang L, Yang X, Zuo J, Wang D, Li L, Tang X. A retrospective review of 101 operatively treated radial neck fractures in children and analysis of risk factors for functional outcomes. Injury. 2022;53:3310–6. https://doi.org/10.1016/j.injury.2022.07.016.
95. Shah MM, Gupta G, Rabbi Q, Bohra V, Wang KK. Close reduction technique for severely displaced radial neck fractures in children. Indian J Orthop. 2020;55:109–15. https://doi.org/10.1007/s43465-020-00168-6.
96. Narang AM, Pandey AA, Bhat M. Management of severely displaced Radial Neck fractures in children: a systematic review and meta-analysis of outcomes. Indian J Orthop. 2020;54(1):60–8.
97. Li XT, Shen XT, Wu X, Wang S. Ultrasound-assisted closed reduction and percutaneous pinning for displaced and rotated lateral condylar humeral fractures in children. J Shoulder Elb Surg. 2021;30:1–7.
98. Chinnock B, Khaletskiy A, Kuo K, Hendey GW. Ultrasound-guided reduction of distal radius fractures. J Emerg Med. 2011;40(3):308–12.
99. Wu J, Shen X, Zhang P, Zhou R, Li Y, Tang B, Wu X. A comparative study: ultrasound-guided leverage reduction with internal fixation using Kirschner wires or elastic stable intramedullary nailing for severely displaced radial neck fractures in children. Medicine. 2023;102(43):e35507.
100. Broberg MA, Morrey BF. Results of delayed excision of the radial head after fracture. J Bone Joint Surg Am. 1986;68:669–74.
101. Karthick SR, Gopinathan NR, Vashisht S, Pattabiraman K. Arthrogram assisted reduction of radial neck fracture in a child with unossified radial head - a case report and review of literature. J Clin Orthop Trauma. 2020;11:324–7.
102. Song KS, Kim BS, Lee SW. Percutaneous leverage reduction for severely displaced radial neck fractures in children. J Pediatr Orthop. 2015;35:e26–30. https://doi.org/10.1097/BPO.0000000000000305.

103. Cha SM, Shin HD, Kim KC, Han SC. Percutaneous reduction and leverage fixation using K-wires in paediatric angulated radial neck fractures. Int Orthop. 2012;36(4):803–9.
104. Ho-Fung VM, Zapala MA, Lee EY. Musculoskeletal traumatic injuries in children: characteristic imaging findings and mimickers. Radiol Clin North Am. 2017;55(4):785–802.
105. Eckert K, Janssen N, Ackermann O, Schweiger B, Radeloff E, Liedgens P. Ultrasound diagnosis of supracondylar fractures in children. Eur J Trauma Emerg Surg. 2014;40(2):159–68.
106. Rowlands R, Rippey J, Tie S, Flynn J. Bedside ultrasound vs X-ray for the diagnosis of forearm fractures in children. J Emerg Med. 2017;52:208–15.
107. Ali AA, Solomon DM, Hoffman RJ. Femur fracture diagnosis and management aided by point-of-care ultrasonography. Pediatr Emerg Care. 2016;32:192–4.
108. Hübner U, Schlicht W, Outzen S, et al. Ultrasound in the diagnosis of fractures in children. J Bone Joint Surg Br. 2000;82(8):1170–3.
109. Maempel JK, Stone OD, Murray AW. Quantificaion of radiation exposure in the operating theatre during management of common fractures of the upper extremity in children[J]. Ann R Coll Surg Engl. 2016;98(7):483–7.
110. Patel N, Mohamed A, Cooper G, McFadyen I. Ionising radiation exposure in paediatric trauma[J]. Ann R Coll Surg Engl. 2014;96(3):190–3.
111. Cha SM, Shin HD, Kim KC, Han SC. Percutaneous reduction and leverage fixation using K-wires in paediatric angulated radial neck fractures. Int Orthop. 2011; https://doi.org/10.1007/s00264-011-1387-3.
112. Bither N, Gupta P, Jindal N. Pediatric displaced radial neck fractures: retrospective results of a modified Metaizeau technique. Eur J Orthop Surg Traumatol. 2014; https://doi.org/10.1007/s00590-014-1452-x.
113. Massetti D, Marinelli M, Facco G, Falcioni D, Giampaolini N, Specchia N, Gigante AP. Percutaneous k-wire leverage reduction and retrograde transphyseal k-wire fixation of angulated radial neck fractures in children. Eur J Orthop Surg Traumatol. 2020; https://doi.org/10.1007/s00590-020-02654-x.
114. Fan YF, Xu WQ, Liu QX, Liu CY, Wang W. Modified Kirschner wire percutaneous rotation prying reduction combined with elastic stable intramedullary nailing in children with Judet IV radial neck fracture. BMC Musculoskelet Disord. 2023; https://doi.org/10.1186/s12891-023-07008-2.
115. Stöckell M, Lampio E, Sagstetter F, Sinikumpu J. Faster healing of radial neck fractures in children treated with the Metaizeau technique compared with percutaneous Kirschner wire fixation: a population-based study. BMC Musculoskelet Disord. 2025; https://doi.org/10.1186/s12891-025-08830-6.
116. Liu Y, Zhu L-Q, Zhang F-Y, Liu Y, Zhen Y-F, Zhao T-T. Open reduction of displaced radial neck fractures in children by internal fixation techniques: comparison of percutaneous Kirschner wiring and elastic stable intramedullary nailing. Indian J Orthop. 2022; https://doi.org/10.1007/s43465-022-00631-6.
117. Xia A, You C, Han J, Wu D, Xia Y, Wang J. Comparison of different treatments for children with radial neck fracture and analysis of prognostic factors. Arch Orthop Trauma Surg. 2021; https://doi.org/10.1007/s00402-021-04178-3.
118. Wu X, Xia J, Li X, Chen X, Wang S, Shen X. Ultrasound-guided vs. fluoroscopy-guided percutaneous leverage reduction for severely displaced radial neck fractures in children: a comparative analysis of clinical and radiological outcomes. BMC Musculoskelet Disord. 2025; https://doi.org/10.1186/s12891-025-08312-9.
119. Lee JE, Kim JB, Choi ES. Ultrasonography-guided reduction of pediatric radial neck fractures. BMC Musculoskelet Disord. 2017; https://doi.org/10.1186/s12891-017-1891-8.

Distal Radius Fracture

9

Introduction by the Author

Distal radius fractures account for up to 35% of all pediatric fractures. They are primarily caused by falling on an outstretched hand or by a direct blow to the arm. It is estimated that wrist fractures represent 25% of all fractures in children.

While these fractures can occur at any age, they are most prevalent during early puberty, when bone mineral density is relatively low. The peak rate of occurrence is observed among individuals between the ages of 11.5 and 14.5. Due to their proximity to the growth plate, distal radius fractures have significant remodeling potential.

Distal radius buckle fractures (less than 1 cm from the growth plate), also known as torus fractures, are a common pediatric injury, especially in younger patients. They are characterized by compression of the radius without cortical disruption or physeal injury. These stable fractures are typically treated with removable splints or braces, minimizing the need for orthopedic follow-up and additional imaging. Torus/buckle fractures are generally easy to diagnose, but greenstick and complete fractures are more difficult, especially for inexperienced surgeons.

Physeal injuries frequently occur during the preadolescent growth spurt when transient cortical porosity is caused by an increase in calcium requirements and bone turnover. Fractures involving the growth plate are often subdivided according to the Salter-Harris classification and are generally treated conservatively since they have the highest remodeling potential.

The treatment of choice for displaced pediatric distal radius fractures is often reduction and immobilization with a cast, although redisplacement rates within the first 2 weeks after initial reduction range from 20% to 40%. To prevent redisplacement, the fracture can be stabilized with Kirschner wires.

© The Author(s), under exclusive license to Springer Nature Switzerland AG 2026
F. Canavese, *Advances in Pediatric Extremity Fracture Management*,
https://doi.org/10.1007/978-3-032-33306-3_9

Overriding distal radius fractures are challenging due to their potential for displacement, though they have high remodeling potential in young patients. Standard treatments for significantly displaced fractures include reduction and casting. However, redisplacement rates remain high, prompting consideration of Kirschner wire fixation, despite its potential complications.

Children with two-bone fractures or complete displacement may benefit from primary Kirschner wire fixation alongside reduction. While anatomical reduction is not necessary for successful treatment of distal radius fractures in children, including overriding fractures, sufficient growth potential for remodeling must be present.

Older children with distal radius fractures pose a significant treatment challenge due to the lack of specific guidelines and the ongoing debate about the optimal approach. Traditional methods, such as closed reduction and casting, are associated with high rates of redisplacement. Alternative techniques, such as Kirschner wire pinning and elastic stable intramedullary nailing, have their own complications and limitations.

9.1 Machine Generated Summaries

Disclaimer: The summaries in this chapter were generated from Springer Nature publications using abstractive AI auto-summarization: An abstraction-based summarizer creates new text based on deep learning. New phrases are created to summarize the content. As the constituted sentences are machine selected, they may not fully reflect the body of the work, so we strongly advise that the original content is read and cited. The auto-generated summaries were curated by the author(s) to meet Springer Nature publication standards.

The Incidence of Distal Radius Fractures in a Swedish Pediatric Population - an Observational Cohort Study of 90 970 Individual Fractures [102]

This is a machine-generated summary of:

Südow, Hanna; Navarro, Cecilia Mellstrand The incidence of distal radius fractures in a Swedish pediatric population - an observational cohort study of 90 970 individual fractures [102]
Published in: BMC Musculoskeletal Disorders (2021)
Link to original: https://doi.org/10.1186/s12891-021-04410-6
Copyright of the summarized publication:
The Author(s) 2021
License: OpenAccess CC BY + CC0 4.0

This article is licensed under a Creative Commons Attribution 4.0 International License, which permits use, sharing, adaptation, distribution and reproduction in any medium or format, as long as you give appropriate credit to the original author(s) and the source, provide a link to the Creative Commons licence, and indicate if changes were made. The images or other third party material in this article are included in the article's Creative Commons licence, unless indicated otherwise in a credit line to the material. If material is not included in the article's Creative Commons licence and your intended use is not permitted by statutory regulation or exceeds the permitted use, you will need to obtain permission directly from the copyright holder. To view a copy of this licence, visit http://creativecommons.org/licenses/by/4.0/. The Creative Commons Public Domain Dedication waiver (http://creativecommons.org/publicdomain/zero/1.0/) applies to the data made available in this article, unless otherwise stated in a credit line to the data.

If you want to cite the papers, please refer to the original.

For technical reasons we could not place the page where the original quote is coming from.

Research Highlights

Fractures are common injuries among children, with a significant proportion experiencing at least one fracture during childhood. Wrist fractures, particularly distal radius fractures, are prevalent and often occur when a child falls on an extended arm. The incidence of these fractures peaks during early puberty when bone mineral density is relatively low. Despite the increasing trend in fracture incidence over the decades, there is limited knowledge about how recent lifestyle changes, such as reduced physical activity due to technological advancements, affect fracture rates in children. Now, a new study by Hanna Südow and colleagues investigates the incidence of distal radius fractures in Swedish children from 2005 to 2014 using nationwide registry data.

The study utilized data from the Swedish National Patient Register, which includes mandatory registrations of all inpatient and outpatient care. Researchers analyzed records of distal radius fractures in individuals aged 0–17 years during the specified period. Fracture events were identified using specific ICD codes, and incidences were calculated per person-years for different age groups and genders. The study found a total of 56,000 distal radius fractures during the study period, with boys experiencing higher rates than girls. The highest incidence was observed in boys aged 10–14 years, while the lowest was in females aged 15 years or older. Seasonal variations were noted, with higher incidences in September and lower in December.

The findings suggest a decrease in fracture incidence over the study period, contrasting with previous reports of increasing trends. This decline may reflect lifestyle changes among children, such as reduced physical activity due to digital entertainment. Future studies could explore whether this trend continues and its long-term implications on children's health. The study highlights the need for further research to understand the relationship between physical activity and fracture risk and to assess potential protective factors that could mitigate fracture occurrences among children.

Distal Radius Fractures in Children Aged 5–12 Years: A Swedish Nationwide Register-Based Study of 25 777 Patients [103]

This is a machine-generated summary of:

Bergkvist, Anna; Lundqvist, Eva; Pantzar-Castilla, Evelina Distal radius fractures in children aged 5–12 years: a Swedish nationwide register-based study of 25 777 patients [103]
Published in: BMC Musculoskeletal Disorders (2023)
Link to original: https://doi.org/10.1186/s12891-023-06680-8
Copyright of the summarized publication:
The Author(s) 2023
License: OpenAccess CC BY + CC0 4.0

This article is licensed under a Creative Commons Attribution 4.0 International License, which permits use, sharing, adaptation, distribution and reproduction in any medium or format, as long as you give appropriate credit to the original author(s) and the source, provide a link to the Creative Commons licence, and indicate if changes were made. The images or other third party material in this article are included in the article's Creative Commons licence, unless indicated otherwise in a credit line to the material. If material is not included in the article's Creative Commons licence and your intended use is not permitted by statutory regulation or exceeds the permitted use, you will need to obtain permission directly from the copyright holder. To view a copy of this licence, visit http://creativecommons.org/licenses/by/4.0/. The Creative Commons Public Domain Dedication waiver (http://creativecommons.org/publicdomain/zero/1.0/) applies to the data made available in this article, unless otherwise stated in a credit line to the data.

If you want to cite the papers, please refer to the original.

For technical reasons we could not place the page where the original quote is coming from.

Research Highlights

Distal radius fractures (DRFs) are the most common type of fracture in children, predominantly affecting boys, often due to falls at home or during sports. These fractures can be managed differently in children than in adults due to the potential for bone remodeling. While simple and incomplete DRFs are typically treated with casting, completely displaced fractures may require more complex interventions such as closed reduction and casting or percutaneous Kirschner wire (K-wire) fixation to prevent redislocation. However, there is no clear consensus on the primary treatment for completely displaced fractures, and nationwide guidelines for K-wire usage are lacking. Now, a new study by Anna Bergkvist and colleagues investigates the epidemiological nature of pediatric DRFs in Sweden, focusing on fracture types, causes of injury, and treatment methods.

The study is a retrospective register analysis using data from the Swedish Fracture Register (SFR), which includes records from all orthopedic departments in

Sweden since 2015. The researchers analyzed data from children aged 0–17 years with DRFs registered between January 2015 and October 2020. They examined variables such as sex, age, type of fracture, cause of injury, and treatment method. The study found that casting was the most common treatment across all fracture types. For complete fractures specifically, casting with or without reduction was used in 67% of cases, while K-wire fixation was employed in 33%. The analysis revealed that boys were more likely than girls to receive K-wire fixation, particularly younger boys with complete fractures.

The study highlights a significant variation in treatment practices for pediatric DRFs in Sweden and underscores the need for further research to establish clear guidelines. It suggests that younger children and boys are more frequently treated with K-wire fixation compared to older children and girls, which contrasts with some previous studies advocating a more conservative approach for younger patients. Future study could focus on understanding the reasons behind these treatment choices and developing a nationwide consensus on managing completely displaced DRFs in children to ensure consistent and effective care across different regions.

Epidemiology of Distal Radius Fractures in Children and Adults During the COVID-19 Pandemic – A Two-Center Study [104]

This is a machine-generated summary of:

Olech, Jarosław; Ciszewski, Mariusz; Morasiewicz, Piotr Epidemiology of distal radius fractures in children and adults during the COVID-19 pandemic – a two-center study [104]
Published in: BMC Musculoskeletal Disorders (2021)
Link to original: https://doi.org/10.1186/s12891-021-04128-5
Copyright of the summarized publication:
The Author(s) 2021
License: OpenAccess CC BY + CC0 4.0

This article is licensed under a Creative Commons Attribution 4.0 International License, which permits use, sharing, adaptation, distribution and reproduction in any medium or format, as long as you give appropriate credit to the original author(s) and the source, provide a link to the Creative Commons licence, and indicate if changes were made. The images or other third party material in this article are included in the article's Creative Commons licence, unless indicated otherwise in a credit line to the material. If material is not included in the article's Creative Commons licence and your intended use is not permitted by statutory regulation or exceeds the permitted use, you will need to obtain permission directly from the copyright holder. To view a copy of this licence, visit http://creativecommons.org/licenses/by/4.0/. The Creative Commons Public Domain Dedication waiver (http://creativecommons.org/publicdomain/zero/1.0/) applies to the data made available in this article, unless otherwise stated in a credit line to the data.

If you want to cite the papers, please refer to the original.

For technical reasons we could not place the page where the original quote is coming from.

Research Highlights

Distal radius fractures (DRFs) are a prevalent type of fracture, particularly among osteoporosis-related injuries, and are treated using various methods in both children and adults. The COVID-19 pandemic significantly disrupted healthcare systems worldwide, altering clinical practices and access to specialist care, which may have impacted the epidemiology and treatment of DRFs. Now, a new study by Jarosław Olech and colleagues provides a comprehensive assessment of the impact of the COVID-19 pandemic on DRF epidemiology in both children and adults across two large trauma centers in Poland.

The study involved a retrospective analysis of medical records from two trauma centers, comparing data from the COVID-19 pandemic period with pre-pandemic figures. Researchers evaluated the total number of DRF cases, treatment methods (surgical vs. conservative), patient demographics, and hospital stay durations. Statistical analyses were conducted using Pearson's chi-square test and Student's t-test to assess differences between the two periods. The findings revealed a significant decrease in the total number of DRF hospitalizations during the pandemic, with a notable reduction in conservative treatments among adults. Conversely, there was an increase in surgical treatments, particularly involving volar plate fixation. The mean age of hospitalized patients decreased, and hospital stays were shorter during the pandemic.

The study highlights important shifts in DRF treatment patterns during the COVID-19 pandemic, suggesting an increase in high-energy fractures requiring surgical intervention. Future study could focus on understanding the long-term implications of these changes on patient outcomes and healthcare resource allocation. Additionally, there is a need to raise awareness about DRF risks among men, as evidenced by an increased male-to-female ratio during this period. These insights could inform strategies for managing fracture care during ongoing or future healthcare disruptions.

Differentiating Stable Buckle Fractures from Other Distal Radius Fractures: The 1-cm Rule [105]

This is a machine-generated summary of:

Iles, Benjamin W.; Samora, Julie B.; Singh, Satbir; Ruess, Lynne Differentiating stable buckle fractures from other distal radius fractures: the 1-cm rule [105]

Published in: Pediatric Radiology (2018)
Link to original: https://doi.org/10.1007/s00247-018-4316-4
Copyright of the summarized publication:
Springer-Verlag GmbH Germany, part of Springer Nature 2018
All rights reserved.

If you want to cite the papers, please refer to the original.

For technical reasons we could not place the page where the original quote is coming from.

Research Highlights

Distal radius buckle fractures, also known as torus fractures, are common pediatric injuries characterized by compression of the radius without cortical disruption or physeal injury. These stable fractures are typically managed with removable splints or braces, minimizing the need for orthopedic follow-up and additional imaging. However, accurate diagnosis is crucial to avoid misclassifying unstable distal radius fractures as buckle fractures, which could lead to inadequate treatment and potential complications. Now, a new study by Benjamin W. Iles and colleagues proposes a measurement rule to help differentiate stable buckle fractures from other potentially unstable distal radius fractures in pediatric patients.

The study was conducted as part of an interdepartmental quality improvement project involving radiology and orthopedic surgery. Researchers retrospectively analyzed radiographs from children who presented with wrist injuries at a tertiary-care center and affiliated clinics. The study included children with isolated buckle or distal radius fractures, excluding those with pathological conditions or prior wrist surgeries. Two senior readers independently reviewed the radiographs to categorize the fractures, achieving near-perfect agreement before reaching a consensus diagnosis. The researchers measured the distance from the fracture to the physis on posteroanterior (PA) and lateral projections to develop a diagnostic aid. Using ROC curves, they identified cut-off values for these measurements to predict buckle fracture diagnoses accurately.

The study found that in children aged 4–12 years, using a cut-off of 20 mm on PA projections provided high sensitivity and specificity for diagnosing buckle fractures. However, diagnostic accuracy was lower for children under 4 years old due to measurement challenges and limited availability of appropriately sized braces. The findings suggest that measuring fracture-to-physis distance can aid in distinguishing stable buckle fractures from potentially unstable ones in older children, reducing unnecessary casting and follow-up appointments. Future studies could focus on refining diagnostic criteria for younger children and exploring alternative imaging techniques to improve accuracy across all age groups.

Classification of Distal Radius Fractures in Children: Good Inter- and Intraobserver Reliability, Which Improves with Clinical Experience [106]

This is a machine-generated summary of:

Randsborg, Per-Henrik; Sivertsen, Einar A Classification of distal radius fractures in children: good inter- and intraobserver reliability, which improves with clinical experience [106]

Published in: BMC Musculoskeletal Disorders (2012)
Link to original: https://doi.org/10.1186/1471-2474-13-6
Copyright of the summarized publication:
Randsborg and Sivertsen; licensee BioMed Central Ltd. 2012
License: OpenAccess CC BY 2.0

This article is published under license to BioMed Central Ltd. This is an Open Access article distributed under the terms of the Creative Commons Attribution License (http://creativecommons.org/licenses/by/2.0), which permits unrestricted use, distribution, and reproduction in any medium, provided the original work is properly cited.

If you want to cite the papers, please refer to the original.

For technical reasons we could not place the page where the original quote is coming from.

Research Highlights

Distal radius fractures are the most common type of fracture in children, typically treated conservatively with plaster casts, and complications are rare. However, the classification of these fractures is crucial for determining appropriate treatment and follow-up strategies, as well as for predicting prognosis. A reliable classification system must account for fracture stability and growth plate involvement to avoid misclassification that could lead to unnecessary follow-ups or complications such as malunion. Now, a new study by Per-Henrik Randsborg and colleagues evaluates the interobserver and intraobserver reliability of a commonly used classification system for distal radius fractures in children, examining how experience influences classification reliability.

The study involved reviewing radiographs of distal radius fractures in children under 18 years old, treated at a single institution. The researchers included only metaphyseal fractures and excluded diaphyseal ones. Observers, including junior orthopedic residents, senior registrars, and experienced orthopedic surgeons, independently classified each fracture into one of four categories: buckle, greenstick, complete, or physeal fracture. Observers were provided with schematics and written instructions but received no further guidance. The classifications were performed twice, months apart, with observers blinded to clinical information. Kappa statistics were used to assess agreement levels among observers.

The study found that interobserver reliability was highest among experienced consultants compared to junior registrars. Buckle fractures had the highest category-specific kappa value, while greenstick and complete fractures were more challenging to classify consistently. Intraobserver reliability was also higher among senior registrars than junior ones. The findings suggest that experience significantly impacts classification accuracy. Future study could focus on improving training for less experienced clinicians to enhance classification reliability further. Additionally, reducing unnecessary follow-ups for stable fractures like buckle fractures could benefit patients and healthcare systems by minimizing costs and resource use without compromising patient outcomes.

2D/3D Ultrasound Diagnosis of Pediatric Distal Radius Fractures by Human Readers vs Artificial Intelligence [107]

This is a machine-generated summary of:

Knight, Jessica; Zhou, Yuyue; Keen, Christopher; Hareendranathan, Abhilash Rakkunedeth; Alves-Pereira, Fatima; Ghasseminia, Siyavesh; Wichuk, Stephanie; Brilz, Alan; Kirschner, David; Jaremko, Jacob 2D/3D ultrasound diagnosis of pediatric distal radius fractures by human readers vs artificial intelligence [107]
Published in: Scientific Reports (2023)
Link to original: https://doi.org/10.1038/s41598-023-41807-w
Copyright of the summarized publication:
The Author(s) 2023
License: OpenAccess CC BY 4.0

This article is licensed under a Creative Commons Attribution 4.0 International License, which permits use, sharing, adaptation, distribution and reproduction in any medium or format, as long as you give appropriate credit to the original author(s) and the source, provide a link to the Creative Commons licence, and indicate if changes were made. The images or other third party material in this article are included in the article's Creative Commons licence, unless indicated otherwise in a credit line to the material. If material is not included in the article's Creative Commons licence and your intended use is not permitted by statutory regulation or exceeds the permitted use, you will need to obtain permission directly from the copyright holder. To view a copy of this licence, visit http://creativecommons.org/licenses/by/4.0/.

If you want to cite the papers, please refer to the original.

For technical reasons we could not place the page where the original quote is coming from.

Research Highlights

Distal radius fractures (DRF) are common injuries in children, often resulting from falls onto an outstretched hand. These fractures occur in a vulnerable area where cortical bone is thinner and reinforced by trabecular bone. Currently, radiographs are the standard diagnostic tool for DRF, but they expose children to radiation and contribute to longer emergency department (ED) wait times. Point-of-care ultrasound (POCUS) offers a radiation-free alternative that can be performed at the bedside, but its effectiveness in diagnosing DRF in children has not been fully established. Now, a new study by Jessica Knight and colleagues explores the feasibility of using POCUS with artificial intelligence (AI) assistance to diagnose DRF in children, potentially reducing radiation exposure and improving ED efficiency.

The study was conducted at Stollery Children's Hospital in Edmonton, Alberta, involving children aged 4–16 years with wrist trauma. Both traditional ultrasound and portable ultrasound devices were used to scan the affected wrists, with images interpreted by readers of varying expertise levels. The study also incorporated AI models trained to recognize fractures from ultrasound images. The AI's performance was compared against human readers and radiographs, which served as the gold standard for diagnosis. The results showed that experienced human readers could detect DRF with high sensitivity using both types of ultrasound devices. Additionally, the AI models demonstrated accuracy comparable to expert human readers, suggesting that AI could assist less experienced users in interpreting ultrasound images.

The study highlights the potential of POCUS combined with AI to improve DRF diagnosis in pediatric patients. By reducing reliance on radiographs, this approach could decrease ED wait times and radiation exposure for children. Future studies could focus on developing app-based AI tools for real-time interpretation of ultrasound images on portable devices, further enhancing accessibility and utility in clinical settings. Expanding the AI model's capabilities to detect other types of upper extremity fractures or assess fracture displacement could also increase its clinical relevance. While promising, these findings need validation through multicenter trials to confirm their generalizability and effectiveness across diverse healthcare settings.

Reference Values for Digital X-Ray Radiogrammetry Parameters in Children and Adolescents in Comparison to Estimates in Patients with Distal Radius Fractures [108]

This is a machine-generated summary of:

Renz, Diane M.; Malich, Ansgar; Ulrich, Andreas; Pfeil, Alexander; Mentzel, Hans-Joachim; Streitparth, Florian; Maurer, Martin H.; Teichgräber, Ulf K.; Böttcher, Joachim Reference values for digital X-ray radiogrammetry parameters in children and adolescents in comparison to estimates in patients with distal radius fractures [108]

Published in: Journal of Bone and Mineral Metabolism (2015)
Link to original: https://doi.org/10.1007/s00774-014-0641-3
Copyright of the summarized publication:
The Japanese Society for Bone and Mineral Research and Springer Japan 2015
All rights reserved.

If you want to cite the papers, please refer to the original.

For technical reasons we could not place the page where the original quote is coming from.

Research Highlights

Fractures in children and adolescents, particularly at the distal forearm, have been on the rise, posing both immediate and long-term health challenges. Traditionally associated with the elderly, osteoporosis is now recognized as having roots in pediatric populations, where failure to achieve optimal peak bone mass can predispose individuals to osteoporosis later in life. Identifying at-risk individuals early is crucial for effective prevention strategies. However, traditional methods like dual-energy X-ray absorptiometry (DXA) pose challenges due to radiation exposure and limitations in pediatric populations. Now, a new study by Diane M. Renz and colleagues explores the potential of digital X-ray radiogrammetry (DXR) as a safer alternative for assessing bone mineral density (BMD) in children.

The study involved a retrospective analysis of digital hand radiographs from Caucasian German children aged 5–18 years, comparing those with distal radius fractures to a reference cohort without fractures. The researchers used DXR to measure cortical BMD and metacarpal index (MCI) from original digital images, avoiding the noise-related issues of previous methods that required printing and scanning. The study established normative DXR-BMD and DXR-MCI values across different age groups and genders. Statistical analyses revealed that children with distal radius fractures had significantly lower DXR-BMD and DXR-MCI values compared to their non-fractured peers, with Z scores indicating reduced bone mineralization in the fracture cohort.

The findings suggest that DXR could be a valuable tool for early identification of children at increased risk of fractures and future osteoporosis. The use of routine hand radiographs minimizes additional radiation exposure, making DXR a promising method for pediatric osteodensitometry. Future studies could focus on refining this technique for younger children and integrating it into routine clinical practice to facilitate early intervention strategies such as dietary modifications and physical activity enhancements. This approach could significantly impact public health by reducing fracture incidence and promoting better bone health from an early age.

Is Reduction Necessary in Overriding Metaphyseal Distal Radius Fractures in Children Under 11 Years: A Systematic Review and Meta-Analysis of Comparative Studies [109]

This is a machine-generated summary of:

Galán-Olleros, María; Mayans-Sanesteban, Jorge; Martínez-Álvarez, Sergio; Miranda-Gorozarri, Carlos; Ramírez-Barragán, Ana; Egea-Gámez, Rosa M.; Alonso-Hernández, Javier; Martínez-Caballero, Ignacio Is reduction necessary in overriding metaphyseal distal radius fractures in children under 11 years: a systematic review and meta-analysis of comparative studies [109]

Published in: European Journal of Orthopaedic Surgery & Traumatology (2024)
Link to original: https://doi.org/10.1007/s00590-024-03936-4
Copyright of the summarized publication:
The Author(s), under exclusive licence to Springer-Verlag France SAS, part of Springer Nature 2024

Copyright comment: Springer Nature or its licensor (e.g. a society or other partner) holds exclusive rights to this article under a publishing agreement with the author(s) or other rightsholder(s); author self-archiving of the accepted manuscript version of this article is solely governed by the terms of such publishing agreement and applicable law.

All rights reserved.

If you want to cite the papers, please refer to the original.

For technical reasons we could not place the page where the original quote is coming from.

Research Highlights

Wrist fractures are the most common type of fracture in children, with complete overriding metaphyseal distal radius fractures posing a particular challenge due to their potential for displacement. While closed reduction is a common treatment, it involves risks such as increased healthcare costs and potential complications from sedation or anesthesia. Despite these concerns, the necessity of anatomical reduction for favorable outcomes remains uncertain. Now, a new study by María Galán-Olleros and colleagues investigates whether reduction is necessary for treating these fractures in children under 12 years old.

The study conducted a systematic review and meta-analysis following PRISMA guidelines, focusing on original studies that compared simple casting without reduction to closed reduction with casting or pin fixation. The researchers searched PubMed, Embase, and Cochrane databases for relevant studies and included three studies involving 159 patients in their analysis. Data were extracted on primary outcomes like radiographic alignment and union, as well as secondary outcomes such as complications and motion limitations. The analysis revealed that simple immobilization resulted in significantly fewer complications compared to reduction methods. Although there was no significant difference in sagittal alignment at final follow-up, the non-reduction group showed a trend towards fewer reinterventions and improved functional outcomes.

The findings suggest that anatomical reduction may not be necessary for successful outcomes in treating overriding distal radius fractures in children, provided there is sufficient growth potential for remodeling. The study highlights the distal radius's exceptional remodeling capacity, which allows for tolerance of initial deformity without compromising healing or function. Future studies should incorporate patient-reported outcome measures (PROMs) to better capture the real-world impact of different treatment approaches. Ongoing randomized controlled trials are expected to provide more robust evidence on this topic, but this meta-analysis offers valuable interim guidance for clinical practice by supporting the use of simple casting as a viable treatment strategy.

Metaphyseal Distal Radius Fractures in Adolescents: Is Closed Reduction and Casting Sufficient for Most? [110]

This is a machine-generated summary of:

Hancock, Daniel William; Barrett-Lee, Joe Jordan Thomas; Abdellatif, Ahmed Mohamed Ahmed; White, Sophie; Liu, Perry; Roberts, Darren Metaphyseal distal radius fractures in adolescents: is closed reduction and casting sufficient for most? [110]
Published in: European Journal of Orthopaedic Surgery & Traumatology (2025)
Link to original: https://doi.org/10.1007/s00590-025-04182-y
Copyright of the summarized publication:
The Author(s), under exclusive licence to Springer-Verlag France SAS, part of Springer Nature 2025

Copyright comment: Springer Nature or its licensor (e.g. a society or other partner) holds exclusive rights to this article under a publishing agreement with the author(s) or other rightsholder(s); author self-archiving of the accepted manuscript version of this article is solely governed by the terms of such publishing agreement and applicable law.

All rights reserved.

If you want to cite the papers, please refer to the original.

For technical reasons we could not place the page where the original quote is coming from.

Research Highlights

Distal radius fractures are the most common type of fracture in the pediatric population, with a notable increase in incidence among adolescents over recent decades. This rise is attributed to factors such as increased sports participation, obesity, and decreased bone density. Traditionally, it was believed that heightened activity levels during puberty were responsible for the increased fracture rates; however, recent studies suggest that the rapid linear growth during puberty outpaces bone mineralization, leading to fractures. Now, a new study by Daniel William Hancock and colleagues investigates the management of metaphyseal distal radius fractures in adolescents, aiming to identify optimal treatment methods and associated complications.

The study conducted a retrospective analysis of patients aged 10–16 years with acute metaphyseal distal radius fractures at Queen Alexandra Hospital over a five-year period. Excluding physeal injuries, the researchers reviewed radiographs and patient records to gather data on demographics, injury mechanisms, management strategies, fracture patterns, outcomes, and complications. Fractures were categorized by displacement type—volar or dorsal—and angulation was measured at initial presentation and final follow-up. Management strategies included non-operative methods like closed reduction and casting under sedation or surgical interventions such as manipulation under anesthesia (MUA) with K-wire fixation or open reduction internal fixation (ORIF). The study used statistical analyses to compare outcomes between non-operative and surgical treatments.

The findings revealed no significant difference in final angulation between fractures managed with closed reduction and casting versus surgical fixation. However, off-ended fractures were more likely to undergo surgical intervention due to higher re-displacement risks. Complications were notably higher in surgically managed cases, particularly those involving K-wire fixation. The study suggests that both MUA with casting in theater and surgical fixation can achieve satisfactory radiographic outcomes for off-ended and angulated fractures if performed under general anesthesia by trained practitioners. Future studies could focus on long-term functional outcomes and explore the impact of rotational malalignment on functionality in this population.

Modified Kapandji Technique in Pediatric Displaced Distal Radius Fractures: Results in 195 Patients [71]

This is a machine-generated summary of:

Bassi, Cristina; Heimann, Alexander F.; Schwab, Joseph M.; Tannast, Moritz; Raabe, Ines Modified Kapandji technique in pediatric displaced distal radius fractures: results in 195 patients [71]
Published in: European Journal of Orthopaedic Surgery & Traumatology (2023)
Link to original: https://doi.org/10.1007/s00590-023-03686-9
Copyright of the summarized publication:
The Author(s) 2023
License: OpenAccess CC BY 4.0

This article is licensed under a Creative Commons Attribution 4.0 International License, which permits use, sharing, adaptation, distribution and reproduction in any medium or format, as long as you give appropriate credit to the original author(s) and the source, provide a link to the Creative Commons licence, and indicate if changes were made. The images or other third party material in this article are included in the article's Creative Commons licence, unless indicated otherwise in a credit line to the material. If material is not included in the article's Creative Commons licence and your intended use is not permitted by statutory regulation or exceeds the permitted use, you will need to obtain permission directly from the copyright holder. To view a copy of this licence, visit http://creativecommons.org/licenses/by/4.0/.

If you want to cite the papers, please refer to the original.

For technical reasons we could not place the page where the original quote is coming from.

Research Highlights

Distal radius fractures are the most common type of fracture in children, often treated conservatively due to the bone's natural corrective potential. However, significant fracture displacement or risk factors like obesity can lead to secondary displacement, necessitating alternative treatment methods. The modified Kapandji technique, a method involving K-wire fracture reduction, has been proposed for pediatric displaced distal radius fractures (DDRFs), but evidence regarding its effectiveness and safety is limited. Now, a new study by Cristina Bassi and colleagues evaluates the outcomes and complications of using the modified Kapandji technique in pediatric DDRFs at their institution.

The study was a retrospective, single-center observational analysis of pediatric patients treated with the modified Kapandji technique between February and October. It included children and adolescents with displaced distal radius fractures who showed skeletal immaturity. The researchers assessed fracture reduction quality using postoperative radiographs and classified reductions as anatomical, good, or fair based on specific criteria. They also evaluated fracture stability by measuring changes in angulation during healing and recorded perioperative complications using a standardized grading system. The surgical procedure involved stab incisions for fracture reduction, followed by stability testing to determine the need for additional pin fixation.

The study found that the modified Kapandji technique resulted in high-quality fracture reduction in most cases, particularly in Salter-Harris fractures. While metaphyseal fractures showed slightly higher changes in angulation during healing, all fixation methods provided adequate stability. The complication rate was comparable to other surgical treatments for pediatric DDRFs, with most complications being transient and resolving without further intervention. The authors recommend extrafocal pinning for unstable metaphyseal fractures to enhance stability. Future studies could explore long-term outcomes and patient-reported measures to further validate these findings and improve treatment protocols for pediatric DDRFs using the modified Kapandji technique.

Antegrade Intrafocal Kapandji Pinning Technique for Volar Displaced Distal Radius Fractures in Older Children [111]

This is a machine-generated summary of:

Jerome, J. Terrence Jose; Matsui, Chihiro Antegrade intrafocal Kapandji pinning technique for volar displaced distal radius fractures in older children [111]
Published in: European Journal of Plastic Surgery (2024)
Link to original: https://doi.org/10.1007/s00238-024-02205-1
Copyright of the summarized publication:
The Author(s), under exclusive licence to Springer-Verlag GmbH Germany, part of Springer Nature 2024

Copyright comment: Springer Nature or its licensor (e.g. a society or other partner) holds exclusive rights to this article under a publishing agreement with the author(s) or other rightsholder(s); author self-archiving of the accepted manuscript version of this article is solely governed by the terms of such publishing agreement and applicable law.

All rights reserved.

If you want to cite the papers, please refer to the original.

For technical reasons we could not place the page where the original quote is coming from.

Research Highlights

Distal radius fractures in older children present a significant treatment challenge due to the absence of specific guidelines and ongoing debates about the optimal approach. Traditional methods like closed reduction and casting are associated with high redisplacement rates, while alternative techniques such as Kirschner wire (K-wire) pinning and elastic stable intramedullary nailing (ESIN) have their own complications and limitations. Now, a new study by J. Terrence Jose Jerome and colleagues explores the outcomes of antegrade intrafocal pinning (AIP) for volar displaced distal radius fractures in older children, offering a potential alternative to more invasive procedures.

The study was conducted retrospectively with twelve patients who had volar displaced distal radius fractures treated using the AIP technique. The procedure involved using a supraclavicular brachial block and making a small dorsal incision to insert a 1.5 mm K-wire antegrade into the fracture site. This method allowed for correction of the fracture alignment, followed by stabilization with two additional K-wires. Postoperatively, patients wore a below-elbow cast for 4 weeks before beginning active wrist exercises. Follow-up assessments included radiographs, MRI, range of motion measurements, grip strength evaluation, and pain assessment using standardized scales. The study reported successful radiological union in all patients without any growth plate injuries or significant complications.

The introduction of antegrade intrafocal pinning offers a promising alternative to volar plate fixation for managing volar displaced distal radius fractures in older children. This technique simplifies the procedure and reduces complication risks compared to traditional methods like plating and screws. While the study's small sample size and retrospective design limit its generalizability, it highlights the potential advantages of AIP in achieving good functional outcomes with lower complication rates. Future studies could focus on larger sample sizes and comparative analyses to further validate these findings and explore cost-effectiveness in clinical practice.

Displaced Distal Radius Fractures in Children, Cast Alone vs Additional K-Wire Fixation: A Meta-Analysis [112]

This is a machine-generated summary of:

Sengab, Alysia; Krijnen, Pieta; Schipper, Inger Birgitta Displaced distal radius fractures in children, cast alone vs additional K-wire fixation: a meta-analysis [112]
Published in: European Journal of Trauma and Emergency Surgery (2018)

Link to original: https://doi.org/10.1007/s00068-018-1011-y
Copyright of the summarized publication:
The Author(s) 2018
License: OpenAccess CC BY 4.0

This article is distributed under the terms of the Creative Commons Attribution 4.0 International License (http://creativecommons.org/licenses/by/4.0/), which permits unrestricted use, distribution, and reproduction in any medium, provided you give appropriate credit to the original author(s) and the source, provide a link to the Creative Commons license, and indicate if changes were made.

If you want to cite the papers, please refer to the original.

For technical reasons we could not place the page where the original quote is coming from.

Research Highlights

Distal radius fractures (DRFs) are among the most prevalent fractures in children, typically managed with reduction and cast immobilization (RCI). However, redisplacement after initial treatment is a common issue, occurring in a significant percentage of cases. To address this, some practitioners use additional percutaneous K-wire fixation (KWF) to stabilize the fracture before cast immobilization. While KWF can reduce redisplacement rates, it also introduces potential complications such as pin-tract infections and neuropraxia. Now, a new study by Alysia Sengab and colleagues conducts a meta-analysis to compare the effectiveness of RCI alone versus RCI with additional KWF in managing displaced DRFs in children.

The study involved a comprehensive literature search across multiple databases, including PubMed and Cochrane, to identify relevant studies comparing RCI alone and RCI with KWF. The authors included studies that met specific criteria regarding patient demographics and fracture characteristics. Data from these studies were extracted and analyzed using Review Manager software, employing a random-effects model to account for variability among studies. The analysis focused on outcomes such as redisplacement rates, secondary reduction rates, range of motion (ROM), and complications. The meta-analysis revealed that while KWF significantly reduced redisplacement rates compared to RCI alone, it was associated with minor complications like superficial infections. Importantly, no significant differences were found in ROM between the two treatment groups.

The findings suggest that while additional KWF effectively reduces redisplacement rates, it does not necessarily improve functional outcomes compared to RCI alone. This indicates that larger degrees of angulation or displacement might be acceptable in pediatric patients without compromising long-term wrist function. Future study could focus on identifying which patients would benefit most from additional KWF by considering factors such as age-related remodeling capacity and acceptable levels of fracture displacement. Additionally, cost considerations and potential complications should be weighed when deciding on the appropriate treatment strategy for DRFs in children.

Risk Factors for Fracture Redisplacement after Reduction and Cast Immobilization of Displaced Distal Radius Fractures in Children: A Meta-Analysis [113]

This is a machine-generated summary of:

Sengab, Alysia; Krijnen, Pieta; Schipper, Inger Birgitta Risk factors for fracture redisplacement after reduction and cast immobilization of displaced distal radius fractures in children: a meta-analysis [113]

Published in: European Journal of Trauma and Emergency Surgery (2019)
Link to original: https://doi.org/10.1007/s00068-019-01227-w

Copyright of the summarized publication:
The Author(s) 2019
License: OpenAccess CC BY 4.0

This article is distributed under the terms of the Creative Commons Attribution 4.0 International License (http://creativecommons.org/licenses/by/4.0/), which permits unrestricted use, distribution, and reproduction in any medium, provided you give appropriate credit to the original author(s) and the source, provide a link to the Creative Commons license, and indicate if changes were made.

If you want to cite the papers, please refer to the original.

For technical reasons we could not place the page where the original quote is coming from.

Research Highlights

Distal radius fractures are common in children, often resulting from falls or direct blows to the arm. While fracture reduction and cast immobilization are standard treatments for significantly displaced fractures, redisplacement rates remain high, prompting consideration of K-wire fixation despite its potential complications. Now, a new study by Alysia Sengab and colleagues conducts a meta-analysis to evaluate risk factors for redisplacement in pediatric distal radius fractures treated with reduction and cast immobilization, aiming to identify which patients might benefit most from primary K-wire fixation.

The study followed systematic review and meta-analysis guidelines, searching multiple databases for relevant literature. Articles were selected based on criteria such as language, treatment method, and availability of odds ratios for redisplacement risk factors. Twelve studies met the inclusion criteria, encompassing various designs and patient demographics. The analysis focused on eight predictors: age, gender, fracture type, displacement completeness, reduction quality, Cast Index, Three-Point Index, and surgeon experience. Results indicated that complete displacement and both-bone fractures significantly increased redisplacement risk. Anatomic reduction reduced this risk, while cast-related indices did not consistently predict outcomes due to data heterogeneity.

The findings suggest that children with both-bone fractures or complete displacement may benefit from primary K-wire fixation alongside reduction. The study highlights the importance of achieving anatomic reduction but notes that physician experience did not significantly impact redisplacement risk. Future study could focus on standardizing criteria for fracture reduction and incorporating remodeling potential into treatment decisions. Additionally, more homogeneous research is needed to clarify the predictive value of cast-related indices, which could be easily adjusted post-reduction to minimize redisplacement risks.

Protecting My Injured Child: A Qualitative Study of Parents' Experience of Caring for a Child with a Displaced Distal Radius Fracture [114]

This is a machine-generated summary of:

Phelps, E. E.; Tutton, E.; Costa, M. L.; Achten, J.; Moscrop, A.; Perry, D. C. Protecting my injured child: a qualitative study of parents' experience of caring for a child with a displaced distal radius fracture [114]
Published in: BMC Pediatrics (2022)
Link to original: https://doi.org/10.1186/s12887-022-03340-z
Copyright of the summarized publication:
The Author(s) 2022
License: OpenAccess CC BY + CC0 4.0

This article is licensed under a Creative Commons Attribution 4.0 International License, which permits use, sharing, adaptation, distribution and reproduction in any medium or format, as long as you give appropriate credit to the original author(s) and the source, provide a link to the Creative Commons licence, and indicate if changes were made. The images or other third party material in this article are included in the article's Creative Commons licence, unless indicated otherwise in a credit line to the material. If material is not included in the article's Creative Commons licence and your intended use is not permitted by statutory regulation or exceeds the permitted use, you will need to obtain permission directly from the copyright holder. To view a copy of this licence, visit http://creativecommons.org/licenses/by/4.0/. The Creative Commons Public Domain Dedication waiver (http://creativecommons.org/publicdomain/zero/1.0/) applies to the data made available in this article, unless otherwise stated in a credit line to the data.

If you want to cite the papers, please refer to the original.

For technical reasons we could not place the page where the original quote is coming from.

Research Highlights

Childhood fractures, particularly wrist fractures, are prevalent and significantly impact families by disrupting daily routines and causing concern over healing and potential complications. In the UK, displaced distal radius fractures in children are often treated surgically, though the necessity of surgery is debated due to children's natural bone remodeling capabilities. Despite the prevalence of these injuries, there is limited understanding of the experiences of parents and children regarding treatment decisions. Now, a new study by E. E. Phelps and colleagues explores these experiences through the Children's Radius Acute Fracture Fixation Trial (CRAFFT), a multicenter randomized non-inferiority trial comparing surgical and non-surgical treatments.

The study employed qualitative methods to delve into the experiences of families approached for participation in CRAFFT. Researchers conducted interviews with a purposive sample of parents who were informed about the trial, aiming to capture diverse perspectives based on factors such as the child's age, injury severity, and treatment choice. The interviews were guided by Heideggerian phenomenology to explore participants' lived experiences in depth. Parents shared their decision-making processes, concerns about their child's recovery, and interactions with clinicians. The analysis revealed themes around parents' efforts to protect their injured child, make informed decisions under pressure, and manage worries about recovery.

The findings underscore the emotional challenges parents face when deciding on trial participation amidst clinical uncertainty and time constraints in emergency settings. Parents expressed a need for more information and reassurance about treatment outcomes to feel confident in their decisions. The study suggests that involving parents more comprehensively in discussions about treatment options and recovery expectations could alleviate anxiety. Future studies could further explore parental experiences of deformity during recovery from wrist fractures to better support families through this process. Additionally, enhancing communication strategies may empower parents to nurture their child's recovery effectively while engaging children in discussions about their care.

Minimal Training Sufficient to Diagnose Pediatric Wrist Fractures with Ultrasound [115]

This is a machine-generated summary of:

Hedelin, Henrik; Tingström, Christian; Hebelka, Hanna; Karlsson, Jon Minimal training sufficient to diagnose pediatric wrist fractures with ultrasound [115]
Published in: The Ultrasound Journal (2017)
Link to original: https://doi.org/10.1186/s13089-017-0066-z
Copyright of the summarized publication:
The Author(s) 2017
License: OpenAccess CC BY 4.0

This article is distributed under the terms of the Creative Commons Attribution 4.0 International License (http://creativecommons.org/licenses/by/4.0/), which permits unrestricted use, distribution, and reproduction in any medium, provided you give appropriate credit to the original author(s) and the source, provide a link to the Creative Commons license, and indicate if changes were made.

If you want to cite the papers, please refer to the original.

For technical reasons we could not place the page where the original quote is coming from.

Research Highlights

Children with wrist trauma represent a significant portion of emergency department visits, with forearm fractures, particularly in the distal radius, being the most common. Radiographs are traditionally used for diagnosis, but treatment guidelines vary widely. The use of ultrasound (US) by non-radiologists has increased, showing promise as a diagnostic tool for fractures. However, its role as a primary screening tool remains debated. Now, a new study by Henrik Hedelin and colleagues investigates whether US can be effectively used as a point-of-care triage tool by non-radiologists with minimal training to differentiate between fractures and non-fractures in children.

The study was conducted at the Queen Silvia Children's Hospital in Sweden, involving six physicians with no prior US experience who underwent a brief intensive training course. They performed US examinations on children aged 3–18 years presenting with wrist trauma. The US findings were compared to standard radiographs interpreted by both the study physicians and independent senior radiologists. The study aimed to determine if US could accurately identify fractures and differentiate between complete and buckle fractures. The results showed that US had a sensitivity of 96% for detecting fractures when compared to radiographic findings, although some complete fractures were misclassified as less severe types.

The study demonstrates that with limited training, emergency physicians can use US to effectively rule out wrist fractures in children, potentially reducing the need for radiographs. However, while US is useful for initial triage, it is less accurate than radiographs for determining specific fracture types requiring follow-up or intervention. Future studies should explore the broader application of point-of-care ultrasound in emergency settings and further refine its use as a triage tool to optimize patient care and resource allocation.

Conclusion

Torus/buckle fractures, physeal injuries, and undisplaced distal radius fractures in older patients can be treated conservatively, with or without reduction. Complete displaced fractures may require surgical stabilization after reduction. Although surgery improves radiographic outcomes, it does not improve functional outcomes. Therefore, surgical fixation is indicated for patients with severely displaced distal radius fractures and limited remodeling potential.

Bibliography

1. Ryan LM, Teach SJ, Searcy K, Singer SA, Wood R, Wright JL, et al. Epidemiology of pediatric forearm fractures in Washington, DC. J Trauma. 2010;69(4 Suppl):S200–5.
2. Hedström EM, Svensson O, Bergström U, Michno P. Epidemiology of fractures in children and adolescents. Acta Orthop. 2010;81(1):148–53. https://doi.org/10.3109/17453671003628780.
3. de Putter CE, van Beeck EF, Looman CW, Toet H, Hovius SE, Selles RW. Trends in wrist fractures in children and adolescents, 1997–2009. J Hand Surg Am. 2011;36(11):1810–5.e2.
4. Khosla S, Melton LJ 3rd, Dekutoski MB, Achenbach SJ, Oberg AL, Riggs BL. Incidence of childhood distal forearm fractures over 30 years: a population-based study. JAMA. 2003;290(11):1479–85.
5. Mamoowala N, Johnson NA, Dias JJ. Trends in paediatric distal radius fractures: an eight-year review from a large UK trauma unit. Ann R Coll Surg Engl. 2019;101(4):297–303.
6. Statistics Sweden 2018. Available from: http://www.statistikdatabasen.scb.se/pxweb/en/ssd/. Accessed 21 Feb 2019.
7. Kanis JA, Odén A, McCloskey EV, Johansson H, Wahl DA, Cooper C. A systematic review of hip fracture incidence and probability of fracture worldwide. Osteoporosis Int. 2012;23(9):2239–56.
8. Körner D, Gonser CE, Bahrs C, Hemmann P. Change in paediatric upper extremity fracture incidences in German Hospitals from 2002 to 2017: an epidemiological study. Arch Orthop Trauma Surg. 2020;140:887–94.
9. Sengab A, Krijnen P, Schipper IB. Risk factors for fracture redisplacement after reduction and cast immobilization of displaced distal radius fractures in children: a meta-analysis. Eur J Trauma Emerg Surg. 2020;46:789–800.
10. Sinikumpu J-J, Nietosvaara Y. Treatment of distal forearm fractures in children. Scand J Surg SAGE Publications Ltd. 2021;110:276–80.
11. Displaced fracture of the distal radius in children. Accessed 29 Sept 2022. Retrieved from : https://online.boneandjoint.org.uk/doi/epub/ https://doi.org/10.1302/0301-620X.87B6.15648
12. Laaksonen T, Puhakka J, Kosola J, Stenroos A, Ahonen M, Nietosvaara Y. Most surgeons still prefer to reduce overriding distal radius fractures in children. Acta Orthop. 2021;92:235–9.
13. Marson BA, Ng JWG, Craxford S, Chell J, Lawniczak D, Price KR. m.fl. Treatment of completely displaced distal radial fractures with a straight plaster or manipulation under anaesthesia. Bone Joint J Br Editorial Soc Bone Joint Surg. 2021;103-B:902–7.
14. Ramoutar DN, Shivji FS, Rodrigues JN, Hunter JB. The outcomes of displaced paediatric distal radius fractures treated with percutaneous Kirschner wire fixation: a review of 248 cases. Eur J Orthop Surg Traumatol. 2015;25:471–6.
15. Prospective A, McLauchlan GJ, Cowan B, Annan IH, Robb JE. Management of completely displaced metaphyseal fractures of the distal radius in children. J Bone Joint Surg. 2002;84:5.
16. Mostafa MF, El-Adl G, Enan A. Percutaneous Kirschner-wire fixation for displaced distal forearm fractures in children. Acta Orthop Belg. 2009;75:8.
17. Möller M, Wolf O, Bergdahl C, Mukka S, Rydberg EM, Hailer NP, m.fl. The Swedish fracture register—ten years of experience and 600,000 fractures collected in a National Quality Register. BMC Musculoskelet Disord. 2022;23:141.
18. Fracture register—purpose and mode of operation. The Swedish Fracture Register. Accessed 8 Dec 2022. Retrieved from: https://sfr.registercentrum.se/om-registret/frakturregistret-syfte-och-funktionssaett/p/BJKP6zs6Q.
19. Baawa-Ameyaw J, Kabariti R, Chandra A, Rhee J. The theoretical impact on corrective upper limb elective services following analysis of distal radius fractures managed nonoperatively during COVID-19 pandemic. Bone Joint Open. 2020;1(10):612–6.
20. Lockey SD, Nelson PC, Kessler MJ, Kessler MW. Approaching "Elective" surgery in the era of COVID-19. J Hand Surg Am. 2021;46(1):60–4.

21. Nabian MH, Vosoughi F, Najafi F, Khabiri SS, Nafisi M, Veisi J. Epidemiological pattern of pediatric trauma in COVID-19 outbreak: data from a tertiary trauma center in Iran. Injury. 2020;S0020–1383(20):30756–7.
22. Bram JT, Johnson MA, Magee LC, Mehta NN, Fazal FZ, Baldwin KD. Where have all the fractures gone? The epidemiology of pediatric fractures during the COVID-19 pandemic. J Pediatr Orthop. 2020;40(8):373–9.
23. Symons S, Rowsell M, Bhowal B, Dias JJ. Hospital versus home management of children with buckle fractures of the distal radius: a prospective, randomised trial. J Bone Joint Surg Br. 2001;83:556–60.
24. Van Bosse HJP, Patel RJ, Thacker M, Sala DAS. Minimalistic approach to treating wrist torus fractures. J Pediatr Orthop. 2005;25:495–500.
25. West S, Andrews J, Bebbington A, et al. Buckle fractures of the distal radius are safely treated in a soft bandage: a randomized prospective trial of bandage versus plaster cast. J Pediatr Orthop. 2005;25:322–5.
26. Randsborg PH, Sivertsen EA. Distal radius fractures in children: substantial difference in stability between buckle and greenstick fractures. Acta Orthop. 2009;80:585–9.
27. Witney-Lagen C, Smith C, Walsh G. Soft cast versus rigid cast for treatment of distal radius buckle fractures in children. Injury. 2012;44:508–13.
28. Koelink E, Schuh S, Howard A, et al. Primary care physician follow-up of distal radius buckle fractures. Pediatrics. 2016;137:1–9.
29. Plint AC, Perry JJ, Correll R, et al. A randomized, controlled trial of removable splinting versus casting for wrist buckle fractures in children. Pediatrics. 2006;117:691–7.
30. TerreBlanche B, Eismann EA, Laor T et al. Overdiagnosis of distal radius buckle fracture in children. American Association for Hand Surgery (abstract), 2016. http://meeting.handsurgery.org/abstracts/2016/P100.cgi. Accessed 12 Oct 2018.
31. Sidor ML, Zuckerman JD, Lyon T, Koval K, Cuomo F, Schoenberg N. The Neer classification system for proximal humeral fractures. An assessment of interobserver reliability and intraobserver reproducibility. J Bone Joint Surg Am. 1993;75:1745–50.
32. van ED, Rhemrev SJ, Meylaerts SA, Roukema GR. The comparison of two classifications for trochanteric femur fractures: the AO/ASIF classification and the Jensen classification. Injury. 2010;41:377–81. https://doi.org/10.1016/j.injury.2009.10.007.
33. Salter RB. Injuries of the epiphyseal plate. Instr Course Lect. 1992;41:351–9.
34. Fleiss JL. Measuring nominal scale agreement among many raters. Psychol Bull. 1971;86:378–82.
35. Barton KL, Kaminsky CK, Green DW, Shean CJ, Kautz SM, Skaggs DL. Reliability of a modified Gartland classification of supracondylar humerus fractures. J Pediatr Orthop. 2001;21:27–30. https://doi.org/10.1097/01241398-200101000-00007.
36. Slongo T, Audigé L, Clavert JM, Nicolas L, Frick S, Hunter J. The AO comprehensive classification of pediatric long-bone fractures: a web-based multicenter agreement study. J Pediatr Orthop. 2007;27:171–80.
37. Slaar A, et al. The role of plain radiography in paediatric wrist trauma. Ins Imag. 2012;3:513–7.
38. van Rijn RR, Grootfaam DS, Lequin MH, Boot AM, van Beek RD, Hop WC, van Kuijk C. Digital radiogrammetry of the hand in a pediatric and adolescent Dutch Caucasian population: normative data and measurements in children with inflammatory bowel disease and juvenile chronic arthritis. Calcif Tissue Int. 2004;74:342–50.
39. Malich A, Freesmeyer MG, Mentzel HJ, Sauner D, Boettcher J, Petrovitch A, Behrendt W, Kaiser WA. Normative values of bone parameters of children and adolescents using digital computer-assisted radiogrammetry (DXR). J Clin Densitom. 2003;6:103–11.
40. van Rijn RR, van der Sluis IM, Link TM, Grampp S, Guglielmi G, Imhof H, Glüer C, Adams JE, van Kuijk C. Bone densitometry in children: a critical appraisal. Eur Radiol. 2003;13:700–10.
41. van Rijn RR, Van Kuijk C. Of small bones and big mistakes; bone densitometry in children revisited. Eur J Radiol. 2009;71:432–9.

42. Leonard MB, Propert KJ, Zemel BS, Stallings VA, Feldman HI. Discrepancies in pediatric bone mineral density reference data: potential for misdiagnosis of osteopenia. J Pediatr. 1999;135:182–8.
43. Rosholm A, Hyldstrup L, Bæcksgaard L, Grunkin M, Thodberg HH. Estimation of bone mineral density by digital X-ray radiogrammetry: theoretical background and clinical testing. Osteoporos Int. 2001;12:961–9.
44. van Rijn RR, Boot A, Wittenberg R, van der Sluis IM, van den Heuvel-Eibrink MM, Lequin MH, de MuinckKeizer-Schrama SM, Van Kuijk C. Direct X-ray radiogrammetry versus dual-energy X-ray absorptiometry: assessment of bone density in children treated for acute lymphoblastic leukaemia and growth hormone deficiency. Pediatr Radiol. 2006;36:227–32.
45. Handoll HH, Elliott J, Iheozor-Ejiofor Z, Hunter J, Karantana A. Interventions for treating wrist fractures in children. Cochrane Database Syst Rev. 2018;12(12):CD012470. https://doi.org/10.1002/14651858.CD012470.pub2.
46. Cooper C, et al. Epidemiology of childhood fractures in Britain: a study using the general practice research database. J Bone Miner Res. 2004;19(12):1976–81.
47. Azad A, Kang HP, Alluri RK, Vakhshori V, Kay HF, Ghiassi A. Epidemiological and treatment trends of distal radius fractures across multiple age groups. J Wrist Surg Thieme Med Publishers. 2019;08:305–11.
48. Proctor MT, Moore DJ, Paterson JM. Redisplacement after manipulation of distal radial fractures in children. J Bone Joint Surg Br. 1993;75(3):453–4. https://doi.org/10.1302/0301-620X.75B3.8496221.
49. Choi KY, Chan WS, Lam TP, Cheng JC. Percutaneous Kirschner-wire pinning for severely displaced distal radial fractures in children. A report of 157 cases. J Bone Joint Surg Br. 1995;77(5):797–801.
50. McLauchlan GJ, Cowan B, Annan IH, Robb JE. Management of completely displaced metaphyseal fractures of the distal radius in children. A prospective, randomised controlled trial. J Bone Joint Surg Br. 2002;84:413–7. https://doi.org/10.1302/0301-620X.84B3.11432.
51. Miller BS, Taylor B, Widmann RF, Bae DS, Snyder BD, Waters PM. Cast immobilization versus percutaneous pin fixation of displaced distal radius fractures in children: a prospective, randomized study. J Pediatr Orthop. 2005;25:490–4. https://doi.org/10.1097/01.bpo.0000158780.52849.39.
52. Colaris JW, Allema JH, Biter LU, de Vries MR, van de Ven CP, Bloem RM, et al. Re-displacement of stable distal both-bone forearm fractures in children: a randomised controlled multicentre trial. Injury. 2013;44(4):498–503. https://doi.org/10.1016/j.injury.2012.11.001.
53. Plánka L, Chalupová P, Skvaril J, Poul J, Gál P. Schopnost remodelace distálního radia pri hojení zlomenin v detském veku [Remodelling ability of the distal radius in fracture healing in childhood]. Rozhledy v chirurgii: mesicnik Ceskoslovenske chirurgicke spolecnosti. 2006;85(10):508–10.
54. Roy DR. Completely displaced distal radius fractures with intact ulnas in children. Orthopedics. 1989;12(8):1089–92. https://doi.org/10.3928/0147-7447-19890801-09.
55. Do TT, Strub WM, Foad SL, Mehlman CT, Crawford AH. Reduction versus remodeling in pediatric distal forearm fractures: a preliminary cost analysis. J Pediatr Orthop B. 2003;12(2):109–15. https://doi.org/10.1097/01.bpb.0000043725.21564.7b.
56. Ploegmakers JJ, Verheyen CC. Acceptance of angulation in the non-operative treatment of paediatric forearm fractures. J Pediatr Orthop B. 2006;15(6):428–32. https://doi.org/10.1097/01.bpb.0000210594.81393.fe.
57. Crawford SN, Lee LS, Izuka BH. Closed treatment of overriding distal radial fractures without reduction in children. J Bone Joint Surg Am. 2012;94(3):246–52. https://doi.org/10.2106/JBJS.K.00163.
58. Digby KH. The measurement of diaphysial growth in proximal and distal directions. J Anat Physiol. 1916;50:187–8.
59. Bae DS. Pediatric distal radius and forearm fractures. J Hand Surg. 2008;33A:1911–23.

60. Greig D, Silva M. Management of distal radius fractures in adolescent patients. J Pediatr Orthop. 2021;41:S1–5. https://doi.org/10.1097/BPO.0000000000001778.
61. van Egmond JC, Selles CA, Cleffken BI, et al. Plate fixation for unstable displaced distal radius fractures in children. J Wrist Surg. 2019;8:384–7. https://doi.org/10.1055/s-0039-1688701.
62. Seefried S, Chin-Goh K, Sahakian V, Lightfoot N, Boyle M. Paediatric forearm fractures manipulated in the emergency department: incidence and risk factors for re-manipulation under general anaesthesia. N Z Med J. 2022;135:60–6. https://doi.org/10.26635/6965.5665.
63. Constantino DMC, Machado L, Carvalho M, et al. Redisplacement of paediatric distal radius fractures: what is the problem? J Child Orthop. 2021;15:532–9. https://doi.org/10.1302/1863-2548.15.210111.
64. Sengab A, Krijnen P, Schipper IB. Displaced distal radius fractures in children, cast alone vs additional K-wire fixation: a meta-analysis. Eur J Trauma Emerg Surg. 2019;45:1003–11.
65. Guichet J, Moller C, Dautel G, Lascombes P. A modified Kapandji procedure for Smith's fracture in children. J Bone Joint Surg Br. 1997;79:734–7. https://doi.org/10.1302/0301-620x.79b5.7620.
66. Parikh S, Jain V, Youngquist J. Intrafocal pinning for distal radius metaphyseal fractures in children. Orthopedics. 2013;36:783–8. https://doi.org/10.3928/01477447-20130523-25.
67. Rubin G, Orbach H, Chezar A, Rozen N. Treatment of physeal fractures of the distal radius by volar intrafocal Kapandji method: surgical technique. Arch Orthop Trauma Surg. 2017;137:49–54. https://doi.org/10.1007/s00402-016-2592-8.
68. Satish B, Vinodkumar M, Suresh M, et al. Closed reduction and *K*-wiring with the Kapandji technique for completely displaced pediatric distal radial fractures. Orthopedics. 2014;37:e810–6. https://doi.org/10.3928/01477447-20140825-58.
69. Terrence Jose Jerome J. Salter-Harris II distal radial fractures treated with the intrafocal *K*-wire technique: a retrospective study of 20 cases. J Hand Surg Eur. 2021;46:471–5. https://doi.org/10.1177/1753193420953078.
70. Valisena S, Gonzalez J, Voumard N, et al. Treatment of paediatric unstable displaced distal radius fractures using Kapandji technique: a case series. Eur J Orthop Surg Traumatol. 2019;29:413–20. https://doi.org/10.1007/s00590-018-2297-5.
71. Bassi C, Heimann AF, Schwab JM, Tannast M, Raabe I. Modified Kapandji technique in pediatric displaced distal radius fractures: results in 195 patients. Eur J Orthop Surg Traumatol. 2023; https://doi.org/10.1007/s00590-023-03686-9. Epub ahead of print. PMID: 37632546
72. Barnes J, Webb MV, Fearon P. Salter-Harris II forearm fracture reduction and fixation using a buttress plate. BMJ Case Rep. 2014;2014:bcr2013202868. https://doi.org/10.1136/bcr-2013-202868. PMID: 24488665; PMCID: PMC3912392
73. Cheng JC, Shen WY. Limb fracture pattern in different pediatric age groups: a study of 3,350 children. J Orthop Trauma. 1993;7(1):15–22.
74. Worlock P, Stower M. Fracture patterns in Nottingham children. J Pediatr Orthop. 1986;6(6):656–60.
75. Rennie L, et al. The epidemiology of fractures in children. Injury. 2007;38(8):913–22.
76. Landin LA. Epidemiology of children's fractures. J Pediatr Orthop B. 1997;6(2):79–83.
77. McQuinn AG, Jaarsma RL. Risk factors for redisplacement of pediatric distal forearm and distal radius fractures. J Pediatr Orthop. 2012;32(7):687–92.
78. Asadollahi S, Ooi KS, Hau RC. Distal radial fractures in children: risk factors for redisplacement following closed reduction. J Pediatr Orthop. 2015;35(3):224–8.
79. McLauchlan GJ, et al. Management of completely displaced metaphyseal fractures of the distal radius in children. A prospective, randomised controlled trial. J Bone Joint Surg Br. 2002;84(3):413–7.
80. Gibbons C, Woods D, Pailthorpe C, et al. The management of isolated distal radius fractures in children. J Pediatr Orthop. 1994;14:207–10. https://doi.org/10.1097/01241398-199403000-00014.
81. Ozcan M, et al. Percutaneous Kirschner Wire fixation in distal radius metaphyseal fractures in children: does it change the overall outcome? Hippokratia. 2010;14(4):265–70.

82. van Egmond PW, Schipper IB, van Luijt PA. Displaced distal forearm fractures in children with an indication for reduction under general anesthesia should be percutaneously fixated. Eur J Orthop Surg Traumatol Orthopedie Traumatologie. 2012;22(3):201–7. https://doi.org/10.1007/s00590-011-0826-6.
83. Proctor MT, Moore DJ, Paterson JM. Redisplacement after manipulation of distal radial fractures in children. J Bone Joint Surg Br. 1993;75(3):453–4.
84. Zamzam MM, Khoshhal KI. Displaced fracture of the distal radius in children: factors responsible for redisplacement after closed reduction. J Bone Joint Surg Br. 2005;87(6):841–3.
85. Jordan RW, Westacott DJ. Displaced paediatric distal radius fractures–when should we use percutaneous wires? Injury. 2012;43(6):908–11.
86. Luscombe KL, et al. Selective Kirschner wiring for displaced distal radial fractures in children. Acta Orthop Traumatol Turc. 2010;44(2):117–23.
87. Arora R, et al. Factors responsible for redisplacement of pediatric forearm fractures treated by closed reduction and cast: role of casting indices and three point index. Indian J Orthop. 2018;52(5):536–47.
88. Ghimire N, Uprety S, Lamichhane A. Risk factors for redisplacement in pediatric distal radius fractures after closed reduction and cast immobilisation. J Inst Med. 2016;38(1):81–4.
89. Haddad FS, Williams RL. Forearm fractures in children: avoiding redisplacement. Injury. 1995;26(10):691–2.
90. Chess DG, et al. Short arm plaster cast for distal pediatric forearm fractures. J Pediatr Orthop. 1994;14(2):211–3.
91. Papiez K, Tutton E, Phelps EE, Baird J, Costa ML, Achten J, et al. A qualitative study of parents' and their child's experience of a medial epicondyle fracture. Bone Joint Open. 2021;2(6):359–64.
92. Feudtner C, Schall T, Hill D. Parental personal sense of duty as a Foundation of Pediatric Medical Decision-making. Pediatrics. 2018;142(Suppl 3):S133–S41.
93. Hedelin H, Goksor LA, Karlsson J, Stjernstrom S. Ultrasound-assisted triage of ankle trauma can decrease the need for radiographic imaging. Am J Emerg Med. 2013;31(12):1686–9. https://doi.org/10.1016/j.ajem.2013.09.005.
94. Douma-den Hamer D, Blanker MH, Edens MA, Buijteweg LN, Boomsma MF, van Helden SH, Mauritz G-J. Ultrasound for distal forearm fracture: a systematic review and diagnostic meta-analysis. PLoS One. 2016;11(5):e0155659. https://doi.org/10.1371/journal.pone.0155659.
95. Joshi N, Lira A, Mehta N, Paladino L, Sinert R. Diagnostic accuracy of history, physical examination, and bedside ultrasound for diagnosis of extremity fractures in the emergency department: a systematic review. Acad Emerg Med. 2013;20(1):1–15.
96. Weinberg ER, Tunik MG, Tsung JW. Accuracy of clinician-performed point-of-care ultrasound for the diagnosis of fractures in children and young adults. Injury. 2010;41(8):862–8.
97. Chen L, Kim Y, Moore CL. Diagnosis and guided reduction of forearm fractures in children using bedside ultrasound. Pediatr Emerg Care. 2007;23(8):528–31. https://doi.org/10.1097/PEC.0b013e318128f85d.
98. Patel DD, Blumberg SM, Crain EF. The utility of bedside ultrasonography in identifying fractures and guiding fracture reduction in children. Pediatr Emerg Care. 2009;25(4):221–5.
99. Chaar-Alvarez FM, Warkentine F, Cross K, et al. Bedside ultrasound diagnosis of nonangulated distal forearm fractures in the pediatric emergency department. Pediatr Emerg Care. 2011;27:1027–32.
100. Eckert K, Ackermann O, Schweiger B, et al. Sonographic diagnosis of metaphyseal forearm fractures in children: a safe and applicable alternative to standard X-rays. Pediatr Emerg Care. 2012;28(9):851–4.
101. Rowlands R, Rippey J, Tie S, Flynn J. Bedside ultrasound vs X-ray for the diagnosis of forearm fractures in children. J Emerg Med. 2017;52:208–15.
102. Südow H, Navarro CM. The incidence of distal radius fractures in a Swedish pediatric population - an observational cohort study of 90 970 individual fractures. BMC Musculoskelet Disord. 2021; https://doi.org/10.1186/s12891-021-04410-6.

103. Bergkvist A, Lundqvist E, Pantzar-Castilla. Evelina Distal radius fractures in children aged 5–12 years: a Swedish nationwide register-based study of 25 777 patients. BMC Musculoskelet Disord. 2023; https://doi.org/10.1186/s12891-023-06680-8.
104. Olech J, Ciszewski M, Morasiewicz P. Epidemiology of distal radius fractures in children and adults during the COVID-19 pandemic—a two-center study. BMC Musculoskelet Disord. 2021; https://doi.org/10.1186/s12891-021-04128-5.
105. Iles BW, Samora JB, Singh S, Lynne R. Differentiating stable buckle fractures from other distal radius fractures: the 1-cm rule. Pediatr Radiol. 2018; https://doi.org/10.1007/s00247-018-4316-4.
106. Randsborg P-H, Sivertsen E. A classification of distal radius fractures in children: good inter- and intraobserver reliability, which improves with clinical experience. BMC Musculoskelet Disord. 2012; https://doi.org/10.1186/1471-2474-13-6.
107. Knight J, Zhou Y, Keen C, Hareendranathan AR, Alves-Pereira F, Ghasseminia S, Wichuk S, Brilz A, Kirschner D, Jaremko J. 2D/3D ultrasound diagnosis of pediatric distal radius fractures by human readers vs artificial intelligence. Sci Rep. 2023; https://doi.org/10.1038/s41598-023-41807-w.
108. Renz DM, Malich A, Ulrich A, Pfeil A, Mentzel H-J, Streitparth F, Maurer MH, Teichgräber UK, Joachim B. Reference values for digital X-ray radiogrammetry parameters in children and adolescents in comparison to estimates in patients with distal radius fractures. J Bone Miner Metab. 2015; https://doi.org/10.1007/s00774-014-0641-3.
109. Galán-Olleros M, Mayans-Sanesteban J, Martínez-Álvarez S, Miranda-Gorozarri C, Ramírez-Barragán A, Egea-Gámez RM, Alonso-Hernández J, Martínez-Caballero I. Is reduction necessary in overriding metaphyseal distal radius fractures in children under 11 years: a systematic review and meta-analysis of comparative studies. Eur J Orthop Surg Traumatol. 2024; https://doi.org/10.1007/s00590-024-03936-4.
110. Hancock DW, Barrett-Lee JJT, Abdellatif AMA, White S, Liu P, Roberts D. Metaphyseal distal radius fractures in adolescents: is closed reduction and casting sufficient for most? Eur J Orthop Surg Traumatol. 2025; https://doi.org/10.1007/s00590-025-04182-y.
111. Jerome JTJ, Matsui C. Antegrade intrafocal Kapandji pinning technique for volar displaced distal radius fractures in older children. Eur J Plast Surg. 2024; https://doi.org/10.1007/s00238-024-02205-1.
112. Sengab A, Krijnen P, Birgitta SI. Displaced distal radius fractures in children, cast alone vs additional K-wire fixation: a meta-analysis. Eur J Trauma Emerg Surg. 2018; https://doi.org/10.1007/s00068-018-1011-y.
113. Sengab A, Krijnen P, Schipper IB. Risk factors for fracture redisplacement after reduction and cast immobilization of displaced distal radius fractures in children: a meta-analysis. Eur J Trauma Emerg Surg. 2019; https://doi.org/10.1007/s00068-019-01227-w.
114. Phelps EE, Tutton E, Costa ML, Achten J, Moscrop A, Perry DC. Protecting my injured child: a qualitative study of parents' experience of caring for a child with a displaced distal radius fracture. BMC Pediatr. 2022; https://doi.org/10.1186/s12887-022-03340-z.
115. Hedelin H, Tingström C, Hebelka H, Karlsson J. Minimal training sufficient to diagnose pediatric wrist fractures with ultrasound. Ultrasound J. 2017; https://doi.org/10.1186/s13089-017-0066-z.

Distal Forearm Fracture 10

Introduction by the Author

A distal forearm fracture is a common type of fracture in children. It is a fracture of the distal third of the forearm or of the distal metaphyseal-diaphyseal junction. In fact, forearm fractures account for 45% of all fractures in children and 62% of all pediatric upper limb fractures. The distal third of the forearm is the location most susceptible to injury. These fractures often occur during puberty when bone fragility and physical activity increase.

Standard radiography is the gold standard for imaging and can easily and consistently diagnose these fractures. It can determine the type of fracture, the degree of angulation, and the degree of displacement. However, ultrasound is a promising alternative for diagnosing pediatric distal forearm fractures. It offers benefits such as reduced radiation exposure and shorter emergency department visits.

Currently, there is no consensus on the best treatment method for these fractures.

Non-displaced fractures are treated non-operatively with cast immobilization due to their rapid healing and remodeling potential. Although long arm casts are traditionally used for better stability, short arm casts have been proposed as a valid alternative. The remodeling potential varies with age: up to 30° of angulation can be accepted in children under 9 years old, up to 25° in children aged 9–12 years, and up to 20° in children 12 years and older.

Displaced fractures are often treated with closed reduction and cast immobilization. However, redisplacement frequently occurs, affecting a significant percentage of cases. Factors associated with loss of reduction include poor casting technique, initial complete displacement, and failure to achieve perfect anatomical reduction after closed reduction. Primary percutaneous fixation significantly reduces the rate of secondary interventions compared to closed reduction alone.

© The Author(s), under exclusive license to Springer Nature Switzerland AG 2026
F. Canavese, *Advances in Pediatric Extremity Fracture Management*,
https://doi.org/10.1007/978-3-032-33306-3_10

Both Kirschner wire and elastic stable intramedullary nailing are effective for treating distal forearm fractures in children; however, elastic stable intramedullary nailing has advantages in terms of reduced operative time and blood loss.

There is some debate about whether to fix both bones when the radius and ulna are fractured. Recent studies have shown no significant differences in perioperative complications, loss of reduction rates, or functional outcomes between patients treated with ulna fixation versus those without. However, radius fixation alone yielded satisfactory clinical outcomes with fewer complications. Meanwhile, operation duration and the number of intraoperative fluoroscopies were significantly higher in patients where both the radius and ulna were stabilized.

10.1 Machine Generated Summaries

Disclaimer: The summaries in this chapter were generated from Springer Nature publications using abstractive AI auto-summarization: An abstraction-based summarizer creates new text based on deep learning. New phrases are created to summarize the content. As the constituted sentences are machine selected, they may not fully reflect the body of the work, so we strongly advise that the original content is read and cited. The auto-generated summaries were curated by the author(s) to meet Springer Nature publication standards.

Diagnostic Accuracy of Ultrasound Versus X-Ray for Distal Forearm Fractures in Children and Adolescents: A Systematic Review and Meta-Analysis [130]

This is a machine-generated summary of:

Delniotis, Ioannis; Bontinis, Vangelis; Ktenidis, Kiriakos; Drakonaki, Elena E.; Galanis, Nikiforos Diagnostic accuracy of ultrasound versus X-ray for distal forearm fractures in children and adolescents: a systematic review and meta-analysis [130]

Published in: European Journal of Trauma and Emergency Surgery (2024)
Link to original: https://doi.org/10.1007/s00068-024-02451-9

Copyright of the summarized publication:
The Author(s), under exclusive licence to Springer-Verlag GmbH Germany 2024
Copyright comment: Springer Nature or its licensor (e.g. a society or other partner) holds exclusive rights to this article under a publishing agreement with the author(s) or other rightsholder(s); author self-archiving of the accepted manuscript version of this article is solely governed by the terms of such publishing agreement and applicable law.
All rights reserved.**If you want to cite the papers, please refer to the original.**

For technical reasons we could not place the page where the original quote is coming from.

Research Highlights

Distal forearm fractures are the most common type of fracture in children, with their incidence rising due to increased sports participation, higher rates of overweight children, and decreased bone mineral density. Traditionally, X-rays have been the gold standard for diagnosing these fractures, but concerns about radiation exposure in children have prompted interest in alternative diagnostic methods. Now, a new study by Ioannis Delniotis and colleagues systematically reviews the diagnostic accuracy of ultrasound for detecting distal forearm fractures in children, comparing it to conventional X-ray imaging.

The study conducted a systematic literature review using databases such as PubMed and Cochrane CENTRAL, following PRISMA guidelines. The authors focused on studies published between January and August that compared ultrasound with X-ray for diagnosing distal forearm fractures in children. They included studies that met specific criteria, such as those published in English or German and those with a sample size greater than 20 patients. Data extraction and quality assessment were performed using the QUADAS-2 tool to evaluate the risk of bias. The analysis involved calculating sensitivity and specificity using a logistic-normal bivariate random-effects meta-analysis model. The results showed that ultrasound has high sensitivity and specificity for detecting distal forearm fractures in children, suggesting it could be a viable alternative to X-rays.

The study highlights several advantages of using ultrasound, including its real-time assessment capability, lack of radiation exposure, and cost-effectiveness compared to X-rays. However, the authors note that variations in sonographer training and scanning methods could affect diagnostic accuracy. Future studies should aim to establish standardized protocols for ultrasound scanning and training to ensure consistent results across different settings. Additionally, further research is needed to evaluate long-term outcomes for children diagnosed with fractures using ultrasound alone. This study suggests that while ultrasound may not entirely replace X-rays, it can significantly reduce unnecessary radiation exposure for many children presenting with potential distal forearm fractures.

Point-of-Care Ultrasound for the Diagnosis of Distal Forearm Fractures in Children and Adolescents: A Scoping Review [131]

This is a machine-generated summary of:

Morello, Rosa; Mariani, Francesco; Snelling, Peter J.; Buonsenso, Danilo Point-of-care ultrasound for the diagnosis of distal forearm fractures in children and adolescents: a scoping review [131]
Published in: European Journal of Pediatrics (2024)
Link to original: https://doi.org/10.1007/s00431-024-05877-w

Copyright of the summarized publication:
The Author(s), under exclusive licence to Springer-Verlag GmbH Germany, part of Springer Nature 2024
Copyright comment: corrected publication 2024
All rights reserved.

If you want to cite the papers, please refer to the original.

For technical reasons we could not place the page where the original quote is coming from.

Research Highlights

Distal forearm fractures are the most common type of pediatric fractures, typically resulting from falls on an outstretched hand. Traditionally, biplanar X-ray has been the standard diagnostic tool for these injuries. However, point-of-care ultrasound (POCUS) has emerged as a potential alternative due to its advantages of being rapid, non-invasive, and radiation-free. Despite its growing use, there has been a lack of randomized controlled trials and orthopedic surgeon involvement in studies assessing POCUS's diagnostic accuracy for pediatric distal forearm fractures. Now, a new study by Rosa Morello and colleagues provides a comprehensive scoping review of the literature on POCUS's diagnostic accuracy and its impact on patient-centered outcomes.

The study conducted a systematic scoping review following the PRISMA Extension for Scoping Reviews guidelines. The authors searched multiple databases, including MEDLINE, SCOPUS, and EMBASE, without date restrictions but limited to English-language publications. They included various study types such as randomized controlled trials and observational studies while excluding systematic reviews and editorials. The primary outcome was the diagnostic accuracy of POCUS compared to standard reference methods like X-ray. The review found that POCUS demonstrated high sensitivity and specificity in detecting distal forearm fractures in children. The studies reviewed varied in methodology but consistently showed that POCUS could be performed by different healthcare providers with good diagnostic accuracy. Additionally, POCUS was associated with reduced emergency department length of stay and was well-tolerated by patients.

The findings suggest that POCUS is a promising alternative for diagnosing pediatric distal forearm fractures, offering benefits such as reduced radiation exposure and shorter emergency department visits. Future study could focus on standardizing scanning protocols and exploring implementation in diverse healthcare settings, including rural or low-resource environments where access to radiography is limited. Additionally, integrating POCUS into routine diagnostic pathways could reduce unnecessary X-rays and streamline patient management. Further research should also consider cost-benefit analyses to support broader adoption of this technology in clinical practice.

A Meta-Analysis on the Diagnostic Utility of Ultrasound in Pediatric Distal Forearm Fractures [132]

This is a machine-generated summary of:

Hassankhani, Amir; Amoukhteh, Melika; Jannatdoust, Payam; Valizadeh, Parya; Ghadimi, Delaram J.; Vasavada, Pauravi S.; Johnston, Jennifer H.; Gholamrezanezhad, Ali A meta-analysis on the diagnostic utility of ultrasound in pediatric distal forearm fractures [132]
Published in: Emergency Radiology (2024)
Link to original: https://doi.org/10.1007/s10140-024-02208-2
Copyright of the summarized publication:
The Author(s) 2024
License: OpenAccess CC BY 4.0

This article is licensed under a Creative Commons Attribution 4.0 International License, which permits use, sharing, adaptation, distribution and reproduction in any medium or format, as long as you give appropriate credit to the original author(s) and the source, provide a link to the Creative Commons licence, and indicate if changes were made. The images or other third party material in this article are included in the article's Creative Commons licence, unless indicated otherwise in a credit line to the material. If material is not included in the article's Creative Commons licence and your intended use is not permitted by statutory regulation or exceeds the permitted use, you will need to obtain permission directly from the copyright holder. To view a copy of this licence, visit http://creativecommons.org/licenses/by/4.0/.

If you want to cite the papers, please refer to the original.

For technical reasons we could not place the page where the original quote is coming from.

Research Highlights

Distal forearm fractures are a common type of musculoskeletal injury in children, traditionally diagnosed using radiography. However, radiography has limitations, such as exposure to ionizing radiation and difficulty in detecting subtle fractures in pediatric bones. Recently, ultrasound has emerged as a promising alternative, offering benefits like the absence of radiation, real-time imaging, and cost-effectiveness. Despite these advantages, the integration of ultrasound into clinical practice for diagnosing pediatric distal forearm fractures remains limited. Now, a new study by Amir Hassankhani and colleagues conducts a meta-analysis to evaluate the diagnostic effectiveness of ultrasound for these fractures in children.

The study employed a systematic review and meta-analysis approach, following PRISMA guidelines. A comprehensive literature search was conducted across four major databases to identify relevant studies. The inclusion criteria focused on studies reporting diagnostic accuracy measures such as sensitivity and specificity for ultrasound in pediatric distal forearm fractures. The quality of included studies was assessed using the QUADAS-2 tool. Statistical analyses involved a random effects diagnostic test accuracy model to generate summary receiver operating characteristic curves and assess heterogeneity. Subgroup analyses were performed based on factors like the training status of ultrasound performers and the specific bone examined (radius or ulna). The study found that ultrasound exhibits high sensitivity and specificity for detecting distal forearm fractures in children, with trained performers achieving notably higher diagnostic accuracy.

The findings highlight ultrasonography as a reliable tool for diagnosing pediatric distal forearm fractures, particularly when performed by trained individuals. The study underscores the importance of training in enhancing diagnostic accuracy, especially for confirming fractures. Future study could explore the role of ultrasound beyond diagnosis, such as its potential to inform surgical decisions and support follow-up assessments. Additionally, further investigation into factors affecting diagnostic accuracy between different forearm bones is warranted to optimize clinical application. While ultrasonography shows promise, clinical judgment remains essential in selecting appropriate imaging modalities based on individual patient characteristics.

Above- or Below-Elbow Casts for Distal Third Forearm Fractures in Children? A Meta-Analysis of the Literature [133]

This is a machine-generated summary of:

Hendrickx, Roel P. M.; Campo, Martin M.; van Lieshout, Arno P. W.; Struijs, Peter A. A.; van den Bekerom, Michel P. J. Above- or below-elbow casts for distal third forearm fractures in children? A meta-analysis of the literature [133]
Published in: Archives of Orthopaedic and Trauma Surgery (2011)
Link to original: https://doi.org/10.1007/s00402-011-1363-9
Copyright of the summarized publication:
Springer-Verlag 2011
All rights reserved.

If you want to cite the papers, please refer to the original.

For technical reasons we could not place the page where the original quote is coming from.

Research Highlights

Fractures of the distal third of the forearm are the most common fractures in childhood, typically treated non-operatively with cast immobilization due to their rapid healing and potential for remodeling. While long arm casts are traditionally used for better stability, short arm casts have been proposed as a valid alternative. Despite a low remanipulation rate reported with short arm casts, many clinicians still prefer long arm casts, believing they minimize forearm movement more effectively. Now, a new study by Roel P. M. Hendrickx and colleagues conducts a meta-analysis to determine the preferred method of immobilization for these fractures, testing the hypothesis that no difference exists in loss of reduction rates between above- and below-elbow casts in children.

The study involved a comprehensive search of Medline, Cochrane Database of Systematic Reviews, and Embase to identify randomized or quasi-randomized controlled trials comparing above- and below-elbow plaster immobilization for distal forearm fractures in children. Three trials with a total of 300 participants were included. Data on loss of reduction, remanipulation, missed school days, return to normal function, cast index, plaster-related complications, and mobility were extracted and analyzed. The meta-analysis revealed that below-elbow casts (BEC) are not inferior to above-elbow casts (AEC), with only 5% loss of reduction and 3% remanipulations necessary. Children treated with BEC missed fewer school days and returned to normal function sooner than those treated with AEC.

The study concludes that BEC is a valid treatment option for distal forearm fractures in children, showing decreased tendency for secondary displacement compared to AEC. Future studies should focus on high-quality randomized clinical trials with larger sample sizes to provide definitive recommendations for clinical practice. These trials should adhere to strict definitions of fracture type and outcome measures while incorporating patient-oriented outcomes like satisfaction and daily functioning limitations. Such research could further clarify the best treatment approach for these common pediatric injuries.

Short and Long-Arm Fiberglass Cast Immobilization for Displaced Distal Forearm Fractures in Children: A Randomized Controlled Trial [134]

This is a machine-generated summary of:

Seiler, Michelle; Heinz, Peter; Callegari, Alessia; Dreher, Thomas; Staubli, Georg; Aufdenblatten, Christoph Short and long-arm fiberglass cast immobilization for displaced distal forearm fractures in children: a randomized controlled trial [134]

Published in: International Orthopaedics (2020)
Link to original: https://doi.org/10.1007/s00264-020-04800-w

Copyright of the summarized publication:
The Author(s) 2020
License: OpenAccess CC BY 4.0

This article is licensed under a Creative Commons Attribution 4.0 International License, which permits use, sharing, adaptation, distribution and reproduction in any medium or format, as long as you give appropriate credit to the original author(s) and the source, provide a link to the Creative Commons licence, and indicate if changes were made. The images or other third party material in this article are included in the article's Creative Commons licence, unless indicated otherwise in a credit line to the material. If material is not included in the article's Creative Commons licence and your intended use is not permitted by statutory regulation or exceeds the permitted use, you will need to obtain permission directly from the copyright holder. To view a copy of this licence, visit http://creativecommons.org/licenses/by/4.0/.

If you want to cite the papers, please refer to the original.

For technical reasons we could not place the page where the original quote is coming from.

Research Highlights

Distal forearm fractures (DFFs) are the most common fractures in children, often managed with non-operative treatments such as closed reduction and splinting. The standard imaging technique for assessing these fractures is projectional radiography, while treatment typically involves casting to stabilize the fracture. However, there is a risk of loss of reduction (LOR) in non-operative treatments, which can occur at a rate of 7–39%. Now, a new study by Michelle Seiler and colleagues investigates whether short-arm fiberglass (FG) casts are as effective as long-arm FG casts in stabilizing displaced forearm fractures in children aged 4 years and older.

The study was a prospective, randomized trial conducted at the authors' institution. Eligible participants were children aged four to 12 years with displaced metaphyseal or epiphyseal DFFs requiring closed reduction. Completely displaced fractures were excluded to avoid variability in treatment opinions regarding osteosynthesis. Participants were randomly assigned to receive either a short-arm or long-arm FG cast after fracture reduction. The study monitored fracture healing through regular follow-up examinations and radiographic assessments at specified intervals. The primary outcome was the rate of LOR, defined by specific angular deviations on radiographs. Secondary outcomes included analgesic needs, restrictions in activities of daily living (ADL), and time to regain unrestricted elbow movement.

The study found that short-arm FG casting was as effective as long-arm casting for immobilizing reduced DFFs, with no significant differences in LOR rates between the two groups. Short-arm casts offered advantages such as less restriction in ADL and quicker recovery of elbow motion post-cast removal. Future studies could explore the generalizability of these findings to other types of forearm fractures and further investigate the impact of age on recovery post-cast removal. The results suggest that short-arm FG casts can be a viable alternative to long-arm casts for treating DFFs in children, providing similar stabilization with added benefits in terms of mobility and daily functioning.

Pediatric Distal Both-Bone Forearm Fractures Treated with Percutaneous Pinning With or Without Ulna Fixation: A Retrospective Cohort Study from Two Centres [135]

This is a machine-generated summary of:

Wang, Biao; Guo, Jiale; Li, Zhenwei; Ji, Zejuan; Liu, Fangna; Sun, Keming; Feng, Wei
Pediatric distal both-bone forearm fractures treated with percutaneous pinning with or without ulna fixation: a retrospective cohort study from two centres [135]

Published in: BMC Musculoskeletal Disorders (2024)
Link to original: https://doi.org/10.1186/s12891-024-07822-2
Copyright of the summarized publication:
The Author(s) 2024
License: OpenAccess CC BY-NC-ND 4.0

This article is licensed under a Creative Commons Attribution-NonCommercial-NoDerivatives 4.0 International License, which permits any non-commercial use, sharing, distribution and reproduction in any medium or format, as long as you give appropriate credit to the original author(s) and the source, provide a link to the Creative Commons licence, and indicate if you modified the licensed material. You do not have permission under this licence to share adapted material derived from this article or parts of it. The images or other third party material in this article are included in the article's Creative Commons licence, unless indicated otherwise in a credit line to the material. If material is not included in the article's Creative Commons licence and your intended use is not permitted by statutory regulation or exceeds the permitted use, you will need to obtain permission directly from the copyright holder. To view a copy of this licence, visit http://creativecommons.org/licenses/by-nc-nd/4.0/.

If you want to cite the papers, please refer to the original.

For technical reasons we could not place the page where the original quote is coming from.

Research Highlights

Distal forearm fractures are prevalent in pediatric populations, often involving both the ulna and radius. While most of these fractures can be managed conservatively due to the bones' remodeling potential, severely displaced fractures may require surgical intervention to restore alignment and optimize wrist function. Closed reduction and percutaneous pinning are common treatments, but fixing distal ulnar fractures is challenging due to their small size and shape. Now, a new study by Biao Wang and colleagues investigates whether surgical fixation of the ulna is necessary in children with distal both-bone forearm fractures by comparing outcomes between those who had only the radius fixed versus those who had both bones fixed.

The study was conducted retrospectively using data from pediatric patients with distal radius and ulnar fractures collected from two hospital databases. Participants were divided into two groups: one receiving fixation of both the radius and ulna (ulna-yes) and another receiving fixation of the radius only (ulna-no). The inclusion criteria included patients aged 5–15 years with unilateral closed displaced distal radius-ulnar fractures treated with closed reduction and percutaneous pinning, followed for at least 1 year. The surgical procedure involved manual fracture reduction under X-ray guidance, followed by K-wire fixation. Postoperative care included regular follow-ups for clinical and radiographic evaluations until bone union was confirmed. Functional outcomes were assessed using the Gartland-Werley score and Mayo Wrist Score, while statistical analyses compared perioperative parameters, complications, and functional results between groups.

The study found no significant differences in peri-operative complications, loss of reduction rates, or functional outcomes between patients treated with ulna fixation versus those without. Fixation of the radius alone yielded satisfactory clinical outcomes with fewer complications. The operation duration and number of intra-operative fluoroscopies were significantly higher in the ulna-yes group. Future studies could explore long-term effects on epiphyseal growth due to pinning techniques. This research suggests that radius-only fixation may be a viable alternative for treating distal both-bone forearm fractures in children, potentially reducing surgical complexity and radiation exposure without compromising outcomes.

Displaced Distal Forearm Fractures in Children with an Indication for Reduction Under General Anesthesia Should Be Percutaneously Fixated [136]

This is a machine-generated summary of:

van Egmond, Pim W.; Schipper, Inger B.; van Luijt, Peter A. Displaced distal forearm fractures in children with an indication for reduction under general anesthesia should be percutaneously fixated [136]
Published in: European Journal of Orthopaedic Surgery & Traumatology (2011)
Link to original: https://doi.org/10.1007/s00590-011-0826-6
Copyright of the summarized publication:
The Author(s) 2011
License: OpenAccess CC BY-NC 2.0

This is an open access article distributed under the terms of the Creative Commons Attribution Noncommercial License (https://creativecommons.org/licenses/by-nc/2.0), which permits any noncommercial use, distribution, and reproduction in any medium, provided the original author(s) and source are credited.

If you want to cite the papers, please refer to the original.

For technical reasons we could not place the page where the original quote is coming from.

Research Highlights

Forearm fractures are among the most common injuries in children, with the distal third of the forearm being particularly susceptible. These fractures are often treated with closed reduction and cast immobilization, but redisplacement is a frequent issue, occurring in a significant percentage of cases. Now, a new study by Pim W. Egmond and colleagues at Leiden University Medical Center investigates the effectiveness of minimally invasive fixation techniques, such as K-wire or Elastic Stable Intramedullary Nailing (ESIN), compared to traditional methods in preventing redisplacement and reducing secondary interventions.

The study was a retrospective cohort analysis involving skeletally immature children with displaced distal forearm fractures treated under general anesthesia.

Patients were categorized based on fracture type and treatment method: closed reduction alone, closed reduction with percutaneous fixation, or open reduction with internal fixation. The researchers analyzed medical records and radiographs to assess outcomes such as the need for secondary reduction and angulation deformity at union. Statistical analysis was conducted using SPSS software to determine the significance of differences between treatment groups.

The findings suggest that primary percutaneous fixation significantly reduces the rate of secondary interventions compared to closed reduction alone. None of the patients who received internal fixation required a second procedure, whereas a substantial proportion of those treated with closed reduction alone did. The study highlights that internal fixation provides better alignment at union without increasing complication rates. Future studies could focus on long-term functional outcomes and further refine treatment protocols to optimize care for pediatric patients with distal forearm fractures.

Think Twice Before Re-Manipulating Distal Metaphyseal Forearm Fractures in Children [137]

This is a machine-generated summary of:

Roth, Kasper C.; Denk, Katharina; Colaris, Joost W.; Jaarsma, Ruurd L. Think twice before re-manipulating distal metaphyseal forearm fractures in children [137]

Published in: Archives of Orthopaedic and Trauma Surgery (2014)

Link to original: https://doi.org/10.1007/s00402-014-2091-8

Copyright of the summarized publication:

Springer-Verlag Berlin Heidelberg 2014

All rights reserved.

If you want to cite the papers, please refer to the original.

For technical reasons we could not place the page where the original quote is coming from.

Research Highlights

Distal forearm fractures are the most common injuries in pediatric traumatology, often requiring reduction and stabilization in a cast. However, re-displacement is a frequent complication, leading to treatment dilemmas regarding re-manipulation versus allowing natural correction through growth. Previous studies have not clarified the long-term outcomes of re-displaced fractures or the necessity of re-manipulations. Now, a new study by Kasper C. Roth and colleagues investigates whether re-manipulation of re-angulated distal forearm fractures in children improves long-term outcomes.

The study was conducted as a retrospective cohort analysis at a trauma institute, including children aged 12 years or younger with distal radius fractures that required closed reduction and later presented with re-angulation. Participants were divided into two groups: those who underwent secondary closed reduction (re-manipulation group) and those managed conservatively with casting alone (conservative group). Radiographic assessments measured true angular deformity, while functional outcomes were evaluated using range of motion tests, grip strength measurements, and patient satisfaction surveys. Statistical analyses compared outcomes between the two groups across different age categories.

The study found no significant differences in long-term radiological or functional outcomes between the re-manipulation and conservative groups. Younger children (<10 years) demonstrated significant remodelling capacity, achieving satisfactory results even with greater residual angulation. In older children (≥10 years), severity of angulation influenced treatment decisions more heavily. The findings suggest that current guidelines for re-manipulating pediatric forearm fractures may be too strict, as satisfactory outcomes were achieved without intervention in many cases. Future studies could explore the potential benefits of below-elbow casting and further investigate the clinical applicability of true angulation measurements to refine treatment protocols for pediatric forearm fractures.

Elastic Stable Intramedullary Nailing Versus Kirschner Wire in the Treatment of Pediatric Metaphyseal–Diaphyseal Junction Fractures of the Distal Radius: A Case-Control Study [138]

This is a machine-generated summary of:

Wu, Rongchang; Wen, Yuwei; Wang, Chunhua; Liu, Tao; Yu, Jiazhi Elastic stable intramedullary nailing versus Kirschner wire in the treatment of pediatric metaphyseal–diaphyseal junction fractures of the distal radius: a case-control study [138]

Published in: BMC Musculoskeletal Disorders (2023)
Link to original: https://doi.org/10.1186/s12891-023-07055-9

Copyright of the summarized publication:
The Author(s) 2023
License: OpenAccess CC BY + CC0 4.0

This article is licensed under a Creative Commons Attribution 4.0 International License, which permits use, sharing, adaptation, distribution and reproduction in any medium or format, as long as you give appropriate credit to the original author(s) and the source, provide a link to the Creative Commons licence, and indicate if changes were made. The images or other third party material in this article are included in the article's Creative Commons licence, unless indicated otherwise in a credit line to the material. If material is not included in the article's Creative Commons licence and your intended use is not permitted by statutory regulation or exceeds the permitted use, you will need to obtain permission directly from the copyright holder. To view a copy of this licence, visit http://creativecommons.org/

licenses/by/4.0/. The Creative Commons Public Domain Dedication waiver (http://creativecommons.org/publicdomain/zero/1.0/) applies to the data made available in this article, unless otherwise stated in a credit line to the data.

If you want to cite the papers, please refer to the original.

For technical reasons we could not place the page where the original quote is coming from.

Research Highlights

Distal radius fractures are the most common type of fracture in children, often occurring during the ages of 10–14 due to increased bone fragility and physical activity during puberty. Treatment of these fractures remains challenging, with no consensus on the best method, particularly for fractures at the metaphyseal–diaphyseal junction (MDJ) of the distal radius. Now, a new study by Rongchang Wu and colleagues retrospectively compares the therapeutic effects of Kirschner wire (K-wire) fixation and elastic stable intramedullary nailing (ESIN) for MDJ fractures in children, hypothesizing that ESIN is the optimal treatment method.

The study analyzed data from children treated at the Children's Hospital Affiliate to Shandong University between August 2018 and January 2021. Inclusion criteria were MDJ fractures with open epiphyseal plates, failed conservative treatment, or unstable fractures. Patients were divided into two groups based on fracture location: those with fracture lines less than 2 cm from the physis underwent K-wire fixation, while those with lines more than 2 cm away were treated with either K-wire or ESIN. The study collected demographic data such as operation time, estimated blood loss (EBL), fluoroscopy time, length of hospital stay, and postoperative complications. At 6 months postoperatively, wrist function was evaluated using the Gartland and Werley scoring system. The results showed that both methods achieved similar wrist function scores; however, ESIN was associated with shorter operation and fluoroscopy times and lower EBL compared to K-wire fixation.

The study concludes that both K-wire and ESIN are effective for treating MDJ fractures in children but highlights ESIN's advantages in terms of reduced operative time and blood loss. Despite these findings, the authors acknowledge limitations such as the retrospective design and small sample size. They suggest that future studies should include larger sample sizes and longer follow-up periods to validate their findings further. Additionally, exploring other minimally invasive techniques could enhance treatment outcomes for pediatric distal radius fractures.

Intramedullary Kirschner Wire Fixation of Displaced Distal Forearm Fractures in Children [139]

This is a machine-generated summary of:

Abulsoud, Mohamed I.; Mohammed, Ahmed Saied; Elmarghany, Mohammed; Elgeushy, Ahmed; Elzahed, Ehab; Moawad, Mohamed; Elshal, Ehab A.; Elhalawany, Mohamed F.; Hassanein, Yahia A.; Fouad, Amr A.; Zakaria, Ahmed

R. Intramedullary Kirschner wire fixation of displaced distal forearm fractures in children [139]

Published in: BMC Musculoskeletal Disorders (2023)
Link to original: https://doi.org/10.1186/s12891-023-06875-z
Copyright of the summarized publication:
The Author(s) 2023
License: OpenAccess CC BY + CC0 4.0

This article is licensed under a Creative Commons Attribution 4.0 International License, which permits use, sharing, adaptation, distribution and reproduction in any medium or format, as long as you give appropriate credit to the original author(s) and the source, provide a link to the Creative Commons licence, and indicate if changes were made. The images or other third party material in this article are included in the article's Creative Commons licence, unless indicated otherwise in a credit line to the material. If material is not included in the article's Creative Commons licence and your intended use is not permitted by statutory regulation or exceeds the permitted use, you will need to obtain permission directly from the copyright holder. To view a copy of this licence, visit http://creativecommons.org/licenses/by/4.0/. The Creative Commons Public Domain Dedication waiver (http://creativecommons.org/publicdomain/zero/1.0/) applies to the data made available in this article, unless otherwise stated in a credit line to the data.

If you want to cite the papers, please refer to the original.

For technical reasons we could not place the page where the original quote is coming from.

Research Highlights

Fractures of the distal radius and forearm are among the most prevalent injuries in children, with boys, particularly in older age groups, being more frequently affected. These fractures account for a significant portion of childhood fractures, with radial metaphyseal fractures being notably common. Treatment approaches vary based on fracture type; while un-displaced fractures can be managed with a splint or cast, displaced fractures often require more invasive interventions such as manipulation and internal fixation. Despite the potential for these fractures to remodel with good functional outcomes, re-displacement remains a concern, often necessitating further corrective surgery. Now, a new study by Mohamed I. Abulsoud and colleagues evaluates the radiographic and functional outcomes of intramedullary K-wire fixation for distal forearm fractures in children, aiming to address complications associated with traditional treatment methods.

The study was conducted prospectively at Al-Azhar University Hospitals in Cairo, Egypt, involving skeletally immature patients with recent displaced distal forearm fractures. Ethical approval was obtained, and informed consent was secured from participants' guardians. The researchers employed intramedullary K-wire fixation under general anesthesia, using a meticulous surgical technique to ensure minimal complications. The procedure involved making a small incision at the distal radius and inserting pre-bent K-wires into both the radius and ulna under fluoroscopic guidance. Postoperative care included applying a sugar-tong splint for 4–6 weeks and regular follow-up visits to monitor healing through serial radiographs. Data analysis focused on preoperative and postoperative angulations, union rates, re-displacement occurrences, and any complications such as infections or nerve damage.

The study's findings suggest that intramedullary K-wire fixation is an effective treatment option for managing displaced distal forearm fractures in children. The technique demonstrated significant improvements in angulation postoperatively compared to preoperative measurements, attributed to the bone's remodeling capacity in patients with open physis. Functional outcomes were favorable, with most patients regaining full range of motion or experiencing only minimal restrictions that resolved spontaneously. Future studies could benefit from larger sample sizes and multi-center trials to further validate these findings and compare them against standard cross-pinning techniques. Additionally, refining outcome measures specific to pediatric wrist fractures could enhance the assessment of treatment efficacy in this population.

Long-Term Results Following Pediatric Distal Forearm Fractures [140]

This is a machine-generated summary of:

Zimmermann, Robert; Gschwentner, Martin; Kralinger, Franz; Arora, Rohit; Gabl, Markus; Pechlaner, Sigurd Long-term results following pediatric distal forearm fractures [140]
Published in: Archives of Orthopaedic and Trauma Surgery (2004)
Link to original: https://doi.org/10.1007/s00402-003-0619-4
Copyright of the summarized publication:
Springer-Verlag 2004
All rights reserved.

If you want to cite the papers, please refer to the original.

For technical reasons we could not place the page where the original quote is coming from.

Research Highlights

Fractures to the distal forearm are among the most common injuries in children, differing significantly from adult fractures due to the unique properties of a child's growing bones. These fractures often heal quickly and can tolerate some degree of displacement, with the expectation that natural bone remodeling will occur. However, despite the generally favorable prognosis, there is limited research on the long-term outcomes and potential complications associated with these injuries. Now, a new study by Robert Zimmermann and colleagues at the University of Innsbruck investigates the frequency and extent of clinical and radiological late sequelae in conservatively treated distal forearm fractures in children, aiming to identify factors that predict long-term outcomes.

The study retrospectively followed children treated for closed distal forearm fractures at the University of Innsbruck's Department of Trauma Surgery and Sports Medicine. Excluding those with other forearm injuries or open fractures, the researchers focused on patients who underwent conservative treatment methods such as cast immobilization or closed reduction under anesthesia. The follow-up examination occurred several years post-injury, assessing pain levels, range of motion, and radiographic findings. Statistical analyses were conducted to evaluate potential predictors of outcomes, including patient age at trauma, fracture type, and presence of concomitant injuries. The results indicated that younger children generally had better outcomes, while older children with significant angular deformities or dislocations experienced poorer long-term results.

Zimmermann and colleagues' study advances our understanding of distal forearm fractures in children by highlighting key factors influencing long-term outcomes. The findings suggest that while younger children can often tolerate some degree of fracture displacement without adverse effects, older children may require more precise anatomical reduction to prevent complications such as ulnocarpal impaction syndrome. Future studies could further explore the impact of specific fracture types on growth disturbances and rotational limitations, as well as refine treatment protocols to optimize recovery across different age groups.

Early Complications of Percutaneous K-Wire Fixation in Pediatric Distal Radius Fractures—A Prospective Cohort Study [92]

This is a machine-generated summary of:

Wasiak, Michał; Piekut, Maciej; Ratajczak, Karol; Waśko, Marcin Early complications of percutaneous K-wire fixation in pediatric distal radius fractures—a prospective cohort study [92]

Published in: Archives of Orthopaedic and Trauma Surgery (2023)
Link to original: https://doi.org/10.1007/s00402-023-04996-7

Copyright of the summarized publication:
The Author(s) 2023
License: OpenAccess CC BY 4.0

This article is licensed under a Creative Commons Attribution 4.0 International License, which permits use, sharing, adaptation, distribution and reproduction in any medium or format, as long as you give appropriate credit to the original author(s) and the source, provide a link to the Creative Commons licence, and indicate if changes were made. The images or other third party material in this article are included in the article's Creative Commons licence, unless indicated otherwise in a credit line to the material. If material is not included in the article's Creative

Commons licence and your intended use is not permitted by statutory regulation or exceeds the permitted use, you will need to obtain permission directly from the copyright holder. To view a copy of this licence, visit http://creativecommons.org/licenses/by/4.0/.

If you want to cite the papers, please refer to the original.

For technical reasons we could not place the page where the original quote is coming from.

Research Highlights

Distal radius fractures are the most common type of fracture in children, often treated with cast immobilization or manipulation under anesthesia. For severely displaced fractures, closed reduction followed by percutaneous pinning (CRPP) is a common approach, though the evidence supporting this method is inconclusive, making treatment decisions challenging for physicians. Now, a new study by Michał Wasiak and colleagues investigates the complications associated with CRPP in pediatric patients with displaced, unstable distal radius fractures, aiming to provide clearer insights into the risks involved.

The study was conducted at a tertiary healthcare center and included 116 pediatric patients who underwent CRPP for distal radius fractures. The researchers used a validated grading scheme to systematically analyze complications over a follow-up period of several months. Patients received antibiotic prophylaxis and were operated on within 24 hours of fracture occurrence. The procedure involved inserting K-wires under fluoroscopic guidance, followed by cast application. Follow-up visits were scheduled at regular intervals to monitor for complications such as pin-site infections and other postoperative issues. Data were collected prospectively and analyzed using statistical methods to assess complication rates and their correlation with various factors.

The study found that while major complications were rare, occurring in less than 2% of cases, minor complications were relatively common, affecting approximately 30% of patients. Most minor issues were related to pin-site inflammation and resolved without additional surgical intervention. The findings suggest that while CRPP is generally safe, there is room for improvement in managing minor complications to reduce patient discomfort. Future studies could focus on developing better wound care protocols and refining criteria for surgical intervention to optimize treatment outcomes for pediatric distal radius fractures.

Treatment of Unstable Forearm Fractures at the Metaphyseal-Diaphyseal Junction in Children: Antegrade ESIN vs. Transepiphyseal Intramedullary K-Wire Fixation [141]

This is a machine-generated summary of:

Dietzel, Markus; Scherer, Simon; Spogis, Jakob; Kirschner, Hans Joachim; Fuchs, Jörg; Lieber, Justus Treatment of unstable forearm fractures at the metaphyseal-diaphyseal junction in children: antegrade ESIN vs. transepiphyseal intramedullary K-wire fixation [141]

Published in: European Journal of Trauma and Emergency Surgery (2024)
Link to original: https://doi.org/10.1007/s00068-024-02562-3
Copyright of the summarized publication:
The Author(s) 2024
License: OpenAccess CC BY 4.0

This article is licensed under a Creative Commons Attribution 4.0 International License, which permits use, sharing, adaptation, distribution and reproduction in any medium or format, as long as you give appropriate credit to the original author(s) and the source, provide a link to the Creative Commons licence, and indicate if changes were made. The images or other third party material in this article are included in the article's Creative Commons licence, unless indicated otherwise in a credit line to the material. If material is not included in the article's Creative Commons licence and your intended use is not permitted by statutory regulation or exceeds the permitted use, you will need to obtain permission directly from the copyright holder. To view a copy of this licence, visit http://creativecommons.org/licenses/by/4.0/.

If you want to cite the papers, please refer to the original.

For technical reasons we could not place the page where the original quote is coming from.

Research Highlights

Fractures in childhood often affect the forearm, with unstable metaphyseal and diaphyseal fractures typically treated using percutaneous bi-cortical Kirschner wire fixation and elastic stable intramedullary nailing (ESIN), respectively. However, the optimal treatment for unstable fractures at the metaphyseal-diaphyseal junction (MDJ) remains debated due to the challenges of balancing invasiveness, technical feasibility, and patient acceptance. Now, a new study by Markus Dietzel and colleagues explores the use of antegrade ESIN (a-ESIN) for treating unstable MDJ forearm fractures in children, comparing it to transepiphyseal intramedullary K-wire (TIK) fixation.

The study retrospectively analyzed children and adolescents with MDJ forearm fractures treated with a-ESIN at the authors' institution. These cases were compared to a cohort treated with TIK prior to the implementation of a-ESIN. Data on demographic characteristics, clinical background, surgical indications, intraoperative findings, and postoperative outcomes were collected from hospital records. The primary endpoints included technical feasibility, fracture stability, and outcomes of fracture reduction and osteosynthesis. The surgical procedure involved using a modified Thompson's approach for nail implantation under general anesthesia. Postoperative care included spontaneous mobilization without plaster cast immobilization for most patients, with follow-up visits scheduled 1 month after surgery.

The study found that a-ESIN is a safe and effective treatment option for unstable MDJ forearm fractures in children, offering advantages such as minimally invasive procedures and early mobilization without additional immobilization. Despite some limitations like a small patient cohort and retrospective design, the results suggest that a-ESIN could replace TIK as the standard care for these fractures. Future studies should focus on including MDJ fractures in pediatric fracture classifications and evaluating biodegradable implants' applicability in these cases. Additionally, further research is needed to define the target population for a-ESIN regarding age limits and fracture types.

Conclusion
Younger children (under 10 years old) can undergo conservative treatment because they have significant remodeling capacity and can achieve satisfactory results, even with greater residual angulation. For older children, reduction under general anesthesia and cast immobilization is the preferred treatment. Using either elastic stable intramedullary nailing or Kirschner wires for fixation avoids secondary displacement, provides a good outcome, and has a low complication rate.

Bibliography

1. Dua K, Abzug JM, Sesko Bauer A, Cornwall R, Wyrick TO. Pediatric distal radius fractures. Instr Course Lect. 2017;66:447–60.
2. Hedström EM, Svensson O, Bergström U, Michno P. Epidemiology of fractures in children and adolescents. Acta Orthop. 2010;81(1):148–53. https://doi.org/10.3109/17453671003628780.
3. Schulte-Uentrop L, Goepfert MS. Anaesthesia or sedation for MRI in children. Curr Opin Anaesthesiol. 2010;23(4):513–7. https://doi.org/10.1097/ACO.0b013e32833bb524.
4. Avci M, Kozaci N, Tulubas G, Caliskan G, Yuksel A, Karaca A, et al. Comparison of Point-of-Care Ultrasonography and radiography in the diagnosis of long bone fractures. Medicina (Kaunas). 2019;55(7):355. https://doi.org/10.3390/medicina55070355.
5. Cross KP, Warkentine FH, Kim IK, Gracely E, Paul RI. Bedside ultrasound diagnosis of clavicle fractures in the pediatric emergency department. Acad Emerg Med. 2010;17(7):687–93.
6. Tsou PY, Ma YK, Wang YH, Gillon JT, Rafael J, Deanehan JK. Diagnostic accuracy of ultrasound for upper extremity fractures in children: a systematic review and meta-analysis. Am J Emerg Med. 2021;44:383–94. https://doi.org/10.1016/j.ajem.2020.04.071.
7. Schmid GL, Lippmann S, Unverzagt S, Hofmann C, Deutsch T, Frese T. The investigation of suspected fracture—a comparison of ultrasound with conventional imaging. Dtsch Arztebl Int. 2017;114(45):757–64. https://doi.org/10.3238/arztebl.2017.0757.
8. Iacob R, Stoicescu ER, Cerbu S, Iacob D, Amaricai E, Catan L, et al. Could ultrasound be used as a triage tool in diagnosing fractures in children? A literature review. Healthcare. 2022;10(5):823. https://doi.org/10.3390/healthcare10050823.
9. Caroselli C, Raffaldi I, Norbedo S, Parri N, Poma F, Blaivas M, et al. Accuracy of point-of-care ultrasound in detecting fractures in children: a validation study. Ultrasound Med Biol. 2021;47(1):68–75. https://doi.org/10.1016/j.ultrasmedbio.2020.09.012.
10. Ackermann O, Liedgens P, Eckert K, Chelangattucheryy E, Ruelander C, Emmanouilidis I, et al. Ultrasound diagnosis of juvenile fractures. J Med Ultrason. 2010;37(3):123–7. https://doi.org/10.1007/s10396-010-0263-x.
11. Eckert K, Ackermann O, Schweiger B, Radeloff E, Liedgens P. Ultrasound as a viable alternative to standard X-rays for the diagnosis of distal forearm fractures in children. Z Orthop Unfall. 2012;150(4):409–14. https://doi.org/10.1055/s-0032-1314974.

12. Herren C, Sobottke R, Ringe MJ, Visel D, Graf M, Müller D, et al. Ultrasound guided diagnosis of fractures of the distal forearm in children. Orthop Traumatol Surg Res. 2015;101(4):501–5. https://doi.org/10.1016/j.otsr.2015.02.010.
13. Galletebeitia Laka I, Samson F, Gorostiza I, Gonzalez A, Gonzalez C. The utility of clinical ultrasonography in identifying distal forearm fractures in the pediatric emergency department. Eur J Emerg Med. 2019;26(2):118–22. https://doi.org/10.1097/MEJ.0000000000000509.
14. Ko C, Baird M, Close M, Cassas KJ. The diagnostic accuracy of ultrasound in detecting distal radius fractures in a pediatric population. Clin J Sport Med. 2019;29(5):426–9. https://doi.org/10.1097/JSM.0000000000000547.
15. Zhang J, Boora N, Melendez S, Rakkunedeth Hareendranathan A, Jaremko J. Diagnostic accuracy of 3D ultrasound and artificial intelligence for detection of pediatric wrist injuries. Children. 2021;8:431.
16. Pountos I, Clegg J, Siddiqui A. Diagnosis and treatment of greenstick and torus fractures of the distal radius in children: a prospective randomised single blind study. J Child Orthop. 2010;4:321–6.
17. Sinha TP, Bhoi S, Kumar S, Ramchandani R, Goswami A, Kurrey L, et al. Diagnostic accuracy of bedside emergency ultrasound screening for fractures in pediatric trauma patients. J Emerg Trauma Shock. 2011;4(4):443–5. https://doi.org/10.4103/0974-2700.86625.
18. Akinmade A, Ikem I, Ayoola O, Orimolade E. Adeyeye comparing ultrasonography with plain radiography in the diagnosis of paediatric long bone fractures. Int Orthop. 2019;43(5):1143–53. https://doi.org/10.1007/s00264-018-4133-2.
19. Snelling PJ, Jones P, Keijzers G, Bade D, Herd DW, Ware RS. Nurse practitioner administered point of care ultrasound compared with X-ray for children with clinically non-angulated distal forearm fractures in the ED: a diagnostic study. Emerg Med J. 2021;38(2):139–45. https://doi.org/10.1136/emermed-2020-209689.
20. Weinberg ER, Tunik MG, Tsung JW. Accuracy of clinician-performed point-of-care ultrasound for the diagnosis of fractures in children and young adults. Injury. 2010;41(8):862–8.
21. Kozaci N, Ay MO, Acimen M, Turhan G, Sasmaz I, Turhan S, et al. Evaluation of the effectiveness of bedside point of care ultrasound in the diagnosis and management of distal radius fractures. Am J Emerg Med. 2015;33(1):67–71. https://doi.org/10.1016/j.ajem.2014.10.022.
22. de Putter CE, van Beeck EF, Looman CW, Toet H, Hovius SE, Selles RW. Trends in wrist fractures in children and adolescents, 1997–2009. J Hand Surg Am. 2011;36(11):1810–5.e2.
23. Goulding A, Jones IE, Taylor RW, Williams SM, Manning PJ. Bone mineral density and body composition in boys with distal forearm fractures: a dual-energy X-ray absorptiometry study. J Pediatr. 2001;139:509–15.
24. Sinikumpu J-J, Nietosvaara Y. Treatment of distal forearm fractures in children. Scand J Surg. SAGE Publications Ltd. 2021;110:276–80.
25. Scheier E, Balla U. Ultrasound-guided distal forearm fracture reduction by pediatric emergency physicians: a single center retrospective study. Pediatr Emerg Care. 2022;38(2):e756–60. https://doi.org/10.1097/PEC.0000000000002464.
26. Katzer C, Wasem J, Eckert K, Ackermann O, Buchberger B. Ultrasound in the diagnostics of metaphyseal forearm fractures in children: a systematic review and cost calculation. Pediatr Emerg Care. 2016;32(6):401–7. https://doi.org/10.1097/PEC.0000000000000446.
27. Douma-den Hamer D, Blanker MH, Edens MA, Buijteweg LN, Boomsma MF, van Helden SH, Mauritz G-J. Ultrasound for distal forearm fracture: a systematic review and diagnostic meta-analysis. PLoS One. 2016;11(5):e0155659. https://doi.org/10.1371/journal.pone.0155659.
28. Ottenhoff J, Kongkatong M, Hewitt M, Phillips J, Thom C. A narrative review of the uses of ultrasound in the evaluation, analgesia, and treatment of distal forearm fractures. J Emerg Med. 2022;63(6):755–65. https://doi.org/10.1016/j.jemermed.2022.09.012.
29. Snelling PJ, Jones P, Bade D, Bindra R, Byrnes J, Davison M, George S, Moore M, Keijzers G, Ware RS, BUCKLED Trial Group. Ultrasonography or radiography for suspected pediatric distal forearm fractures. N Engl J Med. 2023;388(22):2049–57. https://doi.org/10.1056/NEJMoa2213883.

30. Snelling PJ, Jones P, Bade D, Bindra R, Davison M, Gillespie A, McEniery J, Moore M, Keijzers G, Ware RS. Diagnostic accuracy of point-of-care ultrasound versus radiographic imaging for pediatric distal forearm fractures: a randomized controlled trial. Ann Emerg Med. 2024;83(3):198–207. https://doi.org/10.1016/j.annemergmed.2023.10.008.
31. Clark JM, Sanders S, Carter M, et al. Improving the translation of search strategies using the polyglot search translator: a randomized controlled trial. J Med Libr Assoc. 2020;108(2):195–207.
32. Eslick IG, Reid K, Eslick GD, Reid C. Diagnosing a fracture using a smartphone during the COVID-19 pandemic. J Paediatr Child Health. 2022;58(7):1272–3. https://doi.org/10.1111/jpc.16036.
33. Mobasseri A, Noorifard P. Ultrasound in the diagnosis of pediatric distal radius fractures: does it really change the treatment policy? An orthopedic view. J Ultrason. 2022;22(90):e179–82. https://doi.org/10.15557/jou.2022.0029.
34. Eckert K, Ackermann O, Schweiger B, et al. Sonographic diagnosis of metaphyseal forearm fractures in children: a safe and applicable alternative to standard X-rays. Pediatr Emerg Care. 2012;28(9):851–4.
35. Hedelin H, Tingström C, Hebelka H, Karlsson J. Minimal training sufficient to diagnose pediatric wrist fractures with ultrasound. Crit Ultrasound J. 2017;9:11.
36. Reitsma JB, Glas AS, Rutjes AW, Scholten RJ, Bossuyt PM, Zwinderman AH. Bivariate analysis of sensitivity and specificity produces informative summary measures in diagnostic reviews. J Clin Epidemiol. 2005;58:982–90.
37. Haddad FS, Williams RL. Forearm fractures in children: avoiding redisplacement. Injury. 1995;26:691–2.
38. Wenger DR, Pring ME, Rang M. Rang's children's fractures. 3rd ed; 2005. p. 135–50.
39. Hughston JC. Fractures of the forearm in children. J Bone Joint Surg Am. 1962;44:1678–93.
40. Chess DG, Hyndman JC, Leahey JL, Brown DC, Sinclair AM. Short arm plaster cast for distal pediatric forearm fractures. J Pediatr Orthop. 1994;14:211–3.
41. Jadad AR, Moore RA, Carroll D, Jenkinson C, Reynolds DJ, Gavaghan DJ, McQuay HJ. Assessing the quality of reports of randomized clinical trials: is blinding necessary? Control Clin Trials. 1996;17:1–12.
42. Schulz KF, Chalmers I, Grimes DA, Altman DG. Assessing the quality of randomization from reports of controlled trials published in obstetrics and gynecology journals. JAMA. 1994;272:125–8.
43. Verhagen AP, de Vet HC, de Bie RA, Kessels AG, Boers M, Knipschild PG. Balneotherapy and quality assessment: interobserver reliability of the Maastricht criteria list and the need for blinded quality assessment. J Clin Epidemiol. 1998;51:335–41.
44. Bohm ER, Bubbar V, HingK Y, Dzus A. Above and below-the-elbow plaster casts for distal forearm fractures in children. A randomized controlled trial. J Bone Joint Surg Am. 2006;88:1–8.
45. Paneru SR, Raju R, Shrestha BP, Nepal P, Khanal GP, Karn NK, Singh MP, Rai P. Randomized controlled trial comparing above- and below-elbow plaster casts for distal forearm fractures in children. J Child Orthop. 2010;4:233–7.
46. Webb GR, Galpin RD, Armstrong DG. Comparison of short and long arm plaster casts for displaced fractures in the distal third of the forearm in children. J Bone Joint Surg Am. 2006;88:9–17.
47. Sankar WN, Beck NA, Brewer JM, Baldwin KD, Pretell JA. Isolated distal radial metaphyseal fractures with an intact ulna: risk factors for loss of reduction. J Child Orthop. 2011;5:459–64. https://doi.org/10.1007/s11832-011-0373-z.
48. Pretell Mazzini J, Beck N, Brewer J, Baldwin K, Sankar W, Flynn J. Distal metaphyseal radius fractures in children following closed reduction and casting: can loss of reduction be predicted? Int Orthop. 2012;36:1435–40. https://doi.org/10.1007/s00264-012-1493-x.
49. Alemdaroğlu KB, Iltar S, Cimen O, et al. Risk factors in redisplacement of distal radial fractures in children. J Bone Joint Surg Am. 2008;90:1224–30. https://doi.org/10.2106/JBJS.G.00624.

50. Arora R, Mishra P, Aggarwal AN, Anshuman R, Sreenivasan R. Factors responsible for redisplacement of pediatric forearm fractures treated by closed reduction and cast: role of casting indices and three point index. Indian J Orthop. 2018;52:536–47. https://doi.org/10.4103/ortho.IJOrtho_382_17.
51. Bohm ER, Bubbar V, Yong Hing K, Dzus A. Above and below-the-elbow plaster casts for DFF in children. A randomized controlled trial. J Bone Joint Surg Am. 2006;88:1–8. https://doi.org/10.2106/JBJS.E:00320.
52. Maluta T, Dib G, Cengarle M, Bernasconi A, Samaila E, Magnan B. Below- vs above-elbow cast for distal radius fractures: is elbow immobilization really effective for reduction maintenance? Int Orthop. 2019;43:2391–7. https://doi.org/10.1007/s00264-018-4197-z.
53. Kamiloski M, Todorovik L, Memeti S, Jovcevski L, Shuperliska S, Aleksovski Z. The Kapandji technique of closed reduction using Sommer - Pins in the treatment of completely dislocated fractures of the distal radius in children. Open Access Maced J Med Sci. 2018;6:330–5.
54. Caruso G, Caldari E, Sturla FD, Caldaria A, Re DL, Pagetti P, Palummieri F, Massari L. Management of pediatric forearm fractures: what is the best therapeutic choice? A narrative review of the literature. Musculoskelet Surg. 2021;105:225–34.
55. Huang Q, Su F, Wang ZM, Xue HZ, Sun L, Ma T, Wang Q, Lu Y, Li M, Ren C, Zhang CM, Zhang K, Li Z. Prying reduction with mosquito forceps versus limited open reduction for irreducible distal radius-ulna fractures in older children: a retrospective study. BMC Musculoskelet Disord. 2021;22:147.
56. Okoli M, Silverman M, Abboudi J, Jones C, Kirkpatrick W, Liss F, Takei TR, Wang M, Ilyas AM. Radiographic healing and functional outcomes of untreated ulnar styloid fractures following volar plate fixation of distal radius fractures: a prospective analysis. Hand (N Y). 2021;16:332–7.
57. Liebs TR, Lorance A, Berger SM, Kaiser N, Ziebarth K. Health-related quality of life after fractures of the distal forearm in children and adolescents-results from a Center in Switzerland in 432 patients. Children (Basel). 2022;9:1487.
58. Laaksonen T, Stenroos A, Puhakka J, Kosola J, Kautiainen H, Rämö L, Nietosvaara Y. Casting in finger trap traction without reduction versus closed reduction and percutaneous pin fixation of dorsally displaced, over-riding distal metaphyseal radius fractures in children under 11 years old: a study protocol of a randomised controlled trial. BMJ Open. 2021;11(5):e045689. https://doi.org/10.1136/bmjopen-2020-045689.
59. Yuan C, Zhang H, Liu H, Gu J. Does concomitant ulnar styloid fracture and distal radius fracture portend poorer outcomes? A meta-analysis of comparative studies. Injury. 2017;48:2575–81.
60. Sato K, Murakami K, Mimata Y, Numata N, Shiraishi H, Doita M. Conservative treatment of distal ulna metaphyseal fractures associated with distal radius fractures in elderly people. Orthop Traumatol Surg Res. 2018;104:1101–5.
61. Lutsky KF, Lucenti L, Beredjiklian PK. Outcomes of distal ulna fractures associated with operatively treated distal radius fractures. Hand (N Y). 2020;15:418–21.
62. Moloney M, Farnebo S, Adolfsson L. Incidence of distal ulna fractures in a Swedish county: 74/100,000 person-years, most of them treated non-operatively. Acta Orthop. 2020;91:104–8.
63. Nakamura T, Moy OJ, Peimer CA. Relationship between fracture of the Ulnar styloid process and DRUJ instability: a biomechanical study. J Wrist Surg. 2021;10:111–5.
64. Glogovac G, Perry AK, Wigton MD, Stern PJ. Treatment modality of distal ulnar head and neck fractures associated with operatively treated distal radius fractures does not affect outcomes. Hand (N Y). 2022;17:512–8.
65. Graves BR. Editorial commentary: in cases of concurrent triangular fibrocartilage complex tears and ulnar styloid process fracture nonunions, we may neither need to excise nor repair the ulnar styloid fracture nonunion fragment. Arthroscopy. 2023;39:39–40.
66. Moloney M, Farnebo S, Adolfsson L. Distal ulna fractures in adults-subcapitular, transverse fractures did not benefit from surgical treatment. Arch Orthop Trauma Surg. 2023;143:381–7.

67. Velmurugesan PS, Nagashree V, Devendra A, Dheenadhayalan J, Rajasekaran S. Should ulnar styloid be fixed following fixation of a distal radius fracture? Injury. 2023;54:110768.
68. Kocaoglu H, Kalem M, Kavak M, Sahin E, Basarir K, Kinik H. Comparison of operating time, fluoroscopy exposure time, and functional and radiological results of two surgical methods for distal forearm fractures of both-bones in pediatric patients: is it necessary to fix both bones? Acta Orthop Traumatol Turc. 2020;54:155–60.
69. Yung SH, Lam CY, Choi KY, Ng KW, Maffulli N, Cheng JC. Percutaneous intramedullary Kirschner wiring for displaced diaphyseal forearm fractures in children. J Bone Joint Surg Br. 1998;80:91–4.
70. Proctor MT, Moore DJ, Paterson JM. Redisplacement after manipulation of distal radial fractures in children. J Bone Joint Surg Br. 1993;75:453–4.
71. Schmittenbecher PP, Fitze G, Godeke J, Kraus R, Schneidmuller D. Delayed healing of forearm shaft fractures in children after intramedullary nailing. J Pediatr Orthop. 2008;28:303–6.
72. Slongo T, Audigé L, Schlickewei W, Clavert JM, Hunter J. Development and validation of the AO pediatric comprehensive classification of long bone fractures by the pediatric expert group of the AO foundation in collaboration with AO clinical investigation and documentation and the international association for pediatric traumatology. J Pediatr Orthop. 2006;26:43–9.
73. Colaris JW, Allema JH, Biter LU, de Vries MR, van de Ven CP, Bloem RM, et al. Re-displacement of stable distal both-bone forearm fractures in children: a randomised controlled multicentre trial. Injury. 2013;44(4):498–503. https://doi.org/10.1016/j.injury.2012.11.001.
74. Hove LM, Brudvik C. Displaced paediatric fractures of the distal radius. Arch Orthop Trauma Surg. 2007;128:55–60.
75. Johari AN, Sinha M. Remodeling of forearm fractures in children. J Pediatr Orthop B. 1999;8(2):84–7.
76. Franklin CC, Robinson J, Noonan K, Flynn JM. Evidence-based medicine: management of pediatric forearm fractures. J Pediatr Orthop. 2012;32(Suppl 2):S131–4.
77. Valisena S, Gonzalez J, Voumard N, et al. Treatment of paediatric unstable displaced distal radius fractures using Kapandji technique: a case series. Eur J Orthop Surg Traumatol. 2019;29:413–20. https://doi.org/10.1007/s00590-018-2297-5.
78. Lichtman DM, Bindra RR, Boyer MI, Putnam MD, Ring D, Slutsky DJ, et al. Treatment of distal radius fractures. J Am Acad Orthop Surg. 2010;18:180–9.
79. Ramoutar DN, Shivji FS, Rodrigues JN, Hunter JB. The outcomes of displaced paediatric distal radius fractures treated with percutaneous Kirschner wire fixation: a review of 248 cases. Eur J Orthop Surg Traumatol. 2015;25:471–6.
80. Lieber J, Schmid E, Schmittenbecher PP. Unstable diametaphyseal forearm fractures: transepiphyseal intramedullary Kirschner-Wire fixation as a treatment option in children. Eur J Pediatr Surg. 2010;20:395–8.
81. Li J, Rai S, Tang X, Ze R, Liu R, Hong P. Fixation of delayed distal radial fracture involving metaphyseal diaphyseal junction in adolescents: a comparative study of crossed Kirschner-wiring and non-bridging external fixator. BMC Musculoskelet Disord. 2020;21:365.
82. Van der Reis WL, Otsuka NY, Moroz P, Mah J. Intramedullary nailing versus plate fixation for unstable forearm fractures in children. J Pediatr Orthop. 1998;18:9–13.
83. Du M, Han J. Antegrade elastic stable intramedullary nail fixation for paediatric distal radius diaphyseal metaphyseal junction fractures: a new operative approach. Injury. 2019;50:598–601.
84. Cai H, Wang Z, Cai H. Prebending of a titanium elastic intramedullary nail in the treatment of distal radius fractures in children. Int Surg. 2014;99:269–75.
85. Joulié S, Laville JM, Salmeron F. Posteromedial elastic stable intra-medullary nailing (ESIN) in volarly displaced metaphyso-diaphyseal distal radius fractures in child. Orthop Traumatol Surg Res. 2011;97:330–4.
86. Makki D, Matar HE, Webb M, Wright DM, James LA, Ricketts DM. Elastic stable intramedullary nailing in paediatric forearm fractures: the rate of open reduction and complications. J Pediatr Orthop B. 2017;26:412–6.

87. Pace JL. Pediatric and adolescent forearm fractures: current controversies and treatment recommendations. J Am Acad Orthop Surg. 2016;24:780–8.
88. Gibbons C, Woods D, Pailthorpe C, et al. The management of isolated distal radius fractures in children. J Pediatr Orthop. 1994;14:207–10. https://doi.org/10.1097/01241398-199403000-00014.
89. Schneider J, Staubli G, Kubat S, Altermatt S. Treating displaced distal forearm fractures in children. Eur J Trauma Emerg Surg. 2007;33(6):619–25. https://doi.org/10.1007/s00068-007-6204-8.
90. Voto SJ, Weiner DS, Leighley B. Redisplacement after closed reduction of forearm fractures in children. J Pediatr Orthop. 1990;10(1):79–84.
91. Displaced fracture of the distal radius in children. Accessed 29 Sept 29 2022. Retrieved from: https://online.boneandjoint.org.uk/doi/epub/ https://doi.org/10.1302/0301-620X.87B6.15648.
92. Wasiak M, Piekut M, Ratajczak K, Waśko M. Early complications of percutaneous K-wire fixation in pediatric distal radius fractures-a prospective cohort study. Arch Orthop Trauma Surg. 2023;143(11):6649–56. https://doi.org/10.1007/s00402-023-04996-7.
93. Subramanian P, Kantharuban S, Shilston S, Pearce OJ. Complications of Kirschner-wire fixation in distal radius fractures. Tech Hand Up Extrem Surg. 2012;16(3):120–3. https://doi.org/10.1097/BTH.0b013e31824b9ab0.
94. Mani GV, Hui PW, Cheng JC. Translation of the radius as a predictor of outcome in distal radial fractures of children. J Bone Joint Surg. 1993;75(5):808–11. https://doi.org/10.1302/0301-620X.75B5.8376446.
95. Varga M, Józsa G, Fadgyas B, Kassai T, Renner A. Short, double elastic nailing of severely displaced distal pediatric radial fractures: a new method for stable fixation. Medicine. 2017;96(14):e6532. https://doi.org/10.1097/MD.0000000000006532.
96. Chambers H, De La Garza JF, O'Brien E, Price CT, Stanley E, Wilkins KE. Fractures of the radius and ulna. In: Rockwood CA, Wilkins KE, Beaty JH, editors. Fractures in children, vol. 3. 4th ed. Philadelphia: Lippincott-Raven; 1996. p. 449–651.
97. Cheng JCY, Shen WY. Limb fracture pattern in different pediatric age groups: a study of 3350 children. J Orthop Trauma. 1993;7:15–22.
98. Friberg KSI. Remodelling after distal forearm fractures in children. I. The effect of residual angulation on the spatial orientation of the epiphyseal plates. Acta Orthop Scand. 1979;50:537–46.
99. Friberg KSI. Remodelling after distal forearm fractures in children. II. The final orientation of the distal and proximal epiphyseal plates of the radius. Acta Orthop Scand. 1979;50:731–9.
100. Friberg KSI. Remodelling after distal forearm fractures in children. III. Correction of residual angulation in fractures of the radius. Acta Orthop Scand. 1979;50:741–9.
101. Gandhi RK, Wilson P, Mason Brown JJ, MacLeod W. Spontaneous correction of deformity following fractures of the forearm in children. Br J Surg. 1962;50:5–10.
102. Önne L, Sandblom PH. Late results in fractures of the forearm in children. Acta Chir Scand. 1949;98:549–67.
103. Thomas EM, Tuson KWR, Browne PSH. Fractures of the radius and ulna in children. Injury. 1975;7:120–4.
104. Rai P, Haque A, Abraham A. A systematic review of displaced paediatric distal radius fracture management: plaster cast versus Kirschner wiring. J Clin Orthop Trauma. 2020;11:275. https://doi.org/10.1016/J.JCOT.2019.03.021.
105. Miller BS, Taylor B, Widmann RF, Bae DS, Snyder BD, Waters PM. Cast immobilization versus percutaneous pin fixation of displaced distal radius fractures in children: a prospective, randomized study. J Pediatr Orthop. 2005;25:490–4. https://doi.org/10.1097/01.bpo.0000158780.52849.39.
106. Firth GB, Robertson AJF. Treatment of distal radius metaphyseal fractures in children: a case report and literature review. SA Orthop J. 2017;16:59–63. https://doi.org/10.17159/2309-8309/2017/v16n4a10.

107. McLauchlan GJ, Cowan B, Annan IH, Robb JE. Management of completely displaced metaphyseal fractures of the distal radius in children. A prospective, randomised controlled trial. J Bone Joint Surg Br. 2002;84:413–7. https://doi.org/10.1302/0301-620X.84B3.11432.
108. Muratli HH, Yağmurlu MF, Yüksel HY, Aktekin CN, Biçimoğlu A, Tabak AY. Treatment of childhood unstable radius distal methaphysis fractures with closed reduction and percutaneous Kirschner wires. Acta Orthop Traumatol Turc. 2002;36(1):52–7.
109. Ozcan M, Memisoglu S, Copuroglu C, Saridogan K. Percutaneous Kirschner wire fixation in distal radius metaphyseal fractures in children: does it change the overall outcome? Hippokratia. 2010;14:265–70.
110. Tosti R, Foroohar A, Pizzutillo PD, Herman MJ. Kirschner Wire infections in pediatric orthopaedic surgery. J Pediatr Orthop. 2015;35:69–73. https://doi.org/10.1097/BPO.0000000000000208.
111. Van Leemput W, De Ridder K. Distal metaphyseal radius fractures in children : reduction with or without pinning. Acta Orthop Belg. 2009;75:306–9.
112. Battle J, Carmichael KD. Incidence of pin track infections in children's fractures treated with Kirschner wire fixation. J Pediatr Orthop. 2007;27:154–7. https://doi.org/10.1097/BPO.0B013E3180317A22.
113. Choi KY, Chan WS, Lam TP, Cheng JC. Percutaneous Kirschner-wire pinning for severely displaced distal radial fractures in children. A report of 157 cases. J Bone Joint Surg Br. 1995;77(5):797–801.
114. Khandekar S, Tolessa E, Jones S. Displaced distal end radius fractures in children treated with kirschner wires -a systematic review. Acta Orthop Belg. 2016;82:681–9.
115. Luscombe KL, Chaudhry S, Dwyer JS, Shanmugam C, Maffulli N. Selective Kirschner wiring for displaced distal radial fractures in children. Acta Orthop Traumatol Turc. 2010;44(2):117–23. https://doi.org/10.3944/AOTT.2010.2133.
116. Passiatore M, De Vitis R, Perna A, D'Orio M, Cilli V, Taccardo G. Extraphyseal distal radius fracture in children: is the cast always needed? A retrospective analysis comparing Epibloc system and K-wire pinning. Eur J Orthop Surg Traumatol. 2020;30:1243–50.
117. Mostafa MF, El-Adl G, Enan A. Percutaneous Kirschner-wire fixation for displaced distal forearm fractures in children. Acta Orthop Belg. 2009;75:459–66.
118. Waters PM, Alex M. Distal Radius and ulna fraktures. In: Beaty JH, Kasser JR, editors. Rockwood and Wilkins' fractures in children. 6th ed. Philadelphia: Lippincott Williams & Wilkins; 2006. p. 338–95.
119. Kazmers NH, Fragomen AT, Rozbruch SR. Prevention of pin site infection in external fixation: a review of the literature. Strat Traum Limb Recon. 2016;11:75–85. https://doi.org/10.1007/s11751-016-0256-4.
120. Zeng ZK, Liang WD, Sun YQ, Jiang PP, Li D, Shen Z, et al. Is percutaneous pinning needed for the treatment of displaced distal radius metaphyseal fractures in children?: a systematic review. Medicine. 2018;97(36):e12142. https://doi.org/10.1097/MD.0000000000012142.
121. Sengab A, Krijnen P, Schipper IB. Displaced distal radius fractures in children, cast alone vs additional K-wire fixation: a meta-analysis. Eur J Trauma Emerg Surg. 2019;45:1003–11.
122. Lascombes P, Haumont T, Journeau P. Use and abuse of flexible intramedullary nailing in children and adolescents. J Pediatr Orthop. 2006;26:827–34.
123. Kubiak R, Aksakal D, Weiss C, Wessel LM, Lange B. Is there a standard treatment for displaced pediatric diametaphyseal forearm fractures? A STROBE-compliant retrospective study. Medicine (Baltim). 2019;98(28):e16353. https://doi.org/10.1097/MD.0000000000016353.
124. Lieber J, Joeris A, Knorr P, Schalamon J, Schmittenbecher PP. ESIN in forearm fractures: clear indications, often used, but some avoidable complications. Eur J Trauma. 2005;31:3–11.
125. Helber MU, Ulrich C. External fixation in forearm shaft fractures. Injury. 2000;31(Suppl 1):45–7. S0020138399002624 [pii]
126. Murphy M, Teasdall RJ, Comadoll S, Aneja A. Dorsal Thompson: approach to the proximal radial shaft. J Orthop Trauma. 2021;35(Suppl 2):S16–7. https://doi.org/10.1097/BOT.0000000000002162.

127. Lam A, Gordon AM, Thabet AM, Abdelgawad AA. Antegrade flexible nailing for pediatric Metaphyseal-Diaphyseal junction distal radius fracture, is it safe? Tech Hand Up Extrem Surg. 2023;27(3):161–4. https://doi.org/10.1097/BTH.0000000000000430.
128. Dietzel M, Scherer S, Esser M, et al. Fractures of the proximal radius in children: management and results of 100 consecutive cases. Arch Orthop Trauma Surg. 2022;142:1903–10. https://doi.org/10.1007/s00402-021-03917-w.
129. Fernandez FF, Langendorfer M, Wirth T, Eberhardt O. Failures and complications in intramedullary nailing of children's forearm fractures. J Child Orthop. 2010;4(2):159–67. https://doi.org/10.1007/s11832-010-0245-y.
130. Delniotis I, Bontinis V, Ktenidis K, Drakonaki EE, Galanis N. Diagnostic accuracy of ultrasound versus X-ray for distal forearm fractures in children and adolescents: a systematic review and meta-analysis. Eur J Trauma Emerg Surg. 2024; https://doi.org/10.1007/s00068-024-02451-9.
131. Morello R, Mariani F, Snelling PJ, Buonsenso D. Point-of-care ultrasound for the diagnosis of distal forearm fractures in children and adolescents: a scoping review. Eur J Pediatr. 2024; https://doi.org/10.1007/s00431-024-05877-w.
132. Hassankhani A, Amoukhteh M, Jannatdoust P, Valizadeh P, Ghadimi DJ, Vasavada PS, Johnston JH, Gholamrezanezhad A. A meta-analysis on the diagnostic utility of ultrasound in pediatric distal forearm fractures. Emerg Radiol. 2024; https://doi.org/10.1007/s10140-024-02208-2.
133. Hendrickx RPM, Campo MM, van Lieshout APW, Struijs PAA, van den Bekerom MPJ. Above- or below-elbow casts for distal third forearm fractures in children? A meta-analysis of the literature. Arch Orthop Trauma Surg. 2011; https://doi.org/10.1007/s00402-011-1363-9.
134. Seiler M, Heinz P, Callegari A, Dreher T, Staubli G, Aufdenblatten C. Short and long-arm fiberglass cast immobilization for displaced distal forearm fractures in children: a randomized controlled trial. Int Orthop. 2020; https://doi.org/10.1007/s00264-020-04800-w.
135. Wang B, Guo J, Li Z, Ji Z, Liu F, Sun K, Feng W. Pediatric distal both-bone forearm fractures treated with percutaneous pinning with or without ulna fixation: a retrospective cohort study from two centres. BMC Musculoskelet Disord. 2024; https://doi.org/10.1186/s12891-024-07822-2.
136. van Egmond PW, Schipper IB, van Luijt PA. Displaced distal forearm fractures in children with an indication for reduction under general anesthesia should be percutaneously fixated. Eur J Orthop Surg Traumatol. 2011; https://doi.org/10.1007/s00590-011-0826-6.
137. Roth KC, Denk K, Colaris JW, Jaarsma RL. Think twice before re-manipulating distal metaphyseal forearm fractures in children. Arch Orthop Trauma Surg. 2014; https://doi.org/10.1007/s00402-014-2091-8.
138. Wu R, Wen Y, Wang C, Liu T, Yu J. Elastic stable intramedullary nailing versus Kirschner wire in the treatment of pediatric metaphyseal–diaphyseal junction fractures of the distal radius: a case-control study. BMC Musculoskelet Disord. 2023; https://doi.org/10.1186/s12891-023-07055-9.
139. Abulsoud MI, Mohammed AS, Elmarghany M, Elgeushy A, Elzahed E, Moawad M, Elshal EA, Elhalawany MF, Hassanein YA, Fouad AA, Zakaria AR. Intramedullary Kirschner wire fixation of displaced distal forearm fractures in children. BMC Musculoskelet Disord. 2023; https://doi.org/10.1186/s12891-023-06875-z.
140. Zimmermann R, Gschwentner M, Kralinger F, Arora R, Gabl M, Pechlaner S. Long-term results following pediatric distal forearm fractures. Arch Orthop Trauma Surg. 2004; https://doi.org/10.1007/s00402-003-0619-4.
141. Dietzel M, Scherer S, Spogis J, Kirschner HJ, Fuchs J, Lieber J. Treatment of unstable forearm fractures at the metaphyseal-diaphyseal junction in children: antegrade ESIN vs. transepiphyseal intramedullary K-wire fixation. Eur J Trauma Emerg Surg. 2024; https://doi.org/10.1007/s00068-024-02562-3.

Forearm Fracture

11

Introduction by the Author

Two-bone forearm fractures are among the most common types of fractures that orthopedic surgeons encounter in their daily practice. Forearm fractures account for about 20% of all fractures in the pediatric population, affecting males in about two-thirds of cases and involving both bones in half of cases. Specifically, fractures involving both bones account for approximately 3% to 5% of all fractures and 30% of fractures of the upper extremities. Although they can occur at any age, forearm fractures are more frequent in school-age children and adolescents than in infants and preschoolers.

The gold standard treatment for minimally displaced and stable pediatric forearm fractures in younger children is closed reduction and cast immobilization. However, older children (over 9 years old) can tolerate no more than 10° of angular deformation in middle-third fractures, 30° of rotational deformation, and 100% translation, as long as the axis is maintained. A cadaveric study found that 20° of angulation of a middle-third forearm fracture limits pronation-supination. On the other hand, displaced forearm fractures in older children require reduction and surgical stabilization, as their remodeling potential is limited.

Diaphyseal forearm fractures in children and adolescents present a challenge due to their prevalence and the complexity of treatment options. While closed reduction and cast immobilization are viable options for some cases, unstable or irreducible fractures often necessitate surgical intervention. The choice of treatment remains controversial, especially for adolescents, due to varying outcomes related to stability, appearance, and complication rates.

Improper treatment can significantly impact a child's daily life by affecting the forearm's range of motion and function, especially pronation and supination. Several studies have shown that rotational malunions are present in

© The Author(s), under exclusive license to Springer Nature Switzerland AG 2026

F. Canavese, *Advances in Pediatric Extremity Fracture Management*, https://doi.org/10.1007/978-3-032-33306-3_11

children with limited forearm rotation after a fracture. However, soft tissue abnormalities may not play a significant role.

Traditional surgical interventions for diaphyseal fractures of the radius and ulna include plating. However, there has been a shift toward less invasive techniques, such as elastic stable intramedullary nailing. These techniques provide a high healing rate and low postoperative complication rate.

In cases involving both the radius and the ulna, it is important to note that single-bone fixation may not be as effective as two-bone fixation. This is due to higher rates of re-displacement and complications, with no significant gain in intraoperative time. Additionally, single-bone fixation requires a longer period of immobilization in a cast.

Despite the favorable overall prognosis, refracture at the primary fracture site is a concern, especially for diaphyseal fractures of both bones in the forearm. Furthermore, refractures are more likely to occur when elastic nails are removed prematurely before complete fracture healing is achieved. Additionally, although rare, complications such as nonunions can occur. These complications are more likely to occur at specific fracture sites or due to technical errors. Examples of technical errors include open surgery and using screws and plates to fix fractures in skeletally immature patients. In cases of nonunion, conservative management is a feasible option, especially when symptoms are absent. However, surgical treatment is essential for symptomatic cases to ensure proper healing and function.

11.1 Machine Generated Summaries

Disclaimer: The summaries in this chapter were generated from Springer Nature publications using abstractive AI auto-summarization: An abstraction-based summarizer creates new text based on deep learning. New phrases are created to summarize the content. As the constituted sentences are machine selected, they may not fully reflect the body of the work, so we strongly advise that the original content is read and cited. The auto-generated summaries were curated by the author(s) to meet Springer Nature publication standards.

Management of Pediatric Forearm Fractures: What Is the Best Therapeutic Choice? A Narrative Review of the Literature [132]

This is a machine-generated summary of:

Caruso, G.; Caldari, E.; Sturla, F. D.; Caldaria, A.; Re, D. L.; Pagetti, P.; Palummieri, F.; Massari, L. Management of pediatric forearm fractures: what is the best therapeutic choice? A narrative review of the literature [132]

Published in: MUSCULOSKELETAL SURGERY (2020)
Link to original: https://doi.org/10.1007/s12306-020-00684-6
Copyright of the summarized publication:
The Author(s) 2020
License: OpenAccess CC BY 4.0

This article is licensed under a Creative Commons Attribution 4.0 International License, which permits use, sharing, adaptation, distribution and reproduction in any medium or format, as long as you give appropriate credit to the original author(s) and the source, provide a link to the Creative Commons licence, and indicate if changes were made. The images or other third party material in this article are included in the article's Creative Commons licence, unless indicated otherwise in a credit line to the material. If material is not included in the article's Creative Commons licence and your intended use is not permitted by statutory regulation or exceeds the permitted use, you will need to obtain permission directly from the copyright holder. To view a copy of this licence, visit http://creativecommons.org/licenses/by/4.0/.

If you want to cite the papers, please refer to the original.

For technical reasons we could not place the page where the original quote is coming from.

Research Highlights

Forearm fractures are the most common type of fractures in the pediatric population, yet comprehensive overviews of their epidemiology have been lacking. These fractures are particularly prevalent among school-age and preschool children, with a higher incidence in males. Now, a new study by G. Caruso and colleagues provides an extensive analysis of pediatric forearm fractures, examining both conservative and surgical treatment options to offer insights into optimal management strategies.

Caruso et al. utilized data from various studies to explore the anatomy, diagnosis, and treatment of pediatric forearm fractures. The study highlights the importance of understanding the anatomical features of the forearm, such as the role of the ulna in maintaining stability and the growth potential of distal radial and ulnar growth plates. The authors discuss different fracture types, including buckle, greenstick, and complete fractures, and emphasize the need for accurate diagnosis using radiographs or ultrasound. Treatment approaches are stratified by fracture type and patient age, with conservative management being common for stable fractures. Surgical intervention is recommended for unstable or irreducible fractures, with options including intramedullary nailing and plating. The study also examines emerging techniques like hybrid fixation to improve outcomes.

The study by Caruso et al. advances our understanding of pediatric forearm fracture management by providing a detailed comparison of conservative versus surgical treatments. It underscores the need for individualized treatment plans based on patient age, fracture pattern, and potential for bone remodeling. Future study directions could focus on developing standardized guidelines that incorporate new technologies and techniques to optimize treatment outcomes further. The authors call for additional research to establish clear protocols that can guide clinicians in making informed decisions about fracture management in children.

Hand Dominance and Gender in Forearm Fractures in Children [133]

This is a machine-generated summary of:

Hassan, Freih Odeh Abu Hand dominance and gender in forearm fractures in children [133]
Published in: Strategies in Trauma and Limb Reconstruction (2008)
Link to original: https://doi.org/10.1007/s11751-008-0048-6
Copyright of the summarized publication:
Springer-Verlag 2008
All rights reserved.

If you want to cite the papers, please refer to the original.
For technical reasons we could not place the page where the original quote is coming from.

Research Highlights

Pediatric forearm fractures are prevalent injuries managed by orthopedic and trauma surgeons, with existing literature extensively documenting the incidence of hand dominance in children. However, there is a lack of studies exploring the influence of hand dominance on different types of forearm fractures. Notably, upper extremity fractures are more frequently observed on the left side than the right. Now, a new study by Freih Odeh Abu Hassan and colleagues addresses this gap by prospectively evaluating the role of hand dominance, fractured side, and gender in children with various forearm fracture types.

The study involved a cohort of healthy children diagnosed with isolated unilateral forearm fractures over a one-year period. Excluding those with bilateral fractures or multiple injuries from severe accidents, the researchers assessed 200 boys and 100 girls, with a mean age of 8 years. The study meticulously recorded data on age, sex, hand dominance, mechanism of injury, and fracture specifics. Statistical analyses were conducted using Pearson chi-squared tests to evaluate differences among variables. The findings revealed that forearm fractures were significantly more common in boys than girls and predominantly occurred in the non-dominant hand for right-handed children. Greenstick and buckle/torus fractures were prevalent among younger children aged 4–10 years, while complete displaced fractures were more common in older children.

The study advances our understanding of pediatric forearm fractures by highlighting the significant role of hand dominance and gender in fracture patterns. It suggests that non-dominant hands are more susceptible to injury due to their passive role during falls or accidents. Future studies could further explore the biomechanical aspects influencing these patterns or investigate preventive measures tailored to reduce fracture risks in specific demographics. Additionally, understanding the activities leading to such injuries could inform targeted interventions for boys who are at higher risk due to their outdoor activities.

The Effects of Maximal Radial Bowing on Forearm Rotation in Pediatric Diaphyseal Forearm Fractures [134]

This is a machine-generated summary of:

Wongcharoenwatana, J.; Eamsobhana, P.; Chotigavanichaya, C.; Ariyawatkul, T.; Kaewpornsawan, K. The effects of maximal radial bowing on forearm rotation in pediatric diaphyseal forearm fractures [134]
Published in: MUSCULOSKELETAL SURGERY (2021)
Link to original: https://doi.org/10.1007/s12306-021-00728-5
Copyright of the summarized publication:
The Author(s), under exclusive licence to Istituto Ortopedico Rizzoli 2021
All rights reserved.

If you want to cite the papers, please refer to the original.

For technical reasons we could not place the page where the original quote is coming from.

Research Highlights

Forearm rotation is crucial for daily activities, and the radial bow plays a significant role in enabling this motion. In children, fractures of the forearm can alter the normal radial bowing, potentially leading to malunion and impaired forearm function. While many of these fractures are treated nonoperatively, residual deformities, particularly in older children, may not fully remodel, resulting in limited pronation and supination. Now, a new study by J. Wongcharoenwatana and colleagues investigates the effects of radial bowing on forearm rotation in pediatric forearm fractures compared to healthy children.

The study was conducted retrospectively on children aged 5–15 years who had previously sustained diaphyseal forearm fractures. These children were divided into two groups: those with limited forearm rotation (case group) and those with normal rotation (control group). The researchers measured maximal radial bowing (MRB) using radiographs and assessed forearm motion with a goniometer. Statistical analysis was performed to determine the correlation between MRB and limited forearm rotation. The results showed that children with MRB $\leq 5.5\%$ had significantly reduced pronation ($\leq 60°$) and supination ($\leq 60°$), indicating a strong association between decreased MRB and limited forearm motion.

The study highlights the importance of restoring normal radial bowing to ensure optimal forearm function after fracture reduction in children. It suggests that maintaining an MRB of approximately 7–9% is crucial for avoiding limitations in forearm rotation. Future studies could explore age-related differences in remodeling potential and investigate other factors contributing to rotational deficits beyond radial bowing alterations. This research provides valuable insights for surgeons treating pediatric diaphyseal forearm fractures, emphasizing the need to address residual deformities to achieve better functional outcomes.

Forearm Fractures in Overweight—Obese Children and Adolescents: A Matter of Bone Density, Bone Geometry or Body Composition? [135]

This is a machine-generated summary of:

Franceschi, Roberto; Radetti, Giorgio; Soffiati, Massimo; Maines, Evelina Forearm Fractures in Overweight—Obese Children and Adolescents: A Matter of Bone Density, Bone Geometry or Body Composition? [135]
Published in: Calcified Tissue International (2022)
Link to original: https://doi.org/10.1007/s00223-022-00971-3
Copyright of the summarized publication:
The Author(s), under exclusive licence to Springer Science+Business Media, LLC, part of Springer Nature 2022
All rights reserved.

If you want to cite the papers, please refer to the original.

For technical reasons we could not place the page where the original quote is coming from.

Research Highlights

The obesity epidemic poses a significant public health challenge, particularly among children and adolescents. A critical debate exists regarding whether excess body fat negatively or positively impacts skeletal health in this demographic. While some studies suggest that obese children are more prone to extremity fractures than their normal-weight peers, findings are inconsistent across the literature. Dual-Energy X-ray Absorptiometry (DXA) is the most commonly used technique for assessing bone mineral density (BMD) in children, but it has limitations in fracture risk assessment. Now, a new study by Roberto Franceschi and colleagues explores the relationship between obesity and forearm bone health in children, utilizing advanced imaging techniques to provide deeper insights.

The study conducted a comprehensive literature review using PubMed to identify relevant studies on bone indices and body composition assessed by peripheral Quantitative Computed Tomography (pQCT) and/or DXA at the forearm in overweight or obese subjects. The researchers applied the PICOS model to select studies involving children and adolescents, focusing on outcomes such as volumetric BMD, bone strength, and local body composition. After screening numerous studies, they included those that met specific criteria, excluding case reports and studies with insufficient data. The review found that while DXA studies often reported lower areal BMD in overweight and obese children, pQCT studies indicated increased volumetric BMD and normal or increased bone size. However, altered bone geometry with a high fat-to-muscle ratio was negatively associated with bone strength.

The findings suggest that overweight and obese children have increased volumetric BMD and normal or increased bone size at the forearm but may experience altered bone geometry due to a higher proportion of fat relative to muscle. This imbalance could lead to an increased risk of forearm fractures during falls. Future study directions could involve refining clinical practices by incorporating DXA measurements alongside local soft tissue assessments for pediatric patients with significant fracture histories. While pQCT and high-resolution pQCT remain primarily research tools, they offer valuable insights into bone structure and strength when appropriate reference data are available.

Comparison of Ultrasound-Guided Versus Fluoroscopy-Guided Reduction of Forearm Fractures in Children [136]

This is a machine-generated summary of:

Gillon, Jason T.; Gorn, Michael; Wilkinson, Matthew Comparison of ultrasound-guided versus fluoroscopy-guided reduction of forearm fractures in children [136]
Published in: Emergency Radiology (2020)
Link to original: https://doi.org/10.1007/s10140-020-01862-6
Copyright of the summarized publication:
American Society of Emergency Radiology 2020
All rights reserved.

If you want to cite the papers, please refer to the original.

For technical reasons we could not place the page where the original quote is coming from.

Research Highlights

Forearm fractures, particularly those involving the distal radius, are the most common type of fracture in children and have been increasing in incidence, potentially due to heightened sports participation. Traditionally, these fractures are reduced under fluoroscopy in emergency departments (EDs), but this method exposes children to ionizing radiation, which carries a risk of neoplasm. Point-of-care ultrasound (POCUS) has emerged as a promising alternative for diagnosing and managing musculoskeletal injuries in pediatrics, offering excellent diagnostic accuracy without radiation exposure. Now, a new study by Jason T. Gillon and colleagues explores the efficacy of POCUS compared to fluoroscopy for guiding forearm fracture reductions in children, focusing on reduction success rates, ED length of stay, and associated costs.

The study was conducted as a retrospective cohort analysis at a tertiary children's hospital, comparing POCUS-guided and fluoroscopy-guided reduction techniques. Data were extracted from electronic medical records of pediatric patients who presented with forearm fractures over a three-year period. The primary outcome was the success of fracture reduction as determined by post-reduction radiographs reviewed by orthopedic specialists. Secondary outcomes included ED length of stay and cost analysis. POCUS-guided reductions were performed by a single experienced pediatric emergency medicine physician, while fluoroscopy-guided reductions were typically conducted by pediatric orthopedic advanced practice providers. The study found no significant difference in reduction success between the two groups; however, POCUS was associated with a shorter ED length of stay before adjusting for sedation methods.

The findings suggest that POCUS is an effective alternative to fluoroscopy for guiding forearm fracture reductions in children, with comparable success rates and similar costs. The study highlights the potential for POCUS to reduce ED length of stay by freeing up radiologic technologists for other tasks. Future studies could explore the generalizability of these results across different hospital systems and assess how provider experience with POCUS impacts reduction success rates. Additionally, understanding cost implications when billing for POCUS could further inform its integration into clinical practice.

Intramedullary Versus Plate Fixation of Both Bone Forearm Fractures in Skeletally Immature Patients: A Systematic Review and Meta-Analysis [137]

This is a machine-generated summary of:

Ahmed, Ahmed Mohamed; Said, Elsayed; Addosooki, Ahmad; Attya, Hossam Ahmed; Awad, Ahmad Khairy; Ahmed, Emad Hamdy; Tammam, Hamdy Intramedullary versus plate fixation of both bone forearm fractures in skeletally immature patients: a systematic review and meta-analysis [137]
Published in: European Journal of Orthopaedic Surgery & Traumatology (2024)
Link to original: https://doi.org/10.1007/s00590-024-03925-7
Copyright of the summarized publication:
The Author(s) 2024
License: OpenAccess CC BY 4.0

This article is licensed under a Creative Commons Attribution 4.0 International License, which permits use, sharing, adaptation, distribution and reproduction in any medium or format, as long as you give appropriate credit to the original author(s) and the source, provide a link to the Creative Commons licence, and indicate if changes were made. The images or other third party material in this article are included in the article's Creative Commons licence, unless indicated otherwise in a credit line to the material. If material is not included in the article's Creative Commons licence and your intended use is not permitted by statutory regulation or exceeds the permitted use, you will need to obtain permission directly from the copyright holder. To view a copy of this licence, visit http://creativecommons.org/licenses/by/4.0/.

If you want to cite the papers, please refer to the original.

For technical reasons we could not place the page where the original quote is coming from.

Research Highlights

Both bone forearm fractures (BBFFs) are prevalent among the pediatric population, representing a significant portion of upper extremity fractures. The management of these fractures, particularly in unstable cases requiring surgical intervention, remains contentious due to varying opinions on optimal treatment strategies. Now, a new study by Ahmed Mohamed Ahmed and colleagues provides insights into the comparative outcomes of intramedullary fixation (IMF) and plate fixation (PF) for managing unstable pediatric BBFFs. Their systematic review and meta-analysis aim to clarify which surgical technique offers superior outcomes in terms of union rates, complications, and functional recovery.

The study conducted a comprehensive search across multiple databases, adhering to the Preferred Reporting Items for Systematic Reviews and Meta-Analyses guidelines. Sixteen studies were included in the analysis, encompassing both retrospective and one prospective study. The researchers extracted data on union rates, complications, radiographic outcomes, and perioperative parameters from studies comparing IMF and PF in skeletally immature patients. The analysis revealed no significant difference between IMF and PF regarding union time or non-union rates. However, IMF was associated with better cosmetic outcomes but a higher incidence of symptomatic hardware requiring early removal. PF demonstrated longer operating times but allowed for better restoration of radial bow location.

The findings suggest that both IMF and PF are effective for treating BBFFs in children, with each technique offering distinct advantages. While IMF provides shorter surgical times and improved cosmetic results, PF may be preferable for older children due to its potential for earlier union and superior anatomical correction of the radial bow. Future study could focus on high-quality randomized controlled trials to further evaluate these techniques' long-term outcomes and refine treatment guidelines. The choice between IMF and PF should be tailored to individual patient needs, considering factors such as age, fracture characteristics, and family preferences.

Single-Bone Versus Both-Bone Plating of Unstable Paediatric Both-Bone Forearm Fractures. A Randomized Controlled Clinical Trial [138]

This is a machine-generated summary of:

Khaled, Mohamed; Fadle, Amr A.; Attia, Ahmed Khalil; Sami, Andrew; Hafez, Abdelkhalek; Abol Oyoun, Nariman Single-bone versus both-bone plating of unstable paediatric both-bone forearm fractures. A randomized controlled clinical trial [138]

Published in: International Orthopaedics (2021)
Link to original: https://doi.org/10.1007/s00264-021-05097-z
Copyright of the summarized publication:
The Author(s) 2021
License: OpenAccess CC BY 4.0

This article is licensed under a Creative Commons Attribution 4.0 International License, which permits use, sharing, adaptation, distribution and reproduction in any medium or format, as long as you give appropriate credit to the original author(s) and the source, provide a link to the Creative Commons licence, and indicate if changes were made. The images or other third party material in this article are included in the article's Creative Commons licence, unless indicated otherwise in a credit line to the material. If material is not included in the article's Creative Commons licence and your intended use is not permitted by statutory regulation or exceeds the permitted use, you will need to obtain permission directly from the copyright holder. To view a copy of this licence, visit http://creativecommons.org/licenses/by/4.0/.

If you want to cite the papers, please refer to the original.

For technical reasons we could not place the page where the original quote is coming from.

Research Highlights

Radius and ulna fractures, commonly known as both-bone forearm fractures, are among the most frequent injuries in children, particularly affecting the diaphyseal region. The interosseous membrane plays a crucial role in maintaining the structural integrity and function of the forearm by transferring forces between the radius and ulna. While traditional treatment for these fractures involves closed reduction and cast immobilization, especially in younger children, older children often require more stringent criteria for acceptable alignment due to reduced remodeling potential. Now, a new study by Mohamed Khaled and colleagues explores the efficacy of single-bone fixation compared to both-bone fixation in treating unstable diaphyseal both-bone forearm fractures in children.

The study was conducted as a randomized controlled trial at a single academic medical center, involving children aged 9 years and older with unstable diaphyseal forearm fractures. Participants were randomly assigned to either single-bone fixation of the ulna or both-bone fixation. The surgical procedures were standardized, with all operations performed by the same senior pediatric orthopedic surgeon. The primary outcome measures included fracture union, range of motion (ROM), and radiographic parameters such as angulation and displacement. Follow-up assessments were conducted at various intervals up to 6 months post-operatively. Statistical analyses were performed to compare outcomes between the two groups, focusing on operative time, union rates, ROM, and complications.

The study found that single-bone fixation resulted in a significantly shorter operative time compared to both-bone fixation. Although there was a higher risk of radius re-angulation in the single-bone group, this did not translate into clinically significant differences in ROM or functional outcomes. Both groups achieved excellent union rates without complications or refractures. The findings suggest that single-bone fixation may offer advantages such as reduced soft tissue trauma and lower surgical costs while maintaining satisfactory clinical outcomes. Future studies could explore long-term outcomes and compare different fixation methods to further refine treatment strategies for pediatric forearm fractures.

Single-Bone Intramedullary Fixation of Unstable Both-Bone Diaphyseal Forearm Fractures in Children Leads to Increased Re-Displacement: A Multicentre Randomised Controlled Trial [69]

This is a machine-generated summary of:

Colaris, Joost; Reijman, Max; Allema, Jan Hein; Kraan, Gerald; van Winterswijk, Peter; de Vries, Mark; van de Ven, Cees; Verhaar, Jan Single-bone intramedullary fixation of unstable both-bone diaphyseal forearm fractures in children leads to increased re-displacement: a multicentre randomised controlled trial [69]
Published in: Archives of Orthopaedic and Trauma Surgery (2013)
Link to original: https://doi.org/10.1007/s00402-013-1763-0
Copyright of the summarized publication:
Springer-Verlag Berlin Heidelberg 2013
All rights reserved.

If you want to cite the papers, please refer to the original.
For technical reasons we could not place the page where the original quote is coming from.

Research Highlights

Radius and ulna fractures, commonly known as both-bone forearm fractures, are among the most frequent injuries in children, particularly affecting the diaphyseal region. The interosseous membrane plays a crucial role in maintaining the structural integrity and function of the forearm by transferring forces between the radius and ulna. While traditional treatment for these fractures involves closed reduction and cast immobilization, especially in younger children, older children often require more stringent criteria for acceptable alignment due to reduced remodeling potential. Now, a new study by Mohamed Khaled and colleagues explores the efficacy of single-bone fixation compared to both-bone fixation in treating unstable diaphyseal both-bone forearm fractures in children.

The study was conducted as a randomized controlled trial at a single academic medical center, involving children aged 9 years and older with unstable diaphyseal forearm fractures. Participants were randomly assigned to either single-bone fixation of the ulna or both-bone fixation. The surgical procedures were standardized, with all operations performed by the same senior pediatric orthopedic surgeon. The primary outcome measures included fracture union, range of motion (ROM), and radiographic parameters such as angulation and displacement. Follow-up assessments were conducted at various intervals up to 6 months post-operatively. Statistical analyses were performed to compare outcomes between the two groups, focusing on operative time, union rates, ROM, and complications.

The study found that single-bone fixation resulted in a significantly shorter operative time compared to both-bone fixation. Although there was a higher risk of radius re-angulation in the single-bone group, this did not translate into clinically significant differences in ROM or functional outcomes. Both groups achieved excellent union rates without complications or refractures. The findings suggest that single-bone fixation may offer advantages such as reduced soft tissue trauma and lower surgical costs while maintaining satisfactory clinical outcomes. Future studies could explore long-term outcomes and compare different fixation methods to further refine treatment strategies for pediatric forearm fractures.

An Age-Matched Comparative Study on Intramedullary Nailing and Plate Fixation of Both-Bone Diaphyseal Forearm Fracture in Adolescents [139]

This is a machine-generated summary of:

Ishihara, Noriko; Tokutake, Katsuhiro; Takegami, Yasuhiko; Asami, Yuta; Kumagai, Hiroaki; Ota, Hideyuki; Kimura, Yoshihiko; Ohshima, Kazuma; Imagama, Shiro
An age-matched comparative study on intramedullary nailing and plate fixation of both-bone diaphyseal forearm fracture in adolescents [139]
Published in: European Journal of Orthopaedic Surgery & Traumatology (2023)
Link to original: https://doi.org/10.1007/s00590-023-03679-8
Copyright of the summarized publication:
The Author(s), under exclusive licence to Springer-Verlag France SAS, part of Springer Nature 2023

Copyright comment: Springer Nature or its licensor (e.g. a society or other partner) holds exclusive rights to this article under a publishing agreement with the author(s) or other rightsholder(s); author self-archiving of the accepted manuscript version of this article is solely governed by the terms of such publishing agreement and applicable law.

All rights reserved.

If you want to cite the papers, please refer to the original.

For technical reasons we could not place the page where the original quote is coming from.

Research Highlights

Forearm fractures in children, particularly diaphyseal forearm fractures, present a significant challenge in pediatric orthopedics due to their prevalence and the complexity of treatment options. While closed reduction and cast immobilization are viable for some cases, unstable or irreducible fractures often necessitate surgical intervention through intramedullary nailing (IMN) or plate fixation. The choice between these methods remains controversial, especially in adolescents, due to differing outcomes related to stability, cosmesis, and complication rates. Now, a new study by Noriko Ishihara and colleagues investigates the functional and radiological outcomes of IMN versus plate fixation in adolescents with diaphyseal forearm fractures through an age-matched analysis.

The study was conducted as a multicenter retrospective analysis involving hospitals associated with the Department of Orthopedic Surgery in Central Japan. Researchers collected data on surgically treated diaphyseal forearm fractures in patients under 20 years old, focusing on those stabilized with either IMN or plate fixation. The study included 60 patients divided equally into two groups based on the implant type. By employing an age-matched design, the researchers aimed to minimize confounding effects related to age differences. Functional outcomes were assessed using Price criteria and range of motion measurements, while radiological evaluations included fracture classification and angulation assessments. Statistical analyses were performed to compare outcomes between the two groups.

The findings revealed no significant differences in functional outcomes between IMN and plate fixation groups, with both achieving excellent results according to Price criteria. However, IMN demonstrated advantages such as shorter operation times and better cosmesis compared to plate fixation. Despite these benefits, postoperative complications were similar across both groups, although neurological symptoms were more common with plate fixation. Future study could focus on refining surgical indications based on individual patient needs and fracture characteristics to optimize treatment strategies for adolescent diaphyseal forearm fractures. The study highlights the potential of IMN as a viable treatment option even for older pediatric populations while emphasizing the importance of personalized care approaches.

Effectiveness of Hybrid Fixation in the Treatment of Proximal Diaphyseal Both Bone Forearm Fractures in Adolescents [140]

This is a machine-generated summary of:

Romeih, Mohamed Abdelhamed; Khaled, Abdullah Effectiveness of Hybrid Fixation in the Treatment of Proximal Diaphyseal Both Bone Forearm Fractures in Adolescents [140]
Published in: Indian Journal of Orthopaedics (2024)
Link to original: https://doi.org/10.1007/s43465-024-01300-6
Copyright of the summarized publication:
Indian Orthopaedics Association 2024

Copyright comment: Springer Nature or its licensor (e.g. a society or other partner) holds exclusive rights to this article under a publishing agreement with the author(s) or other rightsholder(s); author self-archiving of the accepted manuscript version of this article is solely governed by the terms of such publishing agreement and applicable law.

All rights reserved.

If you want to cite the papers, please refer to the original.

For technical reasons we could not place the page where the original quote is coming from.

Research Highlights

Both-bone forearm fractures are common in pediatric orthopedic practice, and improper treatment can significantly impact a child's daily life by affecting the forearm's range of motion and function. While conservative treatment is often effective for minimally displaced fractures in young children, older children may experience poor remodeling capacity, leading to malunion and functional impairment. Surgical options like elastic stable intramedullary nailing (ESIN) and open reduction with internal fixation (ORIF) have their respective advantages and drawbacks. Now, a new study by Mohamed Abdelhamed Romeih and colleagues explores the efficacy of hybrid fixation—combining ESIN for the radius and ORIF for the ulna—in treating proximal both-bone forearm fractures in adolescents.

The study was conducted as a prospective cohort at Tanta University Hospitals, involving adolescents with closed proximal diaphyseal radius and ulna fractures that met specific clinical criteria. Exclusion criteria included distal third fractures, open fractures, fracture-dislocation injuries, and others. Under general anesthesia, ESIN was used to stabilize the radius through a small incision with fluoroscopic guidance, while the ulna was stabilized using a dynamic compression plate. Postoperative care included immobilization with an above-elbow splint and regular follow-ups to assess clinical and radiographic outcomes. The study found that most patients achieved excellent functional outcomes according to Price et al.'s grading score, with a mean union time of 10 weeks for hybrid fixation.

The study highlights that hybrid fixation offers significant advantages in treating proximal both-bone forearm fractures in adolescents by providing rotational stability and minimizing soft tissue dissection. The authors note that while the technique shows promise, further studies could explore comparative analyses with other surgical methods to validate these findings across different settings. Future study could also investigate long-term outcomes beyond the follow-up period to better understand the durability of this approach in adolescent patients.

Outcome of Elastic Nailing of Diaphyseal Forearm Fractures in Adolescents After Failure of Conservative Management [141]

This is a machine-generated summary of:

Ali, Ayman M. Outcome of elastic nailing of diaphyseal forearm fractures in adolescents after failure of conservative management [141]

Published in: European Journal of Orthopaedic Surgery & Traumatology (2011)
Link to original: https://doi.org/10.1007/s00590-011-0914-7

Copyright of the summarized publication:
Springer-Verlag 2011
All rights reserved.

If you want to cite the papers, please refer to the original.

For technical reasons we could not place the page where the original quote is coming from.

Research Highlights

Orthopedic management of unstable and displaced forearm shaft fractures in children often results in functional restrictions due to axial deviations, leading to limited pronation and supination. Traditional surgical interventions for diaphyseal fractures of the radius and ulna include plating, but there has been a shift towards minimally invasive techniques like intramedullary nailing, despite its complications. Now, a new study by Ayman M. Ali and colleagues evaluates the effectiveness of elastic intramedullary nails for treating diaphyseal forearm fractures in adolescents after conservative management fails.

The study involved 35 patients aged 10–16 years with both-bone forearm fractures treated using elastic intramedullary nails. The procedure was indicated when closed reduction failed or when there was a loss of initial correction during cast treatment. Under general anesthesia, the radius was pinned from distal to proximal, and the ulna from proximal to distal, with nail diameters tailored to each patient's medullary canal size. Postoperatively, an above-elbow plaster cast was applied until sufficient bone healing occurred. Patients were monitored clinically and radiologically every 2 weeks initially, then monthly. The study reported excellent outcomes in most cases, with no poor results and an average union time of 8 weeks. Complications were minimal, including hardware pain in two patients and one case of delayed union in the ulna.

The study advances the understanding of using elastic nailing for adolescent forearm fractures by demonstrating its effectiveness and minimal complications compared to traditional methods. Future studies could explore comparisons with other treatment modalities or refine techniques to further reduce complications such as delayed union or tendon injuries. The findings suggest that elastic nailing is a viable option for managing forearm fractures in adolescents when conservative treatments fail, emphasizing the importance of correct indications and technical precision during surgery.

Early Conversion to Below-Elbow Cast for Non-Reduced Diaphyseal Both-Bone Forearm Fractures in Children Is Safe: Preliminary Results of a Multicentre Randomised Controlled Trial [142]

This is a machine-generated summary of:

Colaris, Joost W.; Reijman, Max; Allema, Jan Hein; Biter, L. Ulas; Bloem, Rolf M.; van de Ven, Cees P.; de Vries, Mark R.; Kerver, Albert J. H.; Verhaar, Jan A. N. Early conversion to below-elbow cast for non-reduced diaphyseal both-bone forearm fractures in children is safe: preliminary results of a multicentre randomised controlled trial [142]

Published in: Archives of Orthopaedic and Trauma Surgery (2013)
Link to original: https://doi.org/10.1007/s00402-013-1812-8
Copyright of the summarized publication:
Springer-Verlag Berlin Heidelberg 2013
All rights reserved.

If you want to cite the papers, please refer to the original.

For technical reasons we could not place the page where the original quote is coming from.

Research Highlights

Both-bone diaphyseal forearm fractures are prevalent in children and are typically managed with above-elbow casts (AEC), intramedullary nails, or plates. While many fractures heal without complications, some children experience limitations in pronation and supination, with an average limitation of 10° reported in about 30% of cases. This limitation is thought to result from malunion of the radius and/or ulna and contracture of surrounding soft tissue. Now, a new study by Joost W. Colaris and colleagues investigates whether early conversion from AEC to below-elbow cast (BEC) affects the limitation of pronation and supination in children with non-reduced both-bone diaphyseal forearm fractures.

The study was a multicenter randomized controlled trial conducted across four Dutch hospitals, involving children under 16 years old with diaphyseal forearm fractures that did not require reduction. Participants were randomly assigned to receive either 6 weeks of AEC or 3 weeks of AEC followed by 3 weeks of BEC. The primary outcome was the limitation of pronation and supination compared to the non-injured arm 6 months post-trauma. Secondary outcomes included fracture re-displacement, complication rates, cast comfort, cosmetic outcomes, and daily life complaints. The study found no significant differences between the two groups in terms of pronation and supination limitations at 6 months follow-up. Both groups showed similar results in secondary outcomes, including fracture displacement rates.

The findings suggest that early conversion to BEC is a safe treatment option for non-reduced diaphyseal both-bone forearm fractures in children and does not significantly impact forearm rotation. However, the study noted a high incidence of fracture displacement during treatment, particularly within the first 3 weeks, indicating a need for careful monitoring during this period. Future studies could explore strategies to minimize displacement risk further and investigate other factors contributing to limitations in pronation and supination beyond malunion and soft tissue contracture.

Three-Dimensional Imaging of Children with Severe Limitation of Pronation/Supination After a Both-Bone Forearm Fracture [143]

This is a machine-generated summary of:

Colaris, Joost W.; Oei, Stanley; Reijman, Max; Holscher, Herma; Allema, Jan Hein; Verhaar, Jan A. N. Three-dimensional imaging of children with severe limitation of pronation/supination after a both-bone forearm fracture [143]
Published in: Archives of Orthopaedic and Trauma Surgery (2014)
Link to original: https://doi.org/10.1007/s00402-014-1922-y
Copyright of the summarized publication:
Springer-Verlag Berlin Heidelberg 2014
All rights reserved.

If you want to cite the papers, please refer to the original.

For technical reasons we could not place the page where the original quote is coming from.

Research Highlights

Both-bone forearm fractures in children typically heal without complications, but some cases result in significant limitations in forearm rotation, affecting daily activities. While malunion is often cited as a primary cause of these limitations, there is no consensus on its role, and other factors such as synostosis or impingement between the radius and ulna have been suggested. The involvement of soft tissue, particularly contractures of the interosseous membrane, remains unclear. Now, a new study by Joost W. Colaris and colleagues aims to evaluate the roles of rotational malunion, bony impingement, and interosseous membrane contractures using three-dimensional imaging techniques.

The study was conducted prospectively with children who sustained both-bone forearm fractures and were treated at four Dutch hospitals. Participants included those aged 4–16 years with significant limitations in pronation/supination post-fracture. The research employed a combination of clinical examinations, conventional radiography, computed tomography (CT), and magnetic resonance imaging (MRI) to assess fracture characteristics and potential causes of rotational limitation. CT scans were used to measure torsion angles of the radius and ulna to identify rotational malunions, while MRI was utilized to detect soft tissue abnormalities such as contractures or bony impingements. The study found rotational malunions in both the radius and ulna but did not detect interosseous membrane contractures or bony impingements.

The findings suggest that while rotational malunions are present in children with limited forearm rotation post-fracture, soft tissue abnormalities may not play a significant role. However, challenges in imaging due to anatomical development issues highlight the need for improved techniques. Future studies could benefit from using CT scans of both whole forearms with bone and soft tissue settings to enhance visualization and accuracy. Additionally, longer follow-up periods may help determine if growth-related corrections influence rotational limitations over time.

Refracture of Pediatric Both-Bone Diaphyseal Forearm Fracture Following Intramedullary Fixation with Kirschner Wires Is Likely to Occur in the Presence of Immature Radiographic Healing [144]

This is a machine-generated summary of:

Tsukamoto, Nobuaki; Mae, Takao; Yamashita, Akihisa; Hamada, Takahiro; Miura, Tatsuhiko; Iguchi, Takahiro; Tokunaga, Masami; Onizuka, Toshihiro; Momii, Kenta; Sadashima, Eiji; Nakashima, Yasuharu Refracture of pediatric both-bone diaphyseal forearm fracture following intramedullary fixation with Kirschner wires is likely to occur in the presence of immature radiographic healing [144]
Published in: European Journal of Orthopaedic Surgery & Traumatology (2020)
Link to original: https://doi.org/10.1007/s00590-020-02689-0
Copyright of the summarized publication:
Springer-Verlag France SAS, part of Springer Nature 2020
All rights reserved.

If you want to cite the papers, please refer to the original.

For technical reasons we could not place the page where the original quote is coming from.

Research Highlights

Diaphyseal forearm fractures are prevalent in children, accounting for a significant portion of pediatric fractures. Traditionally managed conservatively, there is a growing trend towards surgical intervention to minimize postoperative redisplacement risks. Intramedullary nailing, particularly with Kirschner wires (K-wires), is favored over plate fixation due to its minimally invasive nature and the high healing capacity in children. However, refracture at the primary fracture site remains a concern, especially in both-bone diaphyseal forearm fractures (PBDFFs). Now, a new study by Nobuaki Tsukamoto and colleagues investigates the risk factors associated with refracture in pediatric PBDFFs treated with intramedullary K-wires.

The study was conducted as a multicenter retrospective observational analysis across urban hospitals with board-certified orthopedic surgeons. It included patients aged 16 years or younger who sustained traumatic PBDFFs between January 2010 and December 2020. Exclusion criteria were applied to those treated with plate fixation or conservative methods. The researchers extracted demographic data, fracture characteristics, and postoperative outcomes from medical records and radiographs to identify refracture risk factors. Refracture was defined as a fracture occurring at the same site as the primary fracture during follow-up. The study found that refractures occurred in 6% of cases, often within 3 months post-surgery, and were associated with immature radiographic healing at the time of K-wire removal.

The study highlights that refractures are more likely when K-wires are removed prematurely before complete fracture healing is achieved. It suggests that burying K-wires to allow for longer retention may reduce refracture risk by ensuring adequate healing time. Future studies could focus on developing standardized radiographic assessment protocols to better judge fracture consolidation and prevent premature removal of stabilization devices. Additionally, advising patients and families to avoid strenuous activities until full radiographic healing is confirmed could further mitigate refracture risks. This research underscores the importance of careful postoperative management in pediatric forearm fractures treated with intramedullary nailing.

Treatment of Nonunion After Forearm Fractures in Children: A Conservative Approach [145]

This is a machine-generated summary of:

Loose, Oliver; Fernandez, Francisco; Morrison, Stewart; Schneidmüller, Dorien; Schmittenbecher, Peter; Eberhardt, Oliver Treatment of nonunion after forearm fractures in children: a conservative approach [145]
Published in: European Journal of Trauma and Emergency Surgery (2021)
Link to original: https://doi.org/10.1007/s00068-020-01583-y
Copyright of the summarized publication:
Springer-Verlag GmbH, DE part of Springer Nature 2021
All rights reserved.

If you want to cite the papers, please refer to the original.

For technical reasons we could not place the page where the original quote is coming from.

Research Highlights

Childhood forearm fractures are common, with an increasing incidence in recent years. While many fractures can be managed conservatively, displaced unstable fractures often require surgical intervention, typically using elastic stable intramedullary nailing (ESIN). Although complications are rare, nonunions can occur, particularly in specific fracture locations or due to technical errors during surgery. Now, a new study by Oliver Loose and colleagues examines the treatment of pediatric forearm nonunions and explores risk factors and the potential for conservative management.

The study conducted a retrospective analysis of pediatric patients treated for forearm nonunions at their institution. The researchers included cases with open growth plates and nonunion defined as a lack of bony consolidation months after surgery. They analyzed 27 cases, examining fracture types, initial management methods, and subsequent treatments. The study found that over a third of nonunions could be managed conservatively without surgery if there were no clinical symptoms like pain or decreased movement. Surgical intervention was necessary in cases with symptoms or significant misalignment, involving resection of the nonunion, bone grafting, and plate osteosynthesis.

This research highlights that conservative management is feasible for certain pediatric forearm nonunions when symptoms are absent. However, surgical treatment remains essential for symptomatic cases to ensure proper healing and function. The study suggests that factors such as open reduction and technical errors during initial osteosynthesis may contribute to nonunion development. Future studies could further explore these risk factors and refine treatment protocols to prevent nonunions in pediatric forearm fractures. Additionally, understanding the role of fracture location and patient-specific factors could enhance decision-making regarding conservative versus surgical management strategies.

Clinical Consequence of the 4-Week X-Ray Control After ESIN Osteosynthesis of Forearm Fractures in Children [146]

This is a machine-generated summary of:

Wegner, Erik; Laubach, Nora; Schippers, Phillip; Schierjott, Lotte; Shrotriya, Rujuta; Gercek, Erol; Drees, Philipp; Dietz, Sven-Oliver Clinical consequence of the 4-week X-ray control after ESIN osteosynthesis of forearm fractures in children [146]
Published in: European Journal of Trauma and Emergency Surgery (2025)
Link to original: https://doi.org/10.1007/s00068-024-02721-6
Copyright of the summarized publication:
The Author(s) 2025
License: OpenAccess CC BY 4.0

This article is licensed under a Creative Commons Attribution 4.0 International License, which permits use, sharing, adaptation, distribution and reproduction in any medium or format, as long as you give appropriate credit to the original author(s) and the source, provide a link to the Creative Commons licence, and indicate if changes were made. The images or other third party material in this article are included in the article's Creative Commons licence, unless indicated otherwise in a credit line to the material. If material is not included in the article's Creative Commons licence and your intended use is not permitted by statutory regulation or exceeds the permitted use, you will need to obtain permission directly from the copyright holder. To view a copy of this licence, visit http://creativecommons.org/licenses/by/4.0/.

If you want to cite the papers, please refer to the original.

For technical reasons we could not place the page where the original quote is coming from.

Research Highlights

Pediatric forearm fractures, particularly those involving the diaphysis, are common and often require surgical intervention. Elastic stable intramedullary nailing (ESIN) is a preferred treatment due to its minimally invasive nature and favorable outcomes. However, the lack of standardized postoperative guidelines leads to varied practices in radiological follow-ups, raising concerns about unnecessary radiation exposure in children. Now, a new study by Erik Wegner and colleagues investigates the necessity of routine X-ray follow-ups 4 weeks post-ESIN osteosynthesis in pediatric forearm shaft fractures.

The study was conducted at the University Medical Center in Mainz, Germany, involving a retrospective analysis of pediatric patients treated with ESIN for forearm shaft fractures. Patients were selected based on specific criteria, including age and fracture type, and underwent a standardized two-plane radiograph at the four-week follow-up. The researchers analyzed clinical and radiological data to identify any aberrant radiographic findings (ARFs) or non-radiographic deviations (nRDs). Statistical methods, including binary logistic regression, were employed to assess the correlation between nRDs and ARFs. The study found that ARFs were significantly more likely in patients with nRDs, particularly those with irregularities in their medical history.

The findings suggest that routine X-ray follow-ups may not be necessary if the clinical course is uneventful, as ARFs predominantly occurred alongside nRDs. This supports prioritizing thorough medical history and physical examination over indiscriminate radiological assessments. Future study could explore alternative diagnostic tools like fracture ultrasound for safer and cost-effective monitoring. While the study's monocentric and retrospective design may limit generalizability, it highlights the potential for reducing radiation exposure without compromising patient care. Implementing a more cautious approach to postoperative imaging could enhance safety and efficiency in managing pediatric forearm fractures.

Conclusion

Forearm fractures in children, particularly those involving the diaphysis, are common and often require surgery. Elastic stable intramedullary nailing is the preferred treatment for displaced fractures because it is minimally invasive and produces favorable outcomes.

Bibliography

1. Naranje SM, Erali RA, Warner WC, Sawyer JR, Kelly DM. Epidemiology of pediatric fractures presenting to emergency departments in the United States. J Pediatr Orthop. 2016;36(4):e45–8.
2. Ryan LM, Teach SJ, Searcy K, et al. Epidemiology of pediatric forearm fractures in Washington. DC J Trauma. 2010;69(4):200–5.
3. Chia B, Kozin SH, Herman MJ, Safier S, Abzug JM. Complications of pediatric distal radius and forearm fractures. Instr Course Lect. 2015;64:499–507.

4. Pace JL. Pediatric and adolescent forearm fractures: current controversies and treatment recommendations. J Am Acad Orthop Surg. 2016;24(11):780–8.
5. Li Y, James C, Byl N, Sessel J, Caird MS, Farley FA, et al. Obese children have different forearm fracture characteristics compared with normal-weight children. J Pediatr Orthop. 2020;40(2):e127–30.
6. Daruwalla JS. A study of radioulnar movements following fractures of the forearm in children. Clin Orthop. 1979;139:114–20.
7. Morrey BF, Askew LJ, Chao EY. A biomechanical study of normal functional elbow motion. J Bone Joint Surg Am. 1981;63(6):872–7.
8. Valone LC, Waites C, Tartarilla AB, Whited A, Sugimoto D, Bae DS, et al. Functional elbow range of motion in children and adolescents. J Pediatr Orthop. 2019;40(6):304–9. https://doi.org/10.1097/BPO.0000000000001467.
9. Primavesi R. Sticks and stones and broken bones. Can Fam Physician. 2011;57(1):45–6.
10. Barvelink B, Ploegmakers JJW, Harsevoort AGJ, Stevens M, Verheyen CC, Hepping AM, et al. The evolution of hand function during remodelling in nonreduced angulated paediatric forearm fractures: a prospective cohort study. J Pediatr Orthop B. 2020;29(2):172–8.
11. Voto SJ, Weiner DS, Leighley B. Redisplacement after closed reduction of forearm fractures in children. J Pediatr Orthop. 1990;10(1):79–84.
12. Helenius I, Lamberg TS, Kääriäinen S, Impinen A, Pakarinen MP. Operative treatment of fractures in children is increasing. A population-based study from Finland. J Bone Joint Surg Am. 2009;91(11):2612–6.
13. Cruz AI, Kleiner JE, DeFroda SF, Gil JA, Daniels AH, Eberson CP. Increasing rates of surgical treatment for paediatric diaphyseal forearm fractures: a national database study from 2000 to 2012. J Child Orthop. 2017;11(3):201–9.
14. Bowman EN, Mehlman CT, Lindsell CJ, Tamai J. Non-operative treatment of both-bone forearm shaft fractures in children: predictors of early radiographic failure. J Pediatr Orthop. 2011;31(1):23–32.
15. Cumming D, Mfula N, Jones JWM. Paediatric forearm fractures: the increasing use of elastic stable intra-medullary nails. Int Orthop. 2008;32(3):421–3.
16. Wall L, O'Donnell J, Schoenecker P, Keeler K, Dobbs M, Luhmann S, et al. Titanium elastic nailing radius and ulna fractures in adolescents. J Pediatr Orthop B. 2012;21(5):482–8.
17. Herman MJ, Marshall ST. Forearm fractures in children and adolescents: a practical approach. Hand Clin. 2006;22(1):55–67.
18. Zheng W, Tao Z, Chen C, Zhang C, Zhang H, Feng Z, et al. Comparison of three surgical fixation methods for dual-bone forearm fractures in older children: a retrospective cohort study. Int J Surg Lond Engl. 2018;51:10–6.
19. Elhalawany AS, Afifi A, Anbar A, Galal S. Hybrid fixation for adolescent both-bones diaphyseal forearm fractures: preliminary results of a prospective cohort study. J Clin Orthop Trauma. 2020;11(Suppl 1):S46–50.
20. Patel A, Li L, Anand A. Systematic review: functional outcomes and complications of intramedullary nailing versus plate fixation for both-bone diaphyseal forearm fractures in children. Injury. 2014;45(8):1135–43.
21. Baldwin K, Morrison MJ, Tomlinson LA, Ramirez R, Flynn JM. Both bone forearm fractures in children and adolescents, which fixation strategy is superior: plates or nails? A systematic review and meta-analysis of observational studies. J Orthop Trauma. 2014;28(1):e8–14.
22. Freese KP, Faulk LW, Palmer C, Baschal RM, Sibbel SE. A comparison of fixation methods in adolescent patients with diaphyseal forearm fractures. Injury. 2018;49(11):2053–7.
23. Borton D, Masterson E, O'Brien T. Distal forearm fractures in children: the role of hand dominance. J Pediatr Orthop. 1994;14:496–7.
24. Walsh WW, Belding NN, Taylor E, Nunley JA. The effect of upper extremity trauma on handedness. Am J Occup Ther. 1993;47:787–95.
25. Da Paz SN, Stalder A, Berger S, Ziebarth K. Range of motion of the upper extremity in a healthy pediatric population: introduction to normative data. Eur J Pediatr Surg. 2016;26:454–61. https://doi.org/10.1055/s-0035-1563676.

26. Richards RR. Chronic disorders of the forearm. J Bone Joint Surg Am. 1996;78-A:916–30. https://doi.org/10.2106/00004623-199606000-00017.
27. Schemitsch EH, Richards RR. The effect of malunion on functional outcome after plate fixation of fractures of both bones of the forearm in adults. J Bone Joint Surg. 1992;74A:1068–78. https://doi.org/10.2106/00004623-199274070-00014.
28. Price CT, Scott DS, Kurzner ME, Flynn JC. Malunited forearm fractures in children. J Pediatr Orthop. 1990;10(6):705–12. https://doi.org/10.1097/01241398-199011000-00001.
29. Roberts JA. Angulation of the radius in children's fractures. J Bone Joint Surg Br. 1986;68(5):751–4. https://doi.org/10.1302/0301-620X.68B5.3782237.
30. Kuderna H. Connection between deviated axis and impaired function after fractures of the forearm. Unfallchirurgie. 1980;6(1):7–13. https://doi.org/10.1007/bf02589444.
31. Valerio G, Gallè F, Mancusi C, Di Onofrio V, Guida P, Tramontano A, et al. Prevalence of overweight in children with bone fractures: a case control study. BMC Pediatr. 2012;22(12):166.
32. Kessler J, Koebnick C, Smith N, Adams A. Childhood obesity is associated with increased risk of most lower extremity fractures. Clin Orthop Relat Res. 2013;471:1199–207.
33. Goulding A, Jones IE, Taylor RW, Piggot JM, Taylor D. Dynamic and static tests of balance and postural sway in boys: effects of previous wrist bone fractures and high adiposity. Gait Posture. 2003;17:136–41.
34. Lerner ZF, Board WJ, Browning RC. Effects of obesity on lower extremity muscle function during walking at two speeds. Gait Posture. 2014;39:978–84.
35. Davidson PL, Goulding A, Chalmers DJ. Biomechanical analysis of arm fracture in obese boys. J Paediatr Child Health. 2003;39:657–64.
36. Khosla S, Melton LJ 3rd, Dekutoski MB, Achenbach SJ, Oberg AL, Riggs BL. Incidence of childhood distal forearm fractures over 30 years: a population-based study. JAMA. 2003;290(11):1479–85.
37. Farr JN, Dimitri P. The impact of fat and obesity on bone microarchitecture and strength in children. Calcif Tissue Int. 2017;100:500–13.
38. Smotkin-Tangorra M, Purushothaman R, Gupta A, Nejati G, Anhalt H, Ten S. Prevalence of vitamin D insufficiency in obese children and adolescents. J Pediatr Endocrinol Metab. 2007;20:817–23.
39. Manzoni P, Brambilla P, Pietrobelli A, Beccaria L, Bianchessi A, Mora S, et al. Influence of body composition on bone mineral content in children and adolescents. Am J Clin Nutr. 1996;64:603–7.
40. Dimitri P, Jacques RM, Paggiosi M, King D, Walsh J, Taylor ZA, et al. Leptin may play a role in bone microstructural alterations in obese children. J Clin Endocrinol Metab. 2015;100:594–602.
41. Leonard MB, Shults J, Wilson BA, Tershakovec AM, Zemel BS. Obesity during childhood and adolescence augments bone mass and bone dimensions. Am J Clin Nutr. 2004;80:514–23.
42. Goulding A, Jones IE, Taylor RW, Williams SM, Manning PJ. Bone mineral density and body composition in boys with distal forearm fractures: a dual-energy X-ray absorptiometry study. J Pediatr. 2001;139:509–15.
43. Templeton DL, Kelly AS, Steinberger J, Dengel DR. Lower relative bone mineral content in obese adolescents: role of non-weight bearing exercise. Pediatr Exerc Sci. 2010;22:557–68.
44. Dimitri P, Wales JK, Bishop N. Fat and bone in children: differential effects of obesity on bone size and mass according to fracture history. J Bone Miner Res. 2010;25:527–36.
45. Rocher E, El Hage R, Chappard C, Portier H, Rochefort GY, Benhamou CL. Bone mineral density, hip bone geometry, and calcaneus trabecular bone texture in obese and normal-weight children. J Clin Densitom. 2013;16:244–9.
46. Ducher G, Bass SL, Naughton GA, Eser P, Telford RD, Daly RM. Overweight children have a greater proportion of fat mass relative to muscle mass in the upper limbs than in the lower limbs: implications for bone strength at the distal forearm. Am J Clin Nutr. 2009;90:1104–11.
47. Ehehalt S, Binder G, Schurr N, Pfaff C, Ranke MB, Schweizer R, DISKUS-Study Group. The functional muscle-bone unit in obese children - altered bone structure leads to normal strength strain index. Exp Clin Endocrinol Diabetes. 2011;119:321–6.

48. Vandewalle S, Taes Y, Van Helvoirt M, Debode P, Herregods N, Ernst C, et al. Bone size and bone strength are increased in obese male adolescents. J Clin Endocrinol Metab. 2013;98:3019–28.
49. Janicka A, Wren TA, Sanchez MM, Dorey F, Kim PS, Mittelman SD, et al. Fat mass is not beneficial to bone in adolescents and young adults. J Clin Endocrinol Metab. 2007;92:143–7.
50. Wey HE, Binkley TL, Beare TM, Wey CL, Specker BL. Cross-sectional versus longitudinal associations of lean and fat mass with pQCT bone outcomes in children. J Clin Endocrinol Metab. 2011;96:106–14.
51. Rocher E, Chappard C, Jaffre C, Benhamou CL, Courteix D. Bone mineral density in prepubertal obese and control children: relation to body weight, lean mass, and fat mass. J Bone Miner Metab. 2008;26:73–8.
52. Farr JN, Chen Z, Lisse JR, Lohman TG, Going SB. Relationship of total body fat mass to weight- bearing bone volumetric density, geometry, and strength in young girls. Bone. 2010;46:977–84.
53. Yu EW, Thomas BJ, Brown JK, Finkelstein JS. Simulated increases in body fat and errors in bone mineral density measurements by DXA and QCT. J Bone Miner Res. 2012;27:119–24.
54. Liu D, Manske SL, Kontulainen SA, Tang C, Guy P, Oxland TR, et al. Tibial geometry is associated with failure load ex vivo: a MRI, pQCT and DXA study. Osteoporos Int. 2007;18:991–7.
55. Pollock NK, Laing EM, Hamrick MW, Baile CA, Hall DB, Lewis RD. Bone and fat relationships in postadolescent black females: a pQCT study. Osteoporos Int. 2011;22:655–65.
56. Marin JR, Abo AM, Arroyo AC, Doniger SJ, Fischer JW, Rempell R, Gary B, Holmes JF, Kessler DO, Lam SHF, Levine MC, Levy JA, Murray A, Ng L, Noble VE, Ramirez-Schrempp D, Riley DC, Saul T, Shah V, Sivitz AB, Tay ET, Teng D, Chaudoin L, Tsung JW, Vieira RL, Vitberg YM, Lewiss RE. Pediatric emergency medicine point-of-care ultrasound: summary of the evidence. Crit Ultrasound J. 2016;8(1):16.
57. Auten JD, Naheedy JH, Hurst ND, Pennock AT, Hollenbach KA, Kanegaye JT. Comparison of pediatric post-reduction fluoroscopic- and ultrasound forearm fracture images. Am J Emerg Med. 2018;37(5):832–8.
58. Rabiner JE, Khine H, Avner JR, et al. Accuracy of point-of-care ultrasonography for diagnosis of elbow fractures in children. Ann Emerg Med. 2013;61(1):9–17.
59. Hedelin H, Tingström C, Hebelka H, Karlsson J. Minimal training sufficient to diagnose pediatric wrist fractures with ultrasound. Crit Ultrasound J. 2017;9:11.
60. Smith VA, Goodman HJ, Strongwater A, Smith B. Treatment of pediatric both-bone forearm fractures: a comparison of operative techniques. J Pediatr Orthop. 2005;25:309–13. https://doi.org/10.1097/01.bpo.0000153943.45396.22.
61. Slim K, Nini E, Forestier D, et al. Methodological index for non-randomized studies (minors): development and validation of a new instrument. ANZ J Surg. 2003;73(9):712–6. https://doi.org/10.1046/j.1445-2197.2003.02748.x.
62. Yong B, Yuan Z, Li J, Li Y, Southern EP, Canavese F, Xu H. Single bone fixation versus both bone fixation for pediatric unstable forearm fractures: a systematic review and metaanalysis. Indian J Orthop. 2018;52(5):529–35. https://doi.org/10.4103/ortho.IJOrtho_125_17.
63. Sinikumpu JJ, Lautamo A, Pokka T, Serlo W. The increasing incidence of pediatric diaphyseal both-bone forearm fractures and their internal fixation during the last decade. Injury. 2012;43(3):362–6.
64. McGinley JC, Kozin SH. Interosseous membrane anatomy and functional mechanics. Clin Orthop Relat Res. 2001;108–122 https://doi.org/10.1097/00003086-200102000-00013.
65. Younger AS, Tredwell SJ, Mackenzie WG, et al. Accurate prediction of outcome after pediatric forearm fracture. J Pediatr Orthop. 1994;14:200–6. https://doi.org/10.1097/01241398-199403000-00013.

66. Vittas D, Larsen E, Torp-Pedersen S. Angular remodeling of midshaft forearm fractures in children. Clin Orthop Relat Res. 1991;265:261–4.
67. Bhaskar AR, Roberts JA. Treatment of unstable fractures of the forearm in children. Is plating of a single bone adequate? J Bone Joint Surg Br. 2001;83(2):253–8. https://doi.org/10.1302/0301-620x.83b2.10955.
68. Price CT. Acceptable alignment of forearm fractures in children: open reduction indications. J Pediatr Orthop. 2010;30(SUPPL. 2):82–4. https://doi.org/10.1097/BPO.0b013e3181bbf1b4.
69. Colaris J, Reijman M, Allema JH, Kraan G, Van Winterswijk P, De Vries M, Van De Ven C, Verhaar J. Single-bone intramedullary fixation of unstable both-bone diaphyseal forearm fractures in children leads to increased re-displacement: a multicentre randomised controlled trial. Arch Orthop Trauma Surg. 2013;133(8):1079–87. https://doi.org/10.1007/s00402-013-1763-0.
70. Cullen MC, Roy DR, Giza E, Crawford AH. Complications of intramedullary fixation of pediatric forearm fractures. J Pediatr Orthop. 1998;18(1):14–21.
71. Shoemaker SD, Comstock CP, Mubarak SJ, Wenger DR, Chambers HG. Intramedullary Kirschner wire fixation of open or unstable forearm fractures in children. J Pediatr Orthop. 1999;19(3):329–37.
72. Dietz JF, Bae DS, Reiff E, Zurakowski D, Waters PM. Single bone intramedullary fixation of the ulna in pediatric both bone forearm fractures: analysis of short-term clinical and radiographic results. J Pediatr Orthop. 1996;30(5):420–4.
73. Lee S, Nicol RO, Stott NS. Intramedullary fixation for pediatric unstable forearm fractures. Clin Orthop Relat Res. 2002;402:245–50.
74. Yung PS, Lam CY, Ng BK, Lam TP, Cheng JC. Percutaneous transphyseal intramedullary Kirschner wire pinning: a safe and effective procedure for treatment of displaced diaphyseal forearm fracture in children. J Pediatr Orthop. 2004;24:7–12.
75. Meier R, Prommersberger KJ, van Griensven M, Lanz U. Surgical correction of deformities of the distal radius due to fractures in pediatric patients. Arch Orthop Trauma Surg. 2004;124(1):1–9.
76. Boyer BA, Overton B, Schrader W, Riley P, Fleissner P. Position of immobilization for pediatric forearm fractures. J Pediatr Orthop. 2002;22(2):185–7.
77. Zimmermann R, Gabl M, Angermann P, Lutz M, Reinhart C, Kralinger F, Pechlaner S. Spätfolgen nach Frakturen im distalen Unterarmdrittel im Wachstumsalter. Handchir Mikrochir Plast Chir. 2000;32:1–8.
78. Colaris J, van der Linden M, Selles R, Coene N, Allema JH, Verhaar J. Pronation and supination after forearm fractures in children: reliability of visual estimation and conventional goniometry measurement. Injury. 2010;41(6):643–6.
79. Flynn JM, Waters PM. Single-bone fixation of both-bone forearm fractures. J Pediatr Orthop. 1996;16:655–9.
80. Houshian S, Bajaj SK. Forearm fractures in children. Single bone fixation with elastic stable intramedullary nailing in 20 cases. Injury. 2005;36(12):1421–6.
81. Myers GJ, Gibbons PJ, Glithero PR. Nancy nailing of diaphyseal forearm fractures. Single bone fixation for fractures of both bones. J Bone Joint Surg Br. 2004;86(4):581–4.
82. Altay M, Aktekin CN, Ozkurt B, Birinci B, Ozturk AM, Tabak AY. Intramedullary wire fixation for unstable forearm fractures in children. Injury. 2006;37(10):966–73.
83. Richter D, Ostermann PA, Ekkernkamp A, Muhr G, Hahn MP. Elastic intramedullary nailing: a minimally invasive concept in the treatment of unstable forearm fractures in children. J Pediatr Orthop. 1998;18(4):457–61.
84. Rennie L, et al. The epidemiology of fractures in children. Injury. 2007;38(8):913–22.
85. Truntzer J, Vopat ML, Kane PM, et al. Forearm diaphyseal fractures in the adolescent population: treatment and management. Eur J Orthop Surg Traumatol. 2015;25(2):201–9.
86. Teoh KH, Chee YH, Shortt N, Wilkinson G, Porter DE. An age- and sex-matched comparative study on both-bone diaphyseal paediatric forearm fracture. J Child Orthop. 2009;3:367–73. https://doi.org/10.1007/s11832-009-0197-2.

87. Poutoglidou F, Metaxiotis D, Kazas C, et al. Flexible intramedullary nailing in the treatment of forearm fractures in children and adolescents, a systematic review. J Orthop. 2020;20:125–30.
88. Reinhardt KR, Feldman DS, Green DW, Sala DA, Widmann RF, Scher DM. Comparison of intramedullary nailing to plating for both-bone forearm fractures in older children. J Pediatr Orthop. 2008;28:403–9. https://doi.org/10.1097/BPO.0b013e31816d71f2.
89. Abraham A, Kumar S, Chaudhry S, Ibrahim T. Surgical interventions for diaphyseal fractures of the radius and ulna in children. Cochrane Database Syst Rev. 2011; https://doi.org/10.1002/14651858.CD007907.pub2.
90. Garg NK, Ballal MS, Malek IA, Webster RA, Bruce CE. Use of elastic stable intramedullary nailing for treating unstable forearm fractures in children. J Trauma. 2008;65:109–15.
91. Westacott DJ, Jordan RW, Cooke SJ. Functional outcome following intramedullary nailing or plate and screw fixation of paediatric diaphyseal forearm fractures: a systematic review. J Child Orthop. 2012;6(1):75–80.
92. Zhu S, Yang D, Gong C, Chen C, Chen L. A novel hybrid fixation versus dual plating for both-bone forearm fractures in older children: a prospective comparative study. Int J Surg. 2019;70:19–24.
93. Zeybek H, Akti S. Comparison of three different surgical fixation techniques in pediatric forearm double fractures. Cureus. 2021;13:e16931.
94. Schemitsch EH, Jones D, Henley MB, Tencer AF. A comparison of malreduction after plate and intramedullary nail fixation of forearm fractures. J Orthop Trauma. 1995;9:8–16.
95. Flynn JM, Jones KJ, Garner MR, Goebel J. Eleven years experience in the operative management of pediatric forearm fractures. J Pediatr Orthop. 2010;30:313–9.
96. Weinberg A-M, Kasten P, Castellani C, et al. Which axial deviation results in limitations of pro- and supination following diaphyseal lower arm fractures in children. Eur J Trauma. 2001;27:309.
97. Lascombes P, Prevot J, Ligier JN, Metaizeau JP, Poncelet T. Elastic stable intramedullary nailing in forearm shaft fractures in children: 85 cases. J Pediatr Orthop. 1990;10:167–71.
98. Ogden JA. Radius and ulna. In: Skeletal injury in the child. 3rd ed. New York: Springer; 2000. p. 567–649.
99. Nilsson BE, Obrant K. The range of motion following fracture of the shaft of the forearm in children. Acta Orthop Scand. 1977;48(6):600–2.
100. Yasutomi T, Nakatsuchi Y, Koike H, Uchiyama S. Mechanism of limitation of pronation/supination of the forearm in geometric models of deformities of the forearm bones. Clin Biomech. 2002;17(6):456–63. https://doi.org/10.1016/s0268-0033(02)00034-7.
101. Franklin CC, Robinson J, Noonan K, Flynn JM. Evidence-based medicine: management of pediatric forearm fractures. J Pediatr Orthop. 2012;32(Suppl 2):S131–4.
102. Daruwalla JS. A study of radioulnar movements following fractures of the forearm in children. Clin Orthop Relat Res. 1979;139:114–20.
103. Colaris JW, Allema JH, Biter LU, de Vries MR, van de Ven CP, Bloem RM, et al. Re-displacement of stable distal both-bone forearm fractures in children: a randomised controlled multicentre trial. Injury. 2013;44(4):498–503. https://doi.org/10.1016/j.injury.2012.11.001.
104. Colaris J, Reijman M, Allema JH, Kraan G, van Winterswijk P, de Vries M, et al. Single-bone intramedullary fixation of unstable both-bone diaphyseal forearm fractures in children leads to increased re-displacement: a multicentre randomised controlled trial. Arch Orthop Trauma Surg. 2013;133(8):1079–87.
105. Bronstein AJ, Trumble TE, Tencer AF. The effects of distal radius fracture malalignment on forearm rotation: a cadaveric study. J Hand Surg Am. 1997;22(2):258–62.
106. Trousdale RT, Linscheid RL. Operative treatment of malunited fractures of the forearm. J Bone Joint Surg Am. 1995;77(6):894–902.
107. Bindra RR, Cole RJ, Yamaguchi K, Evanoff BA, Pilgram TK, Gilula LA, et al. Quantification of the radial torsion angle with computerized tomography in cadaver specimens. J Bone Joint Surg Am. 1997;79(6):833–7.

108. Aufauvre B, Garcier JM, Boisgard S, Tanguy A. Measurement of the torsion of the two bones of the forearm: evaluation of tomodensitometric reference points. Bull Assoc Anat. 1996;80(248):5–8.
109. Matthews LS, Kaufer H, Garver DF, Sonstegard DA. The effect on supination-pronation of angular malalignment of fractures of both bones of the forearm. J Bone Joint Surg Am. 1982;64(1):14–7.
110. Tarr RR, Garfinkel AI, Sarmiento A. The effects of angular and rotational deformities of both bones of the forearm. An in vitro study. J Bone Joint Surg Am. 1984;66(1):65–70.
111. Nakamura T, Yabe Y, Horiuchi Y. A biomechanical analysis of pronation-supination of the forearm using magnetic resonance imaging: dynamic changes of the interosseous membrane of the forearm during pronation-supination. Nippon Seikeigeka Gakkai Zasshi. 1994;68(1):14–25.
112. Amit Y, Salai M, Chechik A, Blankstein A, Horoszowski H. Closing intramedullary nailing for the treatment of diaphyseal forearm fractures in adolescence: a preliminary report. J Pediatr Orthop. 1985;5(2):S143–6.
113. Griffet J, el Hayek T, Baby M. Intramedullary nailing of forearm fractures in children. J Pediatr Orthop B. 1999;8(2):88–9.
114. Kang SN, Mangwani J, Ramachandran M, Paterson JM, Barry M. Elastic intramedullary nailing of paediatric fractures of the forearm: a decade of experience in a teaching hospital in the United Kingdom. J Bone Joint Surg Br. 2011;93(2):262–5.
115. Schwarz N, Pienaar S, Schwarz AF, Jelen M, Styhler W, Mayr J. Refracture of the forearm in children. J Bone Joint Surg. 1996;78-B:740–4.
116. Bould M, Bannister GC. Refractures of the radius and ulna in children. Injury Int J Care Injured. 1999;30:583–6.
117. Baitner AC, Perry A, Lalonde FD, Bastrom TP, Pawelek J, Newton PO. The healing forearm fracture. A matched comparison of forearm fractures. J Pediatr Orthop. 2007;27(7):743–7.
118. Makki D, Kheiran A, Gadiyar R, Ricketts D. Refractures following removal of plates and elastic nails from paediatric forearms. J Pediatr Orthop B. 2014;23:221–6. https://doi.org/10.1097/BPB.0000000000000041.
119. Martus JE, Preston RK, Schoenecker JG, Lovejoy SA, Green NE, Mencio GA. Complications and outcomes of diaphyseal forearm fracture intramedullary nailing: a comparison of pediatric and adolescent age groups. J Pediatr Orthop. 2013;33:598–607.
120. Kelly BA, Miller P, Shore BJ, Waters PM, Bae DS. Exposed versus buried intramedullary implants for pediatric forearm fractures: a comparison of complications. J Pediatr Orthop. 2014;34(8):749–55.
121. Rousset M, Mansour M, Samba A, Pereira B, Canavese F. Risk factors for re-fracture in children with diaphyseal fracture for the forearm treated with elastic stable intramedullary nailing. Eur J Orthop Surg Traumatol. 2016;26:145–52. https://doi.org/10.1007/s00590-015-1715-1.
122. Franklin CC, Wren T, Ferkel E, Arkader A. Predictors of conversion from conservative to operative treatment of pediatric forearm fractures. J Pediatr Orthop B. 2014;23(2):150–4. https://doi.org/10.1097/BPB.0000000000000018.
123. Fernandez FF, Egenolf M, Carsten C, Holz F, Schneider S, Wentzensen A. Unstable diaphyseal fractures of both bones of the forearm in children: plate fixation versus intramedullary nailing. Injury. 2005;36:1210–6. https://doi.org/10.1016/j.injury.2005.03.004.
124. Barry M, Paterson JMH. Aspects of current management: flexible intramedullary nails for fractures in children. J Bone Joint Surg Br. 2004;86-B:947–53.
125. Di Gennaro GL, Stilli S, Trisolino G. Post-traumatic forearm nonunion in healthy skeletally immature children: a report on 15 cases. Injury. 2017;48(3):724–30. https://doi.org/10.1016/j.injury.2017.01.023.
126. Ogonda L, Wong-Chung J, Wray R, Canavan B. Delayed union and non-union of the ulna following intramedullary nailing in children. J Pediatr Orthop B. 2004;13:330–3.
127. Mehlman CT, Wall EJ. Injuries to the shafts of the radius and ulna. In: Beaty JH, Kessar JR, editors. Rockwood and Wilkins' fractures in children. 6th ed. Philadelphia: Lippincott, Williams & Wilkins; 2006. p. 399–441.

128. Fernandez FF, Eberhardt O, Langendörfer M, Wirth T. Nonunion of forearm shaft fractures in children after intramedullary nailing. J Pediatr Orthop B. 2009;18(6):289–95. https://doi.org/10.1097/BPB.0b013e32832f5b20.
129. Großer K. Behandlung der kindlichen Unterarmschaftfraktur. Trauma Berufskrankheit. 2018;20(1):12–6. https://doi.org/10.1007/s10039-017-0338-7.
130. Oehme F, et al. Routine X-rays after the osteosynthesis of distal radius and ankle fractures. Dtsch Arztebl Int. 2022;119(16):279–84. https://doi.org/10.3238/arztebl.m2022.0099.
131. Schmittenbecher PP, Fitze G, Godeke J, Kraus R, Schneidmuller D. Delayed healing of forearm shaft fractures in children after intramedullary nailing. J Pediatr Orthop. 2008;28:303–6.
132. Caruso G, Caldari E, Sturla FD, Caldaria A, Re DL, Pagetti P, Palummieri F, Massari L. Management of pediatric forearm fractures: what is the best therapeutic choice? A narrative review of the literature. Musculoskelet Surg. 2020; https://doi.org/10.1007/s12306-020-00684-6.
133. Hassan FOA. Hand dominance and gender in forearm fractures in children. Strategies Trauma Limb Reconstr. 2008; https://doi.org/10.1007/s11751-008-0048-6.
134. Wongcharoenwatana J, Eamsobhana P, Chotigavanichaya C, Ariyawatkul T, Kaewpornsawan K. The effects of maximal radial bowing on forearm rotation in pediatric diaphyseal forearm fractures. Musculoskelet Surg. 2021; https://doi.org/10.1007/s12306-021-00728-5.
135. Franceschi R, Radetti G, Soffiati M, Maines E. Forearm fractures in overweight—obese children and adolescents: a matter of bone density, bone geometry or body composition? Calcif Tissue Int. 2022; https://doi.org/10.1007/s00223-022-00971-3.
136. Gillon JT, Gorn M, Wilkinson M. Comparison of ultrasound-guided versus fluoroscopy-guided reduction of forearm fractures in children. Emerg Radiol. 2020; https://doi.org/10.1007/s10140-020-01862-6.
137. Ahmed AM, Said E, Addosooki A, Attya HA, Awad AK, Ahmed EH, Tammam H. Intramedullary versus plate fixation of both bone forearm fractures in skeletally immature patients: a systematic review and meta-analysis. Eur J Orthop Surg Traumatol. 2024; https://doi.org/10.1007/s00590-024-03925-7.
138. Khaled M, Fadle AA, Attia AK, Sami A, Hafez A, Oyoun A, Nariman. Single-bone versus both-bone plating of unstable paediatric both-bone forearm fractures. A randomized controlled clinical trial. Int Orthop. 2021; https://doi.org/10.1007/s00264-021-05097-z.
139. Ishihara N, Tokutake K, Takegami Y, Asami Y, Kumagai H, Ota H, Kimura Y, Ohshima K, Imagama S. An age-matched comparative study on intramedullary nailing and plate fixation of both-bone diaphyseal forearm fracture in adolescents. Eur J Orthop Surg Traumatol. 2023; https://doi.org/10.1007/s00590-023-03679-8.
140. Romeih MA, Khaled A. Effectiveness of hybrid fixation in the treatment of proximal Diaphyseal both bone forearm fractures in adolescents. Indian J Orthop. 2024; https://doi.org/10.1007/s43465-024-01300-6.
141. Ali AM. Outcome of elastic nailing of diaphyseal forearm fractures in adolescents after failure of conservative management. Eur J Orthop Surg Traumatol. 2011; https://doi.org/10.1007/s00590-011-0914-7.
142. Colaris JW, Reijman M, Allema JH, Biter LU, Bloem RM, van de Ven CP, de Vries MR, Kerver AJH, Verhaar JAN. Early conversion to below-elbow cast for non-reduced diaphyseal both-bone forearm fractures in children is safe: preliminary results of a multicentre randomised controlled trial. Arch Orthop Trauma Surg. 2013; https://doi.org/10.1007/s00402-013-1812-8.
143. Colaris JW, Oei S, Reijman M, Holscher H, Allema JH, Verhaar JAN. Three-dimensional imaging of children with severe limitation of pronation/supination after a both-bone forearm fracture. Arch Orthop Trauma Surg. 2014; https://doi.org/10.1007/s00402-014-1922-y.
144. Tsukamoto N, Mae T, Yamashita A, Hamada T, Miura T, Iguchi T, Tokunaga M, Onizuka T, Momii K, Sadashima E, Nakashima Y. Refracture of pediatric both-bone diaphyseal forearm fracture following intramedullary fixation with Kirschner wires is likely to occur in the presence of immature radiographic healing. Eur J Orthop Surg Traumatol. 2020; https://doi.org/10.1007/s00590-020-02689-0.

145. Loose O, Fernandez F, Morrison S, Schneidmüller D, Schmittenbecher P, Eberhardt O. Treatment of nonunion after forearm fractures in children: a conservative approach. Eur J Trauma Emerg Surg. 2021; https://doi.org/10.1007/s00068-020-01583-y.
146. Wegner E, Laubach N, Schippers P, Schierjott L, Shrotriya R, Gercek E, Drees P, Dietz S-O. Clinical consequence of the 4-week X-ray control after ESIN osteosynthesis of forearm fractures in children. Eur J Trauma Emerg Surg. 2025; https://doi.org/10.1007/s00068-024-02721-6.

Acute Monteggia Fracture

12

Introduction by the Author

A Monteggia fracture, first described by Giovanni Battista Monteggia, is an injury involving an ulnar fracture and an associated radial head dislocation. This rare injury usually affects children between the ages of 4 and 10, making up around 1% of all upper limb fractures in this age group. If left undetected or untreated, it can lead to elbow joint dysfunction, chronic pain, and degenerative arthritis. These injuries can be easily overlooked if not properly examined or followed up, posing significant medical and legal issues. The rate of missed or misdiagnosed fractures in children is higher than in adults, ranging from 16% to 33%.

According to the Bado classification system, they can be classified into four types based on the direction of the dislocation (anterior, posterior, or lateral) and whether both bones are fractured (type 4: dislocation of the radial head in any direction with fractures of the radius and ulna).

Treatment options for acute Monteggia fractures in children range from casting to surgical intervention.

Manual reduction and cast immobilization are options, but they often result in failed reduction or redislocation, so surgical intervention is generally recommended. Maintaining the length stability of the ulna and radial head is critical to treatment success.

Elastic stable intramedullary nailing and screw and plate fixation can achieve optimal clinical, functional, and radiographic outcomes, effectively stabilizing the fracture.

Elastic intramedullary nailing results in lower rates of recurrent radial head subluxation and loss of ulnar alignment that require subsequent operative treatment. Plate fixation, on the other hand, provides excellent stability and enables early motion. It can also manage proximal and distal fractures, and it

© The Author(s), under exclusive license to Springer Nature Switzerland AG 2026
F. Canavese, *Advances in Pediatric Extremity Fracture Management*, https://doi.org/10.1007/978-3-032-33306-3_12

does not require a cast during the postoperative period. Patients treated with elastic intramedullary nailing also experience shorter operating times and less blood loss than those treated with screw and plate fixation due to the former's less invasive nature.

Despite these differences in surgical metrics, there are no significant differences in functional outcomes between the two groups. Ultrasound-guided treatment for Monteggia fractures in children offers several advantages, including reduced trauma and radiation exposure while achieving satisfactory clinical outcomes.

12.1 Machine Generated Summaries

Disclaimer: The summaries in this chapter were generated from Springer Nature publications using abstractive AI auto-summarization: An abstraction-based summarizer creates new text based on deep learning. New phrases are created to summarize the content. As the constituted sentences are machine selected, they may not fully reflect the body of the work, so we strongly advise that the original content is read and cited. The auto-generated summaries were curated by the author(s) to meet Springer Nature publication standards.

Ultrasound, a New Adjuvant Method for Treating Acute Monteggia Fracture in Children [32]

This is a machine-generated summary of:

Fan, YongFei; Liu, QiXin; Yu, XueDi; Zhang, JianQiang; Wang, Wei; Liu, ChaoYu Ultrasound, a new adjuvant method for treating acute Monteggia fracture in children [32]
Published in: Journal of Orthopaedic Surgery and Research (2023)
Link to original: https://doi.org/10.1186/s13018-023-04075-y
Copyright of the summarized publication:
The Author(s) 2023
License: OpenAccess CC BY + CC0 4.0

This article is licensed under a Creative Commons Attribution 4.0 International License, which permits use, sharing, adaptation, distribution and reproduction in any medium or format, as long as you give appropriate credit to the original author(s) and the source, provide a link to the Creative Commons licence, and indicate if changes were made. The images or other third-party material in this article is included in the article's Creative Commons licence, unless indicated otherwise in a credit line to the material. If material is not included in the article's Creative Commons licence and your intended use is not permitted by statutory regulation or exceeds the permitted use, you will need to obtain permission directly from the copyright holder. To view a copy of this licence, visit http://creativecommons.org/licenses/by/4.0/. The Creative Commons Public Domain Dedication waiver (http://creativecommons.org/publicdomain/zero/1.0/) applies to the data made available in this article, unless otherwise stated in a credit line to the data.

If you want to cite the papers, please refer to the original.

For technical reasons we could not place the page where the original quote is coming from.

Research Highlights

Monteggia fractures, a rare type of injury primarily affecting children, account for a small percentage of all upper limb fractures in this demographic. If not promptly identified and treated, these fractures can lead to significant complications such as elbow joint dysfunction and chronic pain. Traditional treatment methods involve manual reduction and cast immobilization, but these approaches often result in failure of reduction or redislocation. Surgical intervention is recommended for more complex cases. Now, a new study by YongFei Fan and colleagues explores the use of ultrasound-guided closed reduction and fixation methods in treating acute Monteggia lesions, aiming to improve outcomes while minimizing radiation exposure.

In this retrospective analysis, the authors examined cases of acute Monteggia fractures treated with either Kirschner wire or elastic intramedullary nail fixation under ultrasound guidance. The study included patients aged around 8 years on average, with various types of Monteggia fractures classified according to the Bado system. Surgeries were performed under general anesthesia by a consistent surgical team, utilizing ultrasound to guide fracture reduction and assess soft tissue conditions. This method allowed for precise fracture alignment and minimized radiation exposure compared to traditional fluoroscopy. Postoperative management involved immobilization with a long-arm cast followed by rehabilitation exercises to restore joint function. The study reported excellent outcomes in terms of fracture reduction quality and elbow joint function, with no significant complications observed.

The study by Fan et al. demonstrates that ultrasound-guided treatment for Monteggia fractures in children offers several advantages, including reduced trauma and radiation exposure while achieving satisfactory clinical outcomes. The use of ultrasound allows for dynamic monitoring and precise fracture alignment, potentially expanding its application in pediatric orthopedic surgery. Future studies could focus on larger sample sizes and longer follow-up periods to further validate these findings and explore the integration of ultrasound technology into standard treatment protocols for pediatric fractures.

Correlation Between Inner Epiphysis Ulna Radius Length Ratio and Prognosis of Monteggia Fractures in Children: A Multicenter Study [33]

This is a machine-generated summary of:

Feng, Siyin; Yi, Yangfei; Song, Zhenqi; Lu, Junjie; Zhou, Qingfeng; Wen, Jie; Xiao, Sheng; Li, Yufei Correlation between inner epiphysis ulna radius length ratio and prognosis of Monteggia fractures in children: a multicenter study [33]
Published in: Scientific Reports (2025)
Link to original: https://doi.org/10.1038/s41598-025-89751-1
Copyright of the summarized publication:
The Author(s) 2025
License: OpenAccess CC BY-NC-ND 4.0

This article is licensed under a Creative Commons Attribution-NonCommercial-NoDerivatives 4.0 International License, which permits any non-commercial use, sharing, distribution and reproduction in any medium or format, as long as you give appropriate credit to the original author(s) and the source, provide a link to the Creative Commons licence, and indicate if you modified the licensed material. You do not have permission under this licence to share adapted material derived from this article or parts of it. The images or other third party material in this article are included in the article's Creative Commons licence, unless indicated otherwise in a credit line to the material. If material is not included in the article's Creative Commons licence and your intended use is not permitted by statutory regulation or exceeds the permitted use, you will need to obtain permission directly from the copyright holder. To view a copy of this licence, visit http://creativecommons.org/licenses/by-nc-nd/4.0/.

If you want to cite the papers, please refer to the original.

For technical reasons we could not place the page where the original quote is coming from.

Research Highlights

Among children's fractures, radius and ulna fractures are the most frequently observed, with a higher rate of missed or misdiagnosed cases compared to adults due to the abundance of cartilage that is not fully visible on X-rays. Monteggia fractures, a rare type of forearm fracture in children, involve complex injuries to the ulna and often include dislocation or fracture of the radial head. Incorrect or delayed diagnosis can severely affect bone growth and development, leading to functional impairments and deformities. Now, a new study by Siyin Feng and colleagues aims to identify an appropriate method for evaluating ulna and radius length in healthy children, establish normal values for the inner-epiphysis ulna-radius length ratio, validate this ratio in children with Monteggia fractures, and investigate its role in forearm function.

The study retrospectively analyzed anteroposterior and lateral X-ray images of normal radius and ulna from outpatients suspected of having fractures but with negative results. The researchers collected data from several hospitals between January and December. They calculated the inner-epiphyseal ulna-radius length ratio by measuring the distance from the tip of the olecranon to the midpoint of the distal epiphyseal plate of the ulna and compared it with similar measurements on radiographs from children with Monteggia fractures post-surgery. The study included two groups: Group A with acute Monteggia fractures treated within weeks, and Group B with chronic Monteggia fractures treated after weeks. Surgical techniques involved ulna reduction and internal fixation for acute cases, while chronic cases underwent ulna osteotomy and lengthening. Postoperative follow-ups assessed elbow function using X-rays and Mayo Elbow Performance Scores.

The study found that while both ulna and radius lengths increased with age, their length ratio at the epiphyseal plate remained relatively constant across age groups. Restoring this ratio during surgery resulted in favorable outcomes for elbow joint function in both acute and chronic Monteggia fracture cases. The inner-epiphyseal ulna-radius length ratio can be applied in correcting various pediatric forearm deformities, providing a foundation for extending interosseous distance between the radius and ulna. Future study could involve a prospective multicenter approach to further validate these findings, offering more robust evidence for clinical application in pediatric orthopedic surgery.

Comparison of the Midterm Result Between Locking Plate and Elastic Intramedullary Nail Treating Oblique Ulnar Fracture Bado Type I Acute Monteggia Fracture in Pediatric Patients [34]

This is a machine-generated summary of:

Vithran, Djandan Tadum Arthur; Song, Zhenqi; Wang, Kongjian; Tang, Zhongwen; Xiang, Feng; Wen, Jie; Xiao, Sheng Comparison of the midterm result between locking plate and elastic intramedullary nail treating oblique ulnar fracture Bado type I acute monteggia fracture in pediatric patients [34]
Published in: BMC Musculoskeletal Disorders (2022)
Link to original: https://doi.org/10.1186/s12891-022-05809-5
Copyright of the summarized publication:
The Author(s) 2022
License: OpenAccess CC BY + CC0 4.0

This article is licensed under a Creative Commons Attribution 4.0 International License, which permits use, sharing, adaptation, distribution and reproduction in any medium or format, as long as you give appropriate credit to the original author(s) and the source, provide a link to the Creative Commons licence, and indicate if changes were made. The images or other third party material in this article are included in the article's Creative Commons licence, unless indicated otherwise in a credit line to the material. If material is not included in the article's Creative Commons licence and your intended use is not permitted by statutory regulation or exceeds the permitted use, you will need to obtain permission directly from the copyright holder. To view a copy of this licence, visit http://creativecommons.org/licenses/by/4.0/. The Creative Commons Public Domain Dedication waiver (http://creativecommons.org/publicdomain/zero/1.0/) applies to the data made available in this article, unless otherwise stated in a credit line to the data.

If you want to cite the papers, please refer to the original.

For technical reasons we could not place the page where the original quote is coming from.

Research Highlights

Monteggia fractures, first described by Giovanni Batista Monteggia, involve an ulnar fracture with an associated radial head dislocation and are classified into four types by Bado. These fractures are rare, predominantly affecting children aged 4–10 years, and require acute management to ensure proper healing. Treatment options for Bado type I acute Monteggia fractures in children range from conservative casting to surgical interventions. The critical aspect of treatment is maintaining the length stability of the ulna and radial head. Now, a new study by Djandan Tadum Arthur Vithran and colleagues compares two surgical methods—elastic intramedullary nailing (EIN) and locking compression plate (LCP) fixation—to improve understanding of the optimal therapeutic approach for these fractures.

The study enrolled children with Bado type I acute Monteggia fractures treated at their department between January and August. Participants were divided into two groups based on the surgical method used: EIN or LCP. The EIN group underwent a minimally invasive procedure involving a small incision and insertion of an elastic nail into the ulna, while the LCP group received open reduction and plate fixation through a larger incision. Both procedures aimed to achieve stable ulnar alignment and concentric reduction of the radial head, confirmed via fluoroscopy. Post-surgery, patients were immobilized with a splint or cast for 3–4 weeks. Data on operation time, blood loss, Mayo Elbow Performance Score (MEPS), range of motion (ROM), and range of rotation (ROR) were collected pre-operation, 3 months post-operation, and at the last follow-up.

The study found that both EIN and LCP methods resulted in significant improvements in MEPS, ROM, and ROR at follow-up points, indicating effective stabilization of the fracture. However, the EIN group experienced shorter operation times and less blood loss compared to the LCP group due to its less invasive nature. Despite these differences in surgical metrics, there were no significant differences in functional outcomes between the two groups. This suggests that EIN can provide similar stability to LCP for oblique ulnar fractures while offering advantages in terms of reduced surgical time and blood loss. Future study could focus on long-term outcomes and further refine criteria for choosing between these surgical options based on fracture characteristics.

Simultaneous Monteggia Type I Fracture Equivalent with Ipsilateral Fracture of the Distal Radius and Ulna in a Child: A Case Report [31]

This is a machine-generated summary of:

Sood, Asheesh; Khan, Osman; Bagga, Tajesh Simultaneous monteggia type I fracture equivalent with ipsilateral fracture of the distal radius and ulna in a child: a case report [31]
Published in: Journal of Medical Case Reports (2008)
Link to original: https://doi.org/10.1186/1752-1947-2-190
Copyright of the summarized publication:
Sood et al.; licensee BioMed Central Ltd. 2008
License: OpenAccess CC BY 2.0

This article is published under license to BioMed Central Ltd. This is an Open Access article distributed under the terms of the Creative Commons Attribution License (http://creativecommons.org/licenses/by/2.0), which permits unrestricted use, distribution, and reproduction in any medium, provided the original work is properly cited.

If you want to cite the papers, please refer to the original.

For technical reasons we could not place the page where the original quote is coming from.

Research Highlights

Monteggia lesions, characterized by a dislocation of the radial head and fracture of the ulna, are uncommon in children. These injuries become even rarer when combined with fractures of the distal radius and ulna. Now, a new study by Asheesh Sood and colleagues reports a unique case of a type I Monteggia fracture equivalent with an ipsilateral fracture of the distal radius and ulna in a child, marking the first documented instance of this specific injury combination.

The study details the case of an 8-year-old girl who sustained these injuries after falling from a swing. Initial examination revealed severe deformities in her wrist and elbow, but no neurovascular deficits. Radiographs confirmed complex fractures, including a complete fracture of the olecranon and radial neck, along with a Salter-Harris type II fracture of the distal radius and ulna. The treatment involved surgical intervention under general anesthesia: open reduction and internal fixation of the ulna using a dynamic compression plate, reduction of the radial neck under direct vision, and manipulation of the wrist fracture under image intensifier control. Postoperatively, the patient developed symptoms of median nerve compression, which were resolved through urgent carpal tunnel decompression and Kirschner-wire stabilization.

The successful management of this rare injury combination underscores the importance of thorough clinical and radiological examination to avoid missing associated injuries. The study highlights that early recognition and prompt surgical intervention can lead to favorable outcomes despite the complexity and rarity of such cases. Future study could focus on understanding the mechanisms leading to simultaneous two-level forearm fractures in children to improve diagnostic protocols and treatment strategies. Additionally, exploring minimally invasive techniques for similar cases could enhance recovery times and reduce complications.

Type III Monteggia Injury with Ipsilateral Type II Salter Harris Injury of the Distal Radius and Ulna in a Child: A Case Report [35]

This is a machine-generated summary of:

Williams, Huw LM; Madhusudhan, Thayur R; Sinha, Amit Type III monteggia injury with ipsilateral type II Salter Harris injury of the distal radius and ulna in a child: a case report [35]

Published in: BMC Research Notes (2014)
Link to original: https://doi.org/10.1186/1756-0500-7-156

Copyright of the summarized publication:
Williams et al.; licensee BioMed Central Ltd. 2014

Copyright comment: This article is published under license to BioMed Central Ltd. This is an Open Access article distributed under the terms of the Creative Commons Attribution License (http://creativecommons.org/licenses/by/2.0), which permits unrestricted use, distribution, and reproduction in any medium, provided the original work is properly credited. The Creative Commons Public Domain Dedication waiver (http://creativecommons.org/publicdomain/zero/1.0/) applies to the data made available in this article, unless otherwise stated.

If you want to cite the papers, please refer to the original.

For technical reasons we could not place the page where the original quote is coming from.

Research Highlights

Monteggia fracture patterns, though rare in children, require appropriate treatment to prevent long-term disability of the elbow and forearm. These injuries can be easily overlooked if not properly examined or followed up. Both operative and non-operative treatments are viable, with the choice depending on the injury pattern and stability of reduction. Now, a new study by Huw LM Williams and colleagues highlights a rare case of Monteggia fracture with associated distal radius and ulna injury in a child, emphasizing the importance of thorough clinical examination and full-length radiographs to avoid misdiagnosis, especially by junior doctors in emergency settings.

In this case study, a 5-year-old boy presented with pain and swelling in his right wrist after falling from a height. Initial examination revealed deformity and tenderness in the wrist and forearm, but no neurovascular deficits or other skeletal injuries. Radiographs confirmed a Type II Salter Harris injury to the distal radius and ulna, along with an angulated ulna fracture and anterolateral dislocation of the radial head. The patient underwent anesthesia for manipulation of the distal radius fracture, which was stabilized with K-wires. The radial head was relocated using a closed method and stabilized with radio-capitellar wiring due to instability. The ulna fracture was treated non-operatively with immobilization in a plaster cast. Post-operative monitoring for compartment syndrome was conducted, followed by weekly clinic visits for radiographic follow-up. After wire removal and physiotherapy, the patient regained full range of motion except for slight limitations in supination.

The study underscores the critical need for careful clinical assessment and appropriate imaging to identify Monteggia fractures in children accurately. It highlights that while non-operative methods can be successful for stable fractures, operative intervention is necessary for unstable patterns like those seen in this case. Future study could focus on long-term outcomes of percutaneous radial head pinning to assess potential complications such as capitellar or physeal damage. This case reinforces the importance of vigilance among healthcare providers to prevent missed diagnoses and ensure optimal recovery in pediatric patients with complex forearm injuries.

Conclusion
Though rare in children, Monteggia fracture patterns require proper treatment to prevent long-term disability of the elbow and forearm. Depending on the injury pattern and reduction stability, both operative and non-operative treatments are viable options.

Bibliography

1. Vithran DTA, Song Z, Wang K, Tang Z, Xiang F, Wen J, et al. Comparison of the midterm result between locking plate and elastic intramedullary nail treating oblique ulnar fracture Bado type I acute monteggia fracture in pediatric patients. BMC Musculoskelet Disord. 2022;23:858.
2. Yuan Z, Xu HW, Liu YZ, Li YQ, Li JC, Canavese F. The use of external fixation for the management of acute and chronic Monteggia fractures in children. J Child Orthop. 2019;13:551–9.
3. Lightdale-Miric NR, Obana KK, Fan BB, Padilla AN, Lin AJ, Bennett JT, et al. Exposed intramedullary fixation produces similar outcomes to buried fixation for acute pediatric Monteggia fractures. J Pediatr Orthop. 2023;43:129–34.
4. Liu W, Sui X, Ye L, Zhao L. Ultrasonographic evaluation of radial nerve injuries associated with pediatric chronic Monteggia lesions. Muscle Nerve. 2019;59:326–30.
5. Mathur N, Lau KK. Monteggia fracture: an easy fracture to miss. Emerg Radiol. 2020;27:377–81.
6. Beutel BG. Monteggia fractures in pediatric and adult populations. Orthopedics. 2012;35:138–44.
7. Loder RT, Johnson BA. Changes in pediatric fracture patterns presenting to US emergency departments before, during, and after the COVID-19 pandemic. Heliyon. 2023;9(11):e20953. https://doi.org/10.1016/j.heliyon.2023.e20953.
8. Antoon SF, Russo SA, Kozin SH, Zlotolow DA. Evaluation of Monteggia fracture outcomes: acute to chronic. Hand. 2024;19(6):961–6.
9. Gopinathan NR, et al. Management of missed Type-2 Monteggia fracture equivalent in a 9-year-old child: a case report. JBJS Case Connect. 2021;11(1):e2000179.
10. Ring D, Jupiter JB, Waters PM. Monteggia fractures in children and adults. J Am Acad Orthop Surg. 1998;6(4):215–24.

11. Monteggia GB. Lussazioni delle ossa delle estremita superiori. Instituzioni Chirurgiches. 1814;5:131–3.
12. Bado JL. The Monteggia lesion. Clin Orthop. 1967;50:71–86. PubMed: 6029027
13. Ring D. Monteggia fractures. Orthop Clin North Am. 2013;44:59–66.
14. Kontakis GM, Pasku D, Pagkalos J, Katonis PG. The natural history of a mistreated ipsilateral Galeazzi and Monteggia lesion: report of a case 39 years post-injury. Acta Orthop Belg. 2008;74:546–9.
15. Lädermann A, Ceroni D, Lefèvre Y, De Rosa V, De Coulon G, Kaelin A. Surgical treatment of missed Monteggia lesions in children. J Child Orthop. 2007;1(4):237–42.
16. Ramski DE, Hennrikus WP, Bae DS, Baldwin KD, Patel NM, Waters PM, Flynn JM. Pediatric monteggia fractures: a multicenter examination of treatment strategy and early clinical and radiographic results. J Pediatr Orthop. 2015;35(2):115–20.
17. Leonidou A, Pagkalos J, Lepetsos P, Antonis K, Flieger I, Tsiridis E, Leonidou O. Pediatric Monteggia fractures: a single-center study of the management of 40 patients. J Pediatr Orthop. 2012;32(4):352–6.
18. He JP, Hao Y, Shao JF. Comparison of treatment methods for pediatric Monteggia fracture: met vs missed radial head dislocation. Medicine. 2019;98:e13942.
19. Ring D, Waters PM. Operative fixation of Monteggia fractures in children. J Bone Joint Surg Br. 1996;78:734–9.
20. Sinha S, Chang WR, Campbell AC, Hussein SM. Type III Monteggia injury with ipsilateral distal radius and ulna fracture. Internet J Orthop Surg. 2003;1(2). https://ispub.com/IJOS/1/2.
21. Papavasiliou H, Neuropoulos B. Ipsilateral injuries of the elbow and forearm in children. J Pediatr Orthop. 1993;13:561–6.
22. Kristiansen B, Erikson AF. Simultaneous type II Monteggia lesion and fracture separation of the lower radial epiphysis. Injury. 1986;17:51–2. https://doi.org/10.1016/0020-1383(86)90019-7.
23. Rodgers WB, Smith B. A type IV Monteggia injury with a distal diaphyseal fracture in a child. J Orthop Trauma. 1993;7:84–6. https://doi.org/10.1097/00005131-199302000-00015.
24. Theodorou SD, Ierodiaconou MD, Roussis MD. Fracture of the upper end of the ulna associated with dislocation of the head of the radius in children. Clin Orthop Relat Res. 1988;228:240–9.
25. Osada D, Tamai K, Kuramochi T, Saotome K. Three epiphyseal fractures (distal radius and ulna and proximal radius) and a diaphyseal ulnar fracture in a seven-year-old child's forearm. J Orthop Trauma. 2001;15:375–7. https://doi.org/10.1097/00005131-200106000-00015.
26. Peter N, Myint S. Type I Monteggia lesion and associated fracture of the distal radius and ulna metaphysis in a child. Can J Emerg Med. 2007;9(5):383–6.
27. Letts M, Locht R, Wiens J. Monteggia fracture-dislocation in children. J Bone Joint Surg. 1985;67B:724–7.
28. Sen RK, Tripathy SK, Kumar S, Aggarwal S, Tamuk T. Ipsilateral proximal and distal forearm fracture/fracture dislocation in children. J Pediatr Orthop B. 2011;20(3):129–37. https://doi.org/10.1097/BPB.0b013e328341df92.
29. Peiro A, Andres F, Fernandez-Esteve F. Acute Monteggia lesions in children. J Bone Joint Surg Am. 1977;59(1):92–7.
30. Gleeson AP, Beattie TF. Monteggia fracture–disclocation in children. J Accid Emerg Med. 1994;11:192–4. https://doi.org/10.1136/emj.11.3.192.
31. Sood A, Khan O, Bagga T. Simultaneous Monteggia type I fracture equivalent with ipsilateral fracture of the distal radius and ulna in a child: a case report. J Med Case Rep. 2008;2:190. https://doi.org/10.1186/1752-1947-2-190.
32. Fan YF, Liu QX, Yu XD, Zhang JQ, Wang W, Liu CY. Ultrasound, a new adjuvant method for treating acute Monteggia fracture in children. J Orthop Surg Res. 2023;18:595. https://doi.org/10.1186/s13018-023-04075-y.
33. Feng S, Yi Y, Song Z, Lu J, Zhou Q, Wen J, Xiao S, Li Y. Correlation between inner epiphysis ulna radius length ratio and prognosis of Monteggia fractures in children: a multicenter study. Sci Rep. 2025;15:5195. https://doi.org/10.1038/s41598-025-89751-1.

34. Vithran DTA, Song Z, Wang K, Tang Z, Xiang F, Wen J, Xiao S. Comparison of the mid-term result between locking plate and elastic intramedullary nail treating oblique ulnar fracture Bado type I acute monteggia fracture in pediatric patients. BMC Musculoskelet Disord. 2022;23:858. https://doi.org/10.1186/s12891-022-05809-5.
35. Williams HLM, Madhusudhan TR, Sinha A. Type III monteggia injury with ipsilateral type II salter Harris injury of the distal radius and ulna in a child: a case report. BMC Res Notes. 2014;7:156. https://doi.org/10.1186/1756-0500-7-156.

Missed Monteggia Fracture

13

Introduction by the Author

A Monteggia fracture is an injury that is often overlooked and becomes increasingly difficult to treat if not addressed promptly. Acute injuries that go undiagnosed for more than four weeks after the initial trauma can progress to chronic (or missed) Monteggia fractures.

Historically, missed cases have been treated conservatively. However, recent studies have highlighted the adverse outcomes of untreated dislocations, including limited elbow motion and forearm rotation, valgus deformity, osteoarthritis, and pain. Additionally, mechanical stimulation from a chronically unstable radius contributes to the formation of heterotopic ossifications at the elbow joint, particularly in cases of anterior dislocations. Notably, no heterotopic ossification is observed in patients who undergo timely surgical intervention for acute fractures, underscoring the importance of early treatment.

Missed cases often require open reduction of the radial head and ulnar osteotomy to restore proper alignment. The literature describes a series of surgical options, including open reduction of the radial head and ulnar osteotomy, with or without annular ligament reconstruction; indirect radial head reduction by ulnar overcorrection; nonoperative treatment; and radial head resection at skeletal maturity. However, preventing redislocation of the radiocapitellar joint remains challenging despite the development of various stabilization techniques. The redislocation rate after surgical treatment of missed Monteggia fractures averages 20%, and time from injury to surgery is a critical predictor. There is still debate over whether reconstructing the annular ligament reduces redislocation rates.

© The Author(s), under exclusive license to Springer Nature Switzerland AG 2026

F. Canavese, *Advances in Pediatric Extremity Fracture Management*,
https://doi.org/10.1007/978-3-032-33306-3_13

Reconstructive surgery can significantly improve elbow function in children with chronic radial head dislocation due to Monteggia lesions. However, precise surgical techniques are needed to effectively address ulnar malalignment because excessive ulnar angulation may contribute to instability. Some authors have suggested that reduction of the radial head is not recommended for patients who are more than 12 years old and for whom the interval between injury and operation is more than three years.

13.1 Machine Generated Summaries

Disclaimer: The summaries in this chapter were generated from Springer Nature publications using abstractive AI auto-summarization: An abstraction-based summarizer creates new text based on deep learning. New phrases are created to summarize the content. As the constituted sentences are machine selected, they may not fully reflect the body of the work, so we strongly advise that the original content is read and cited. The auto-generated summaries were curated by the author(s) to meet Springer Nature publication standards.

Outcomes After Surgical Treatment of Missed Monteggia Fractures in Children [54]

This is a machine-generated summary of:

Di Gennaro, Giovanni L.; Martinelli, Alessandro; Bettuzzi, Camilla; Antonioli, Diego; Rotini, Roberto Outcomes after surgical treatment of missed Monteggia fractures in children [54]
Published in: MUSCULOSKELETAL SURGERY (2015)
Link to original: https://doi.org/10.1007/s12306-015-0362-3
Copyright of the summarized publication:
Istituto Ortopedico Rizzoli 2015
All rights reserved.

If you want to cite the papers, please refer to the original.

For technical reasons we could not place the page where the original quote is coming from.

Research Highlights

Chronic dislocation of the radial head in children, often resulting from Monteggia lesions, presents a significant challenge in pediatric orthopedics. Historically, a conservative approach was favored, but recent studies have highlighted the adverse outcomes of untreated dislocations, such as limited elbow motion and forearm rotation, valgus deformity, and pain. Despite advancements in understanding these sequelae, there remains a lack of consensus on the optimal treatment for skeletally immature patients. Now, a new study by Giovanni L. Di Gennaro and colleagues explores the clinical outcomes of surgical interventions in one of the largest case series of pediatric patients with chronic Monteggia lesions.

The study reviewed records and radiographs of 22 children with chronic Monteggia lesions treated operatively at a single center. The patients, aged between 3.5 and 12 years, underwent various surgical procedures based on individual needs and surgeon preference. These included open reduction with annular ligament reconstruction using the Bell-Tawse procedure, ulnar osteotomy with gradual lengthening and angulation via external fixators, and in one case, radial head excision. The surgeries aimed to restore joint stability and improve range of motion while minimizing complications. Postoperative care involved immobilization with long-arm casts followed by gradual mobilization. Outcomes were assessed using Kim's elbow performance score and radiographic evaluations to determine joint congruency and detect any deformities or arthritic changes.

The study highlights that reconstructive surgery can significantly improve elbow function in children with chronic radial head dislocation due to Monteggia lesions. However, it emphasizes the need for precise surgical techniques to address ulnar malalignment effectively. Future study directions could focus on refining surgical algorithms and exploring advanced imaging techniques like MRI for better preoperative planning. While the results are promising, the authors acknowledge limitations such as variability in surgical approaches and the need for long-term follow-up to assess persistent subluxation outcomes in skeletally immature patients.

Risk Factors for Redislocation of Chronic Monteggia Fracture-Dislocation in Children After Reconstruction Surgery [55]

This is a machine-generated summary of:

Dai, Zhen-Zhen; Xu, Jing; Zhang, Zhi-Qiang; Li, Hai; Jin, Fang-Chun Risk factors for redislocation of chronic Monteggia fracture-dislocation in children after reconstruction surgery [55]
Published in: International Orthopaedics (2022)
Link to original: https://doi.org/10.1007/s00264-022-05473-3
Copyright of the summarized publication:
The Author(s) under exclusive licence to SICOT aisbl 2022
All rights reserved.

If you want to cite the papers, please refer to the original.

For technical reasons we could not place the page where the original quote is coming from.

Research Highlights

Monteggia fracture-dislocation, characterized by traumatic ulnar fractures and dislocation of the radial head, is a frequently overlooked injury that becomes increasingly complex to treat if not addressed promptly. Chronic cases often require open reduction of the radial head and ulnar osteotomy to restore proper alignment. However, preventing redislocation of the radiocapitellar joint remains a challenge, with various stabilization techniques such as annular ligament reconstruction and radiocapitellar pinning being debated. Now, a new study by Zhen-Zhen Dai and colleagues investigates the benefits of these surgical interventions and identifies risk factors for redislocation in pediatric patients with chronic Monteggia lesions.

The study retrospectively reviewed 62 pediatric patients who underwent surgical treatment for chronic Monteggia fracture-dislocation at their institution. Inclusion criteria focused on patients under 18 years old with specific injury causes and at least two years of follow-up post-operation. The surgical approach involved ulnar osteotomy with plate and screw fixation, removal of fibrotic tissue hindering radial head reduction, and annular ligament repair or reconstruction using forearm or triceps fascia. Radiocapitellar joint stability was assessed intraoperatively, with Kirschner wire fixation used in cases of instability. Postoperative evaluations included radiographic assessments and clinical outcomes measured by the Kim Elbow Performance Score. Statistical analyses identified age, time from injury to surgery, and radial osteotomy as significant risk factors for redislocation.

The study found that redislocation occurred in 16% of cases, with time from injury to surgery being a critical predictor. A nonlinear relationship was observed, where each month delay within the first year post-injury increased redislocation risk by 1.5-fold; beyond one year, this risk plateaued. The findings suggest that early surgical intervention is crucial for successful outcomes in chronic Monteggia cases. While annular ligament reconstruction and radiocapitellar pinning did not significantly reduce redislocation rates, future studies could explore alternative stabilization techniques or refine existing methods to improve joint stability post-surgery.

Risk Factors for the Development of Heterotopic Ossification of the Elbow in Children with Untreated Chronic Monteggia Fractures: A Radiographic Review of 274 Cases [56]

This is a machine-generated summary of:

Wang, WenTao; Mei, QianQian; Zhao, ChongZhi; Andreacchio, Antonio; Tang, ShengPing; Liu, Hang; Chen, ShunYou; Xiong, Zhu; Canavese, Federico; He, ShengHua Risk factors for the development of heterotopic ossification of the elbow in children with untreated chronic Monteggia fractures: a radiographic review of 274 cases [56]

Published in: Journal of Orthopaedics and Traumatology (2025)

Link to original: https://doi.org/10.1186/s10195-025-00842-1
Copyright of the summarized publication:
The Author(s) 2025
License: OpenAccess CC BY-NC-ND 4.0

This article is licensed under a Creative Commons Attribution-NonCommercial-NoDerivatives 4.0 International License, which permits any non-commercial use, sharing, distribution and reproduction in any medium or format, as long as you give appropriate credit to the original author(s) and the source, provide a link to the Creative Commons licence, and indicate if you modified the licensed material. You do not have permission under this licence to share adapted material derived from this article or parts of it. The images or other third party material in this article are included in the article's Creative Commons licence, unless indicated otherwise in a credit line to the material. If material is not included in the article's Creative Commons licence and your intended use is not permitted by statutory regulation or exceeds the permitted use, you will need to obtain permission directly from the copyright holder. To view a copy of this licence, visit http://creativecommons.org/licenses/by-nc-nd/4.0/.

If you want to cite the papers, please refer to the original.

For technical reasons we could not place the page where the original quote is coming from.

Research Highlights

Heterotopic ossification (HO) is the abnormal formation of bone in non-skeletal tissues, such as muscles and ligaments, and is associated with adverse outcomes like pain and restricted joint movement. It has been observed in children with untreated chronic Monteggia fractures (UCMFs), but the rarity of these fractures and lack of comprehensive studies have left gaps in understanding the risk factors for HO development. Now, a new study by WenTao Wang and colleagues addresses these gaps by examining radiographic data from pediatric patients with UCMFs to identify risk factors for HO formation.

The study involved a retrospective review of clinical data from children diagnosed with UCMFs more than three weeks post-injury, across four institutions. The researchers included patients who had not undergone previous attempts to reduce the dislocated radial head (RH) or received surgical treatment. They classified the direction of RH dislocation into subtypes and measured the distance of the dislocated RH from its anatomical position using radiographs. Statistical analyses, including logistic regression, were conducted to identify risk factors for HO, focusing on variables such as age at injury, laterality, and distance of RH dislocation. The study also compared these findings with a control group of patients with acute Monteggia fractures treated within 24 h.

The study found that age at injury greater than 6.5 years and a smaller distance of RH dislocation were significant risk factors for HO development in UCMFs. The findings suggest that mechanical stimulation from an unstable RH contributes to HO formation, particularly in anterior dislocations. Interestingly, no HO was observed in patients who underwent timely surgical intervention for acute fractures, highlighting the importance of early treatment. Future studies could further explore the molecular mechanisms underlying HO development and its clinical implications on patient outcomes. These insights could inform strategies to prevent HO in pediatric patients with UCMFs.

Risk Factors for Proximal Radial Abnormalities in Children with Untreated Chronic Monteggia Fractures: A Review of 142 Cases [57]

This is a machine-generated summary of:

Wang, WenTao; Mei, QianQian; Liu, Hang; Guo, YueMing; Mei, HaiBo; Canavese, Federico; Andreacchio, Antonio; Lyu, HanQing; Chen, ShunYou; He, ShengHua Risk factors for proximal radial abnormalities in children with untreated chronic Monteggia fractures: a review of 142 cases [57]
Published in: Journal of Orthopaedics and Traumatology (2024)
Link to original: https://doi.org/10.1186/s10195-024-00793-z
Copyright of the summarized publication:
The Author(s) 2024
License: OpenAccess CC BY 4.0

This article is licensed under a Creative Commons Attribution 4.0 International License, which permits use, sharing, adaptation, distribution and reproduction in any medium or format, as long as you give appropriate credit to the original author(s) and the source, provide a link to the Creative Commons licence, and indicate if changes were made. The images or other third party material in this article are included in the article's Creative Commons licence, unless indicated otherwise in a credit line to the material. If material is not included in the article's Creative Commons licence and your intended use is not permitted by statutory regulation or exceeds the permitted use, you will need to obtain permission directly from the copyright holder. To view a copy of this licence, visit http://creativecommons.org/licenses/by/4.0/.

If you want to cite the papers, please refer to the original.

For technical reasons we could not place the page where the original quote is coming from.

Research Highlights

Monteggia fractures, characterized by an ulnar fracture with associated radial head dislocation, present a diagnostic challenge in pediatric patients. These fractures can progress to chronic Monteggia fractures (CMFs) if not diagnosed promptly, leading to potential complications such as proximal radial anomalies (PRA). Despite previous observations of enlarged radial heads (RH) during surgery for CMFs, the lack of comparative and statistical analyses has left the relationship between PRA and surgical outcomes unclear. Now, a new study by WenTao Wang and colleagues aims to elucidate the radiographic characteristics of PRA and identify risk factors associated with surgical reduction failure in pediatric patients with untreated CMFs.

The study involved a retrospective review of clinical data from pediatric patients diagnosed with unilateral CMFs more than three weeks post-trauma. Patients were treated across four institutions, and those with congenital dislocations or other complicating conditions were excluded. Radiographic measurements focused on the RNS AP angle and RH L size to assess PRA severity. Statistical analyses, including paired-sample t-tests and multiple linear regression, were conducted to compare injured and uninjured elbows and identify risk factors for increased En-RH L size. The study found that age at injury, time from injury to diagnosis, and DD-RH were significant risk factors for increased En-RH L size.

The findings suggest that PRA in untreated CMFs is primarily due to RH enlargement or radial neck narrowing rather than valgus deformities. The study highlights the importance of early diagnosis and intervention to prevent severe PRA, which could lead to surgical reduction failure. Future studies could focus on prospective trials and molecular investigations to further understand the mechanisms underlying PRA development and its impact on surgical outcomes. This research provides valuable insights into managing pediatric CMFs and underscores the need for timely diagnosis to improve treatment success rates.

Does Overcorrection Cause any Negative Effect on Pediatric Missed Monteggia Lesion? [58]

This is a machine-generated summary of:

Musikachart, Piyanuch; Tisavipat, Nanthaya; Eamsobhana, Perajit Does overcorrection cause any negative effect on pediatric missed Monteggia lesion? [58]
Published in: European Journal of Orthopaedic Surgery & Traumatology (2020)
Link to original: https://doi.org/10.1007/s00590-020-02660-z
Copyright of the summarized publication:
Springer-Verlag France SAS, part of Springer Nature 2020
All rights reserved.

If you want to cite the papers, please refer to the original.

For technical reasons we could not place the page where the original quote is coming from.

Research Highlights

Monteggia fractures, characterized by a fracture of the ulna and dislocation of the radial head, are often missed in young patients, leading to complications such as valgus deformity and elbow instability. The prevalence of these fractures is significant among forearm injuries, yet the dislocation of the radial head is frequently overlooked due to factors like soft tissue swelling and inadequate radiographs.

Despite the known benefits of overcorrection in ulnar osteotomy for treating missed Monteggia fractures, there is limited research directly comparing clinical and radiologic outcomes between anatomical correction and overcorrection techniques. Now, a new study by Piyanuch Musikachart and colleagues aims to fill this gap by comparing these two surgical approaches.

The study retrospectively reviewed medical records of patients with missed Monteggia fractures who underwent surgery between January and June. Patients were divided into two groups based on postoperative ulnar angulation: anatomical correction and overcorrection. The surgical procedure involved open reduction osteotomy with or without annular ligament reconstruction (ALR), depending on intraoperative stability. Clinical outcomes were assessed using the Kim elbow performance score, while radiological outcomes were evaluated through standard elbow radiographs. Statistical analyses were conducted to compare outcomes between the two groups, focusing on parameters such as range of motion and radiological alignment.

The findings revealed that while clinical outcomes did not significantly differ between the groups, radiological results were inferior in the overcorrection group, with a higher incidence of posterior radial head dislocation. This suggests that excessive ulnar angulation may contribute to instability. The study highlights the need for careful consideration of ulnar angulation during surgery to avoid complications. Future studies should aim to determine the optimal degree of ulnar angulation to minimize postoperative issues, as well as explore other factors influencing surgical outcomes in missed Monteggia fractures.

The Treatment of Chronic Radial Head Dislocation in Monteggia Fracture Without Annular Ligament Reconstruction [59]

This is a machine-generated summary of:

Chen, Hsuan-Yu; Wu, Kuan-Wen; Dong, Zheng-Ren; Huang, Shier-Chieg; Kuo, Ken N.; Wang, Ting-Ming The treatment of chronic radial head dislocation in Monteggia fracture without annular ligament reconstruction [59]
Published in: International Orthopaedics (2018)
Link to original: https://doi.org/10.1007/s00264-018-3943-6
Copyright of the summarized publication:
SICOT aisbl 2018
All rights reserved.

If you want to cite the papers, please refer to the original.

For technical reasons we could not place the page where the original quote is coming from.

Research Highlights

Monteggia fractures, particularly in children, often present diagnostic challenges due to their subtle presentation, which can lead to chronic conditions if untreated.

These injuries typically involve an ulnar fracture with radial head subluxation or dislocation, which may be overlooked on initial radiographs. Untreated cases can result in complications such as loss of motion, arthritis, and pain, necessitating complex reconstructive surgeries with variable outcomes. Now a new study by Hsuan-Yu Chen and colleagues explores an alternative surgical approach for neglected isolated radial head dislocation in children, focusing on ulnar dorsal angulation lengthening osteotomy without annular ligament reconstruction.

The study conducted a retrospective review of patients treated for neglected radial head dislocation at the National Taiwan University Hospital. The researchers utilized a novel pre-operative templating technique using Microsoft® Office PowerPoint® to plan the surgery. This involved creating a template from radiographs to determine the optimal site and angle for ulnar osteotomy. The surgical procedure included open reduction of the radial head and dorsal angulation osteotomy of the ulna, with or without trans-capitellar K wire fixation depending on stability. Post-operative care involved casting and monitoring for complications such as compartment syndrome. The study evaluated functional outcomes using the Mayo Elbow Performance Index and range-of-motion assessments.

The findings suggest that this surgical strategy effectively maintains radial head reduction with satisfactory functional outcomes, even without annular ligament reconstruction. The pre-operative templating technique proved useful in planning the osteotomy accurately, although some intraoperative adjustments were necessary. Future study could focus on refining this approach with three-dimensional imaging or printing to enhance precision. Despite limitations such as a small sample size and retrospective design, this study provides valuable insights into managing neglected Monteggia fractures in children and highlights potential areas for further research and development in surgical techniques.

Missed Monteggia Fractures in Children Treated by Open Reduction of the Radial Head and Corrective Osteotomy of the Ulna [60]

This is a machine-generated summary of:

Cao, Shu; Dong, Zhong-Gen; Liu, Li-Hong; Wei, Jian-Wei; Luo, Zhao-Biao; Peng, Ping Missed Monteggia fractures in children treated by open reduction of the radial head and corrective osteotomy of the ulna [60]

Published in: Scientific Reports (2022)
Link to original: https://doi.org/10.1038/s41598-022-21019-4
Copyright of the summarized publication:
The Author(s) 2022
License: OpenAccess CC BY 4.0

This article is licensed under a Creative Commons Attribution 4.0 International License, which permits use, sharing, adaptation, distribution and reproduction in

any medium or format, as long as you give appropriate credit to the original author(s) and the source, provide a link to the Creative Commons licence, and indicate if changes were made. The images or other third party material in this article are included in the article's Creative Commons licence, unless indicated otherwise in a credit line to the material. If material is not included in the article's Creative Commons licence and your intended use is not permitted by statutory regulation or exceeds the permitted use, you will need to obtain permission directly from the copyright holder. To view a copy of this licence, visit http://creativecommons.org/licenses/by/4.0/.

If you want to cite the papers, please refer to the original.

For technical reasons we could not place the page where the original quote is coming from.

Research Highlights

Monteggia lesions, a type of forearm fracture, are often overlooked due to non-standard radiographs and the subtlety of ulnar plastic deformation. Missed Monteggia lesions, defined as those identified weeks after injury, can lead to severe long-term complications such as pain and dysfunction. Current treatment options include surgical interventions like open reduction and ulnar osteotomy. However, the role of preoperative imaging, particularly MRI, in assessing the proximal radioulnar joint's morphology has been underexplored. Now, a new study by Shu Cao and colleagues investigates the effectiveness of using MRI alongside traditional X-rays to evaluate missed Monteggia lesions and guide surgical treatment.

In this retrospective study conducted at Hunan Provincial People's Hospital, 12 children with missed Monteggia fractures underwent preoperative MRI and X-ray evaluations before receiving open reduction of the radial head and ulnar osteotomy. The researchers aimed to assess clinical and radiographic outcomes post-surgery and identify factors influencing these results. The study found that all patients had radial head dislocation visible on MRI, with some showing deformities in the radial notch or annular ligament tears. Surgical intervention included reconstruction of the annular ligament and use of a transcapitellar K-wire in cases of instability. Postoperative assessments revealed significant improvements in elbow function scores, with most patients achieving excellent or good outcomes.

The study highlights that preoperative MRI provides valuable insights into the condition of the radial head and notch, which are crucial for predicting surgical success. It was observed that a longer interval between injury and surgery correlated with more severe abnormalities and poorer outcomes. Future studies could focus on refining surgical techniques based on MRI findings to enhance patient outcomes further. The authors suggest that addressing severe hyperplasia of the radial head and notch is essential for successful reconstruction, emphasizing the importance of timely intervention in managing missed Monteggia fractures effectively.

Influence of Ulnar Bow Sign on Surgical Treatment of Missed Bado Type I Monteggia Fracture in Children [61]

This is a machine-generated summary of:

Liao, Shijie; Wang, Tiantian; Huang, Qian; Liu, Yun; Lu, Rongbin; Xu, Yaofeng; Ding, Xiaofei Influence of ulnar bow sign on surgical treatment of missed Bado type I Monteggia fracture in children [61]
Published in: Scientific Reports (2022)
Link to original: https://doi.org/10.1038/s41598-022-14513-2
Copyright of the summarized publication:
The Author(s) 2022
License: OpenAccess CC BY 4.0

This article is licensed under a Creative Commons Attribution 4.0 International License, which permits use, sharing, adaptation, distribution and reproduction in any medium or format, as long as you give appropriate credit to the original author(s) and the source, provide a link to the Creative Commons licence, and indicate if changes were made. The images or other third party material in this article are included in the article's Creative Commons licence, unless indicated otherwise in a credit line to the material. If material is not included in the article's Creative Commons licence and your intended use is not permitted by statutory regulation or exceeds the permitted use, you will need to obtain permission directly from the copyright holder. To view a copy of this licence, visit http://creativecommons.org/licenses/by/4.0/.

If you want to cite the papers, please refer to the original.

For technical reasons we could not place the page where the original quote is coming from.

Research Highlights

Missed Bado type I Monteggia fractures in children are characterized by an arcuate curvature of the ulna and anterior dislocation of the radial head, often leading to complications such as elbow deformity, limited movement, and nerve paralysis. Surgical intervention is typically recommended to address these issues, with humeroradial joint open reduction and ulnar osteotomy being common treatments. However, complications such as radial head re-dislocation and limited forearm rotation remain prevalent. Now, a new study by Shijie Liao and colleagues explores the relationship between the ulnar bow sign and ulnar osteotomy angle to improve surgical outcomes for these fractures.

The study involved 32 children with missed Bado type I Monteggia fractures who underwent open radial head reduction and ulnar osteotomy without annular ligament reconstruction. The researchers measured the maximum ulnar bow (MUB) on lateral radiographs and divided patients into two groups based on the position of the MUB: middle and distal. The surgical procedure included combined anterior and posterior approaches for radial head reduction and ulnar osteotomy. Postoperative management involved immobilization followed by periodic X-ray evaluations to monitor healing. Statistical analyses were conducted to assess elbow joint function improvements and correlations between MUB position, osteotomy angle, and surgical outcomes.

The study found that a larger ulnar osteotomy angle was necessary for stable radial head reduction when the MUB was located more proximally. This approach improved elbow flexion and extension functions significantly, although forearm rotation slightly decreased without statistical significance. Future study could focus on refining surgical techniques to further enhance forearm rotation outcomes. The findings suggest that considering the position of the maximum ulnar bow sign can be crucial in preoperative planning, potentially reducing complications such as subluxation or instability post-surgery.

Conclusion

If not diagnosed within four weeks of the initial trauma, acute Monteggia fractures progress to chronic, or missed, Monteggia fractures. Missed Monteggia fractures are not uncommon and require surgery to restore the anatomy, alignment, and function of the elbow joint. Although ulnar osteotomy is an essential part of each procedure, the need for annular ligament reconstruction is still debated.

Bibliography

1. Koslowsky TC, Mader K, Wulke AP, et al. Operative treatment of chronic Monteggia lesion in younger children: a report of three cases. J Shoulder Elb Surg. 2006;15:119–21. https://doi.org/10.1016/j.jse.2004.12.002.
2. Bell Tawse AJ. The treatment of malunited anterior Monteggia fractures in children. J Bone Joint Surg (Br). 1965;47-B:718–23. PMID: 5846773; ISSN: 0301620X
3. Stelling FH, Cote RH. Traumatic dislocation of the head of radius in children. JAMA J Am Med Assoc. 1956;160:732–6. https://doi.org/10.1001/jama.1956.02960440004002.
4. Kalamchi A. Monteggia fracture-dislocation in children. Late treatment in two cases. J Bone Joint Surg. 1968;68-A:615–9. PMID: 3957989
5. Hui JHP, Sulaiman AR, Lee HC, et al. Open reduction and annular ligament reconstruction with fascia of the forearm in chronic Monteggia lesions in children. J Pediatr Orthop. 2005;25(4):501–6.
6. Lädermann A, Ceroni D, Lefèvre Y, De Rosa V, De Coulon G, Kaelin A. Surgical treatment of missed Monteggia lesions in children. J Child Orthop. 2007;1(4):237–42.
7. Seel MJ, Peterson HA. Management of chronic posttraumatic radial head dislocation in children. J Pediatr Orthop. 1999;19(3):306–12. https://doi.org/10.1097/01241398-199905000-00006.
8. Nakamura K, Hirachi K, Uchiyama S, et al. Long-term clinical and radiographic outcomes after open reduction for missed Monteggia fracture-dislocations in children. J Bone Joint Surg Am. 2009;91:1394–404. https://doi.org/10.2106/JBJS.H.00644.
9. Bae DS. Successful strategies for managing Monteggia injuries. J Pediatr Orthop. 2016;36(suppl 1):S67–70.

10. Xu Z, Li Y, Wang Z, Cai H. Open reduction combined with CORA-based osteotomy of the ulna in the treatment of missed Bado type I Monteggia injury: a retrospective study of 5 cases. Medicine (Baltimore). 2017;96:e8609. https://doi.org/10.1097/md.0000000000008609.
11. Shinohara D, Yasuda T, Arai M, Sato K, Arima T, Kanzaki K. A long-standing Monteggia fracture in a child who underwent bone lengthening and annular ligament reconstruction: a case report. J Orthop Case Rep. 2019;9:30–3. https://doi.org/10.13107/jocr.2250-0685.1406.
12. Liao S, Pan J, Lin H, Xu Y, Lu R, Wu J, Zhao M, Chen H, Cai M, Ding X, Zhao J. A new approach for surgical treatment of chronic Monteggia fracture in children. Injury. 2019;50:1237–41. https://doi.org/10.1016/j.injury.2019.04.017.
13. Chen HY, Wu KW, Dong ZR, Huang SC, Kuo KN, Wang TM. The treatment of chronic radial head dislocation in Monteggia fracture without annular ligament reconstruction. Int Orthop. 2018;42:2165–72. https://doi.org/10.1007/s00264-018-3943-6.
14. Kamble P, Prabhakar A, Wankhade A. Heterotopic ossification of annular ligament: a case report and review of literature. J Clin Orthop Trauma. 2021;21:101511. https://doi.org/10.1016/j.jcot.2021.101511.
15. Earwaker J. Posttraumatic calcification of the annular ligament of the radius. Skeletal Radiol. 1992;21:149–54. https://doi.org/10.1007/BF00242127.
16. Prabhu J, Faqi MK, Al Khalifa F, Awad RK. Angulating-distraction ulnar osteotomy and interpositional phosphocalcic ceramic wedge graft for a chronic Monteggia lesion. Open Orthop J. 2017;11:263–7. https://doi.org/10.2174/1874325001711010263.
17. Kay RM, Skaggs DL. The pediatric Monteggia fracture. Am J Orthop. 1998;27:606–9.
18. Barfield WR, Holmes RE, Hartsock LA. Heterotopic ossification in trauma. Orthop Clin North Am. 2017;48:35–46. https://doi.org/10.1016/j.ocl.2016.08.009.
19. Nauth A, Giles E, Potter BK, Nesti LJ, O'brien FP, Bosse MJ, et al. Heterotopic ossification in orthopaedic trauma. J Orthop Trauma. 2012;26:684–8. https://doi.org/10.1097/BOT.0b013e3182724624.
20. Potter BK, Forsberg JA, Davis TA, Evans KN, Hawksworth JS, Tadaki D, et al. Heterotopic ossification following combat-related trauma. J Bone Joint Surg Am. 2010;92(Suppl 2):74–89. https://doi.org/10.2106/JBJS.J.00776.
21. Goyal T, Arora SS, Banerjee S, Kandwal P. Neglected Monteggia fracture dislocations in children: a systematic review. J Pediatr Orthop B. 2015;24:191–9.
22. Wang W, Xiong Z, Huang D, Li Y, Huang Y, Guo Y, et al. Risk factors for unsuccessful reduction of chronic Monteggia fractures in children treated surgically. Bone Jt Open. 2024;5:581–91. https://doi.org/10.1302/2633-1462.57.BJO-2024-0004.R2.
23. Anthonissen J, Steffen CT, Hofmann A, Victor J. The pathogenesis of heterotopic ossification after traumatic brain injury: a review of current literature. Acta Orthop Belg. 2020;86:369–77.
24. Lu W, Yan J, Wang C, Qin W, Han X, Qin Z, et al. Interorgan communication in neurogenic heterotopic ossification: the role of brain-derived extracellular vesicles. Bone Res. 2024;12:11. https://doi.org/10.1038/s41413-023-00310-8.
25. Huang H, Cheng WX, Hu YP, Chen JH, Zheng ZT, Zhang P. Relationship between heterotopic ossification and traumatic brain injury: why severe traumatic brain injury increases the risk of heterotopic ossification. J Orthop Translat. 2017;12:16–25. https://doi.org/10.1016/j.jot.2017.10.002.
26. Rahbek O, Deutch SR, Kold S, Sojbjerg JO, Moller-Madsen B. Long-term outcome after ulnar osteotomy for missed Monteggia fracture dislocation in children. J Child Orthop. 2011;5:449–57. https://doi.org/10.1007/s11832-011-0372-0.
27. Ko KR, Shim JS, Park J, Won J. Predictors of ideal outcomes after reconstructive surgery for chronic Monteggia fracture in children. J Orthop Sci. 2022;27:1025–31.
28. Cao S, Dong ZG, Liu LH, Wei JW, Luo ZB, Peng P. Missed Monteggia fractures in children treated by open reduction of the radial head and corrective osteotomy of the ulna. Sci Rep. 2022;12:16819.
29. Kim HT, Conjares JNV, Suh JT, et al. Chronic radial head dislocation in children, Part 1: Pathologic changes preventing stable reduction and surgical correction. J Pediatr Orthop. 2002;22:583–90. https://doi.org/10.1097/01241398-200209000-00004.

30. Kim HT, Can LV, Ahn TY, Kim IH. Analysis of radiographic parameters of the forearm in traumatic radial head dislocation. Clin Orthop Surg. 2017;9:521–8. https://doi.org/10.4055/cios.2017.9.4.521.
31. Gleeson AP, Beattie TF. Monteggia fracture–disclocation in children. J Accid Emerg Med. 1994;11:192–4. https://doi.org/10.1136/emj.11.3.192.
32. Lu X, Kun Wang Y, Zhang J, Zhu Z, Guo Y, Lu M. Management of missed Monteggia fractures with ulnar osteotomy, open reduction, and dual-socket external fixation. J Pediatr Orthop. 2013;33(4):398–402. https://doi.org/10.1097/BPO.0b013e3182812762.
33. Tajima T, Yoshizu T. Treatment of long-standing dislocation of the radial head in neglected Monteggia fractures. J Hand Surg Am. 1995;20(3 Pt 2):S91–4. https://doi.org/10.1016/s0363-5023(95)80177-4.
34. Eamsobhana P, Kaewpornsawan K. Chronic Monteggia lesions treatment with open reduction and Z-lengthening technique with annular ligament reconstruction. J Med Assoc Thail. 2012;95(Suppl 9):S47–53.
35. Hirayama T, Takemitsu Y, Yagihara K, Mikita A. Operation for chronic dislocation of the radial head in children. Reduction by osteotomy of the ulna. J Bone Joint Surg Br. 1987;69(4):639–42. https://doi.org/10.1302/0301-620X.69B4.3611173.
36. Inoue G, Shionoya K. Corrective ulnar osteotomy for malunited anterior Monteggia lesions in children. Acta Orthop Scand. 1998;69(1):73–6. https://doi.org/10.3109/17453679809002361.
37. Gyr BM, Stevens PM, Smith JT. Chronic Monteggia fractures in children: outcome after treatment with the Bell-Tawse procedure. J Pediatr Orthop B. 2004;13:402–6. https://doi.org/10.1097/01202412-200411000-00011.
38. Lloyd-Roberts GC, Bucknill TM. Anterior dislocation of the radial head in children: aetiology, natural history and management. J Bone Joint Surg (Br). 1977;59-B(4):402–7.
39. Kim HT, et al. Chronic radial head dislocation in children, Part 1: Pathologic changes preventing stable reduction and surgical correction. J Pediatr Orthop. 2002;22(5):583–90.
40. Rodgers WB, Waters PM, Hall JE. Chronic Monteggia lesions in children. Complications and results of reconstruction. J Bone Joint Surg Am. 1996;78(9):1322–9. https://doi.org/10.2106/00004623-199609000-00005.
41. Best TN. Management of old unreduced Monteggia fracture dislocations of the elbow in children. J Pediatr Orthop. 1994;14:193–9. https://doi.org/10.1097/01241398-199403000-00012.
42. Kim HT, et al. Chronic radial head dislocation in children, Part 2: Results of open treatment and factors affecting final outcome. J Pediatr Orthop. 2002;22(5):591–7.
43. Wang MN, Chang WN. Chronic posttraumatic anterior dislocation of the radial head in children. Thirteen cases treated by open reduction, ulnar osteotomy, and annular ligament reconstruction through a Boyd incision. J Orthop Trauma. 2006;20(1):1–5. https://doi.org/10.1097/01.bot.0000189881.75421.92.
44. Kawoosa AA, Dhar SA, Butt MF, Wani SA, Mir MR, Dar TA. Stable relocation of the radial head without annular ligament reconstruction using the Ilizarov technique to treat neglected Monteggia fracture: two case reports. J Med Case Rep. 2010;4:344. https://doi.org/10.1186/1752-1947-4-344.
45. Osamura N, et al. Posterior interosseous nerve injury complicating ulnar osteotomy for a missed Monteggia fracture. Scand J Plast Reconstr Surg Hand Surg. 2004;38(6):376–8.
46. Oka K, Murase T, Moritomo H, Sugamoto K, Yoshikawa H. Morphologic evaluation of chronic radial head dislocation: three-dimensional and quantitative analyses. Clin Orthop Relat Res. 2010;468(9):2410–8.
47. Chen WS. Late neuropathy in chronic dislocation of the radial head. Report of two cases. Acta Orthop Scand. 1992;63:343–4. https://doi.org/10.3109/17453679209154798.
48. Eamsobhana P, Chalayon O, Kaewpornsawan K, Ariyawatkul T. Missed Monteggia fracture dislocations treated by open reduction of the radial head. Bone Joint J. 2018;100-B(8):1117–24.
49. Langenberg LC, Beumer A, The B, Koenraadt K, Eygendaal D. Surgical treatment of chronic anterior radial head dislocations in missed Monteggia lesions in children: a rationale for treatment and pearls and pitfalls of surgery. Shoulder Elbow. 2019;12:1–10.

50. Refsland S, Kozin SH, Zlotolow DA. Ulnar distraction osteogenesis in the treatment of forearm deformities in children with multiple hereditary exostoses. J Hand Surg. 2016;41(9):888–95.
51. Stoll TM, Willis RB, Paterson DC. Treatment of the missed Monteggia fracture in the child. J Bone Joint Surg Br. 1992;74:436–40.
52. Lincoln T, Mubarak S. "Isolated" traumatic radial-head dislocation. J Pediatr Orthop. 1994;14:454–7.
53. Park H, Park KW, Park KB, Kim HW, Eom NK, Lee DH. Impact of open reduction on surgical strategies for missed Monteggia fracture in children. Yonsei Med J. 2017;58:829–36. https://doi.org/10.3349/ymj.2017.58.4.829.
54. Di Gennaro GL, Martinelli A, Bettuzzi C, Antonioli D, Rotini R. Outcomes after surgical treatment of missed Monteggia fractures in children. Musculoskelet Surg. 2015; https://doi.org/10.1007/s12306-015-0362-3.
55. Dai Z-Z, Xu J, Zhang Z-Q, Li H, Jin F-C. Risk factors for redislocation of chronic Monteggia fracture-dislocation in children after reconstruction surgery. Int Orthop. 2022; https://doi.org/10.1007/s00264-022-05473-3.
56. Wang WT, Mei QQ, Zhao CZ, Andreacchio A, Tang SP, Liu H, Chen SY, Xiong Z, Canavese F, He SH. Risk factors for the development of heterotopic ossification of the elbow in children with untreated chronic Monteggia fractures: a radiographic review of 274 cases. J Orthop Traumatol. 2025; https://doi.org/10.1186/s10195-025-00842-1.
57. Wang WT, Mei QQ, Liu H, Guo YM, Mei HB, Canavese F, Andreacchio A, Lyu HQ, Chen SY, He SH. Risk factors for proximal radial abnormalities in children with untreated chronic Monteggia fractures: a review of 142 cases. J Orthop Traumatol. 2024; https://doi.org/10.1186/s10195-024-00793-z.
58. Musikachart P, Tisavipat N, Eamsobhana P. Does overcorrection cause any negative effect on pediatric missed Monteggia lesion? Eur J Orthop Surg Traumatol. 2020; https://doi.org/10.1007/s00590-020-02660-z.
59. Chen H-Y, Wu K-W, Dong Z-R, Huang S-C, Kuo KN, Wang T-M. The treatment of chronic radial head dislocation in Monteggia fracture without annular ligament reconstruction. Int Orthop. 2018; https://doi.org/10.1007/s00264-018-3943-6.
60. Cao S, Dong Z-G, Liu L-H, Wei J-W, Luo Z-B, Peng P. Missed Monteggia fractures in children treated by open reduction of the radial head and corrective osteotomy of the ulna. Sci Rep. 2022; https://doi.org/10.1038/s41598-022-21019-4.
61. Liao S, Wang T, Huang Q, Liu Y, Lu R, Xu Y, Ding X. Influence of ulnar bow sign on surgical treatment of missed Bado type I Monteggia fracture in children. Sci Rep. 2022; https://doi.org/10.1038/s41598-022-14513-2.

Proximal Femur Fracture

14

Introduction by the Author

Femoral neck fractures account for less than 0.5% of all childhood fractures per year. There is a male preponderance, peaking between 11 and 12 years of age. Unlike osteoporotic proximal femur fractures in the elderly, most cases in children result from high-energy trauma, such as road traffic accidents or falls from a great height.

Pediatric femoral neck fractures are generally treated surgically in all age groups, though younger patients with undisplaced, stable fractures may benefit from conservative treatment involving immobilization in a spica cast.

Recent trends toward aggressive surgical intervention and improved implant technology have led to fewer complications and better outcomes for patients with displaced and unstable fractures. Reduction can be achieved using closed or open techniques, and various types of hardware are available to stabilize fractures. The type of hardware used depends on the location of the fracture, as well as the patient's age and weight.

The broad classification of pediatric femoral neck fractures as displaced versus non-displaced has prognostic significance; displaced fractures are more likely to result in major complications.

Currently, femoral neck fractures in children are classified according to the Delbet classification, which correlates with the most serious complication of such injuries, avascular necrosis of the femoral head. This is due to the unique blood supply characteristics of the pediatric femur, which has less anastomosis and collateral circulation than the adult femur. Other complications include coxa vara, premature physeal closure, and nonunion.

Total hip replacement surgery can effectively address avascular necrosis of the femoral head when the femoral head is completely affected by

© The Author(s), under exclusive license to Springer Nature Switzerland AG 2026
F. Canavese, *Advances in Pediatric Extremity Fracture Management*,
https://doi.org/10.1007/978-3-032-33306-3_14

compensating for limb shortening and preserving hip function. In cases of partial necrosis, valgus osteotomy of the proximal femur has been shown to be beneficial in moving the necrotic segment away from weight-bearing zones and correcting leg shortening.

14.1 Machine Generated Summaries

Disclaimer: The summaries in this chapter were generated from Springer Nature publications using abstractive AI auto-summarization: An abstraction-based summarizer creates new text based on deep learning. New phrases are created to summarize the content. As the constituted sentences are machine selected, they may not fully reflect the body of the work, so we strongly advise that the original content is read and cited. The auto-generated summaries were curated by the author(s) to meet Springer Nature publication standards.

Fractures of the Proximal Femur in Childhood: A Review [38]

This is a machine-generated summary of:

Pinto, Deepika A.; Aroojis, Alaric Fractures of the Proximal Femur in Childhood: A Review [38]
Published in: Indian Journal of Orthopaedics (2020)
Link to original: https://doi.org/10.1007/s43465-020-00259-4
Copyright of the summarized publication:
Indian Orthopaedics Association 2020
All rights reserved.

If you want to cite the papers, please refer to the original.

For technical reasons we could not place the page where the original quote is coming from.

Research Highlights

Fractures of the femoral neck in children are rare, accounting for less than 1% of all childhood fractures annually. Traditionally, these injuries have been linked to high complication rates and poor outcomes. However, recent trends towards aggressive surgical intervention and improved implant technology have led to reduced complications and better outcomes. Despite these advances, appropriate and timely management remains crucial to prevent long-term disability from hip osteoarthritis. Now, a new study by Deepika A. Pinto and colleagues reviews the current knowledge on pediatric proximal femoral fractures, highlighting the importance of classification systems and surgical techniques in improving patient outcomes.

The study conducted by Pinto et al. involved a comprehensive review of literature sourced from databases such as the Cochrane Database of Systematic Reviews, EMBASE, and Google Scholar. The authors included systematic reviews, meta-analyses, clinical trials, cohort studies, and case series that met specific inclusion criteria. They focused on the epidemiology, classification, pathophysiology, diagnosis, and management of pediatric femoral neck fractures. The study emphasizes the significance of accurate classification systems like Delbet's for guiding treatment decisions. It also discusses various surgical approaches such as closed versus open reduction and the role of internal fixation in achieving stable fracture repair. The authors highlight that while non-operative treatments are largely obsolete for displaced fractures, they may still be applicable in specific cases involving very young children with undisplaced fractures.

The study by Pinto et al. advances our understanding of pediatric femoral neck fractures by synthesizing existing knowledge and identifying areas needing further research. It underscores the need for large-scale prospective studies with long-term follow-up to address unanswered questions about optimal treatment strategies. Future study directions could include multi-centered research efforts due to the rarity of these fractures in children. The authors also point out that while complications like osteonecrosis remain a significant concern, advancements in surgical techniques and implant technology offer promising avenues for improving patient outcomes.

Research on the Analysis of Morphological Characteristics in Pediatric Femoral Neck Fractures Utilizing 3D CT Mapping [39]

This is a machine-generated summary of:

Zhao, Niu-Niu; Gu, Xue-Lian; Dai, Zhen-Zhen; Wu, Chen-Chen; Zhang, Tian-Yi; Li, Hai Research on the analysis of morphological characteristics in pediatric femoral neck fractures utilizing 3D CT mapping [39]

Published in: Medical & Biological Engineering & Computing (2025)

Link to original: https://doi.org/10.1007/s11517-024-03260-3

Copyright of the summarized publication:

International Federation for Medical and Biological Engineering 2024

Copyright comment: Springer Nature or its licensor (e.g. a society or other partner) holds exclusive rights to this article under a publishing agreement with the author(s) or other rightsholder(s); author self-archiving of the accepted manuscript version of this article is solely governed by the terms of such publishing agreement and applicable law.

All rights reserved.

If you want to cite the papers, please refer to the original.

For technical reasons we could not place the page where the original quote is coming from.

Research Highlights

Femoral neck fractures (FNF) in children, though rare, pose significant treatment challenges due to potential complications such as avascular necrosis and nonunion. These complications are influenced by the fracture's morphology and the stability of surgical fixation. Traditional X-ray imaging often falls short in accurately determining fracture lines, leading to the increased use of computed tomography (CT) and fracture mapping technology. Now, a new study by Niu-Niu Zhao and colleagues utilizes CT-based fracture mapping to analyze pediatric FNF morphology and its relationship with age, providing insights into optimal treatment strategies.

The study conducted a retrospective review of pediatric patients diagnosed with FNF, using CT data to create three-dimensional models of fractured femurs. The researchers employed image processing software to align fractured femurs with a standard template, delineating fracture lines to produce a distribution map and heat map. The femoral neck was divided into four zones to identify concentrated fracture areas. The study also measured Pauwels angles to assess fracture stability and used Delbet classification for categorizing fractures based on location. Statistical analyses were performed to explore the relationship between fracture types and patient age.

The findings reveal that pediatric FNFs predominantly occur in the mid to lower regions of the femoral neck, with Delbet type III fractures more common in younger children and type II more prevalent in those over 10 years old. Pauwels angle type III fractures, indicating instability, were frequent among older children. These insights suggest that age-specific internal fixation strategies are crucial for effective treatment. Future studies could focus on multi-center collaborations to address sample size limitations and further refine fracture mapping techniques for enhanced accuracy in diverse pediatric populations.

Retrospective Analysis of 35 Pediatric Femoral Neck Fractures [40]

This is a machine-generated summary of:

Yerli, Mustafa; Ocak, Olcayto; Yüce, Ali; Bayraktar, Tahsin Olgun; Kir, Mustafa Çağlar; İmren, Yunus; Dedeoğlu, Süleyman Semih; Gürbüz, Hakan Retrospective analysis of 35 pediatric femoral neck fractures [40]
Published in: European Journal of Orthopaedic Surgery & Traumatology (2021)
Link to original: https://doi.org/10.1007/s00590-021-03126-6
Copyright of the summarized publication:
The Author(s), under exclusive licence to Springer-Verlag France SAS, part of Springer Nature 2021
All rights reserved.

If you want to cite the papers, please refer to the original.

For technical reasons we could not place the page where the original quote is coming from.

Research Highlights

Pediatric proximal femur fractures are rare but serious injuries that often occur alongside other traumatic conditions, such as neurological or abdominal trauma. These fractures are prone to complications due to the unique blood supply characteristics of the pediatric femur, which has less anastomosis and collateral circulation compared to adults. Now, a new study by Mustafa Yerli and colleagues investigates the incidence of early complications and outcomes of pediatric proximal femur fractures, focusing on different fracture types as classified by the Delbet system.

The study was conducted retrospectively and included patients under a certain age with proximal femur fractures, excluding those with tumoral, rheumatologic, or metabolic conditions. The fractures were classified using the Delbet system, and treatment modalities varied from conservative management to surgical interventions like open or closed reduction with internal fixation. Surgical decisions were made by senior attending physicians, and all procedures were performed under general anesthesia. The outcomes were assessed using Ratliff's method, categorizing results as satisfactory or unsatisfactory based on complications such as avascular necrosis (AVN), coxa vara, and premature physeal closure. Statistical analyses were performed using SPSS software to evaluate the data.

The study highlights that while pediatric femoral neck fractures are rare, they can be managed with relatively low complication rates if treated early and with precise anatomical reduction. The findings suggest that AVN remains a significant complication but was observed at lower rates in this study compared to previous literature, possibly due to the distribution of fracture types. Future study could focus on larger sample sizes and standardized surgical approaches to further validate these findings. Additionally, understanding the factors contributing to complications like coxa vara could improve treatment protocols and patient outcomes in pediatric orthopedic trauma care.

Operative Treatment of Avascular Necrosis of the Femoral Head After Proximal Femur Fractures in Adolescents [41]

This is a machine-generated summary of:

Bartoníček, Jan; Vávra, Jaroslav; Bartoška, Radek; Havránek, Petr Operative treatment of avascular necrosis of the femoral head after proximal femur fractures in adolescents [41]

Published in: International Orthopaedics (2011)

Link to original: https://doi.org/10.1007/s00264-011-1272-0

Copyright of the summarized publication:

Springer-Verlag 2011

All rights reserved.

If you want to cite the papers, please refer to the original.

For technical reasons we could not place the page where the original quote is coming from.

Research Highlights

Proximal femoral fractures in adolescents, though rare, pose significant challenges due to their severe complications, particularly avascular necrosis of the femoral head (ANFH). While the incidence of these complications is well-documented, there is limited consensus on their optimal treatment, especially for ANFH. Now, a new study by Jan Bartoníček and colleagues explores the outcomes of reconstructive surgery for ANFH with a follow-up period of 4–6 years, providing valuable insights into operative treatments for this condition.

The study involved 11 patients who underwent surgery for ANFH following proximal femur fractures. The patients were divided into two groups based on the type of necrosis: total ANFH and partial ANFH. Total hip replacement (THR) was performed in patients with total ANFH, while valgus intertrochanteric osteotomy (VITO) was used for those with partial ANFH. The surgical procedures were meticulously planned using preoperative radiographic and MRI assessments to ensure precise correction and optimal outcomes. The study also included additional procedures like Bosworth hip-shelf arthroplasty in cases where further coverage of the femoral head was necessary. Postoperative assessments were conducted using the Harris Hip Score and MRI scans to evaluate healing and resorption of the necrotic segment.

The findings suggest that THR effectively addresses total ANFH by compensating for limb shortening and preserving hip function. For partial ANFH, VITO proved beneficial in relocating the necrotic segment away from weight-bearing zones and correcting leg shortening. The study highlights that while VITO does not fully restore the femoral head's biological integrity, it significantly delays premature osteoarthritis development. Future studies could focus on long-term outcomes and further refine surgical techniques to enhance treatment efficacy for adolescent patients with post-traumatic ANFH.

Extra-Articular Proximal Femur Fractures in Children and Adolescents Treated by Elastic Stable Intramedullary Nailing [42]

This is a machine-generated summary of:

Alberghina, Flavia; Andreacchio, Antonio; Cravino, Mattia; Paonessa, Matteo; Canavese, Federico Extra-articular proximal femur fractures in children and adolescents treated by elastic stable intramedullary nailing [42]
Published in: International Orthopaedics (2019)
Link to original: https://doi.org/10.1007/s00264-019-04379-x
Copyright of the summarized publication:
SICOT aisbl 2019
All rights reserved.

If you want to cite the papers, please refer to the original.

For technical reasons we could not place the page where the original quote is coming from.

Research Highlights

Extra-articular proximal femur fractures (EPFF) in children are rare, accounting for a small percentage of pediatric femoral fractures. These fractures present a significant challenge due to their intrinsic instability and the complex forces acting on the fracture fragments. Despite various classification systems, there is no consensus on the definition of EPFF, particularly in pediatric patients. Now, a new study by Flavia Alberghina and colleagues evaluates the clinical and radiological outcomes of children with EPFF managed by elastic stable intramedullary nailing (ESIN), providing insights into its effectiveness as a treatment option.

The study conducted a retrospective analysis of pediatric patients with EPFF treated using ESIN between January 2010 and June 2020. The researchers included patients who were admitted through the emergency department and met specific criteria, such as having complete radiographic data and being treated within 5 days following trauma. Exclusion criteria included poly-traumatized patients, open or pathological fractures, and incomplete data. The treatment involved closed reduction and internal fixation using two retrograde titanium elastic nails, followed by spica casting in younger patients to maintain alignment and control pain. Radiographic evaluations were performed at multiple intervals post-surgery to assess fracture healing and alignment.

The study found that ESIN is an effective treatment for EPFF in children, resulting in excellent radiological and clinical outcomes in most cases. The procedure was associated with a low complication rate and relatively short hospital stays. However, the authors note that heavier children may require more stable fixation methods due to a higher risk of complications with ESIN. Future studies could focus on comparing different treatment methods to establish best practices for managing EPFF in various patient subgroups. Despite its limitations, this study provides valuable evidence supporting the use of ESIN for treating EPFF in pediatric populations.

Conclusion

Although femoral neck fractures in children are rare, they present significant treatment challenges due to the risk of complications. Most of these fractures are treated surgically. While complications such as avascular necrosis of the femoral head are a major concern, advancements in surgical techniques and implant technology offer hope for improved patient outcomes.

Bibliography

1. Patterson JT, Tangtiphaiboontana J, Pandya NK. Management of pediatric femoral neck fracture. J Am Acad Orthop Surg. 2018;26(12):411–9.
2. Ratliff AH. Fractures of the neck of the femur in children. J Bone Joint Surg Br. 1962;44B(3):528–42.
3. Mirdad T. Fractures of the neck of femur in children: an experience at the Aseer Central Hospital, Abha, Saudi Arabia. Injury. 2002;33(9):823–7.

4. Azouz EM, Karamitsos C, Reed MH, Baker L, Kozlowski K, Hoeffel J-C. Types and complications of femoral neck fractures in children. Pediatr Radiol. 1993;23(6):415–20.
5. Hughes LO, Beaty JH. Fractures of the head and neck of the femur in children. J Bone Joint Surg. 1994;76(2):283–92.
6. Colonna PC. Fracture of the neck of the femur in children. Am J Surg. 1929;6(6):793–7.
7. Moon ES, Mehlman CT. Risk factors for avascular necrosis after femoral neck fractures in children: 25 Cincinnati cases and meta-analysis of 360 cases. J Orthop Trauma. 2006;20(5):323–9.
8. Panigrahi R, Sahu B, Mahapatra AK, Palo N, Priyadarshi A, Biswal MR. Treatment analysis of paediatric femoral neck fractures: a prospective multicenter theraupetic study in Indian scenario. Int Orthop. 2015;39(6):1121–7.
9. Gautier E, Ganz K, Krügel N, Gill T, Ganz R. Anatomy of the medial femoral circumflex artery and its surgical implications. J Bone Joint Surg. 2000;82(5):679–83.
10. Boardman MJ, Herman MJ, Buck B, Pizzutillo PD. Hip fractures in children. J Am Acad Orthop Surg. 2009;17(3):162–73.
11. Dial BL, Lark RK. Pediatric proximal femur fractures. J Orthop. 2018;15(2):529–35.
12. Bali K, Sudesh P, Patel S, Kumar V, Saini U, Dhillon MS. Pediatric femoral neck fractures: our 10 years of experience. Clin Orthop Surg. 2011;3(4):302–8.
13. Bukva B, Abramović D, Vrgoč G, Marinović M, Bakota B, Dučić S, et al. Femoral neck fractures in children and the role of early hip decompression in final outcome. Injury. 2015;46:S44–7.
14. Ng GPK, Cole WG. Effect of early hip decompression on the frequency of avascular necrosis in children with fractures of the neck of the femur. Injury. 1996;27(6):419–21.
15. Yeranosian M, Horneff JG, Baldwin K, Hosalkar HS. Factors affecting the outcome of fractures of the femoral neck in children and adolescents. Bone Joint J. 2013;95-B(1):135–42.
16. AlKhatib N, Younis MH, Hegazy A, Ibrahim T. Early versus late treatment of paediatric femoral neck fractures: a systematic review and meta-analysis. Int Orthop. 2019;43(3):677–85.
17. Qi B, Yu A, Zhang G, Yu G, Shi Y, Zhu S, et al. The treatment of displaced femoral neck fractures with vascularized great trochanter periosteal flap transposition in children. Microsurgery. 2008;28(1):21–4.
18. Gurnea TP, Nielsen RC, Althausen PL. Use of proximal humerus locking plates for fixation of pediatric femoral neck fractures: technical trick. J Orthop Trauma. 2020;34:e312–5. https://doi.org/10.1097/BOT.0000000000001765.
19. Pavone V, Testa G, Riccioli M, et al. Surgical treatment with cannulated screws for pediatric femoral neck fractures: a case series. Injury. 2019;50:S40–4. https://doi.org/10.1016/j.injury.2019.01.043.
20. Wang S-H, Yang J-J, Shen H-C, et al. Using a modified Pauwels method to predict the outcome of femoral neck fracture in relatively young patients. Injury. 2015;46:1969–74. https://doi.org/10.1016/j.injury.2015.06.016.
21. Wu S, Zhu X, Wang W, et al. Three-dimensional computed tomography mapping and clinical predictive factors for morphologic characterization of displaced femoral neck fractures. Ann Transl Med. 2022;10:1096. https://doi.org/10.21037/atm-22-1213.
22. Djuric M, Milovanovic P, Djonic D, et al. Morphological characteristics of the developing proximal femur: a biomechanical perspective. Srp Arh Celok Lek. 2012;140:738–45. https://doi.org/10.2298/SARH1212738D.
23. Pape H-C, Krettek C, Friedrich A, Pohlemann T, Simon R, Tscherne H. Long-term outcome in children with fractures of the proximal femur after high-energy trauma. J Trauma. 1999;46:58–64.
24. Ratliff AHC. Fractures of the neck of the femur in children. J Bone Joint Surg Br. 1962;44-B:528–42.
25. Axhausen G. Epiphyseonekrose und arthritis deformans. Arch Klin Chir. 1924;126:341–63.
26. Canale ST, Bourland WL. Fracture of the neck and intertrochanteric region of the femur in children. J Bone Joint Surg Am. 1977;59-A:431–43.
27. Swiontkowski MF. Complications of hip fractures in children. Complicat Orthop. 1989;4:58–64.
28. Boitzy A. La fracture du col du femur chez l'enfant et l'adolescent. Paris: Mason; 1971.

29. Abbas AA, Yoon TR, Lee JH, Hur CI. Posttraumatic avascular necrosis of the femoral head in teenagers treated by a modified transtrochanteric rotational osteotomy: a report of three cases. J Orthop Trauma. 2008;22:63–9.
30. Nötzli HP, Chou LB, Ganz R. Open-reduction and intertrochanteric osteotomy for osteonecrosis and extrusion of the femoral head in adolescents. J Pediatr Orthop. 1995;15:16–20.
31. Canavese F, Marengo L, Andreacchio A, Mansour M, Paonessa M, Rousset M, Samba A, Dimeglio A. Complications of elastic stable intramedullary nailing of femoral shaft fractures in children weighing fifty kilograms (one hundred and ten pounds) and more. Int Orthop. 2016;40(12):2627–34. https://doi.org/10.1007/s00264-016-3259-3.
32. Andreacchio A, Alberghina F, Marengo L, Canavese F. Pediatric tibia and femur fractures in patients weighing more than 50 kg (110 lb): mini-review on current treatment options and outcome. Musculoskelet Surg. 2019;103(1):23–30. https://doi.org/10.1007/s12306-018-0570-8.
33. Jarvis J, Davidson D, Letts M. Management of subtrochanteric fractures in skeletally immature adolescents. J Trauma. 2006;60(3):613–9. https://doi.org/10.1097/01.ta.0000197606.63124.9e.
34. Hajdu S, Oberleitner G, Schwendenwein E, Ringl H, Vécsei V. Fracture of the head and neck of the femur in children: an outcome study. Int Orthop. 2011;35(6):883–8. https://doi.org/10.1007/s00264-010-1039-z.
35. Maruenda-Paulino JI, Sanchis-Alfonso V, Gomar-Sancho F, Darder-Prats A, Gasco-Gomez de Membrillera J. Kuntscher nailing of femoral shaft fractures in children and adolescents. Int Orthop. 1993;17(3):158–61.
36. Pombo MW, Shilt JS. The definition and treatment of pediatric subtrochanteric femur fractures with titanium elastic nails. J Pediatr Orthop. 2006;26(3):364–70. https://doi.org/10.1097/01.bpo.0000203005.50906.41.
37. Parikh SN, Nathan ST, Priola MJ, Eismann EA. Elastic nailing for pediatric subtrochanteric abd supracondylar femur fractures. Clin Orthop Relat Res. 2014;472(9):2735–44. https://doi.org/10.1007/s11999-013-3240-z.
38. Pinto DA, Aroojis A. Fractures of the proximal femur in childhood: a review. Indian J Orthop. 2020;55:23–34. https://doi.org/10.1007/s43465-020-00259-4.
39. Niu-Niu Z, Xue-Lian G, Zhen-Zhen D, Chen-Chen W, Tian-Yi Z, Hai L. Research on the analysis of morphological characteristics in pediatric femoral neck fractures utilizing 3D CT mapping. Med Biol Eng Comput. 2025;63:1497–505. https://doi.org/10.1007/s11517-024-03260-3.
40. Yerli M, Ocak O, Yüce A, Bayraktar TO, Kir MÇ, İmren Y, Dedeoğlu SS, Gürbüz H. Retrospective analysis of 35 pediatric femoral neck fractures. Eur J Orthop Surg Traumatol. 2021;32:1385–90. https://doi.org/10.1007/s00590-021-03126-6.
41. Bartoníček J, Vávra J, Bartoška R, Havránek P. Operative treatment of avascular necrosis of the femoral head after proximal femur fractures in adolescents. Int Orthop. 2011;36:149–57. https://doi.org/10.1007/s00264-011-1272-0.
42. Alberghina F, Andreacchio A, Cravino M, Paonessa M, Canavese F. Extra-articular proximal femur fractures in children and adolescents treated by elastic stable intramedullary nailing. Int Orthop. 2019;43:2849–56. https://doi.org/10.1007/s00264-019-04379-x.

Diaphyseal Femur Fracture

15

Introduction by the Author

Fractures of the femoral diaphysis account for 1–2% of all fractures in children and are the second most common type of fracture affecting the lower extremities, affecting approximately 25 out of 100,000 children per year. Although these fractures can occur at any age, they are more prevalent in children over 6 years old. These injuries often result from sports or motor vehicle accidents and are more prevalent in males. Though fractures at the junction of the distal diaphysis and metaphysis are rare, it has been reported that such fractures in non-walking children caused by abuse account for 50% of these fractures.

Treatment options for pediatric femoral fractures vary depending on the patient's age and weight. Infants are usually treated conservatively, while those aged 6 and older typically undergo elastic stable intramedullary nailing. However, complications such as instability have been reported, particularly in complex fractures and in older children weighing over 110 pounds (50 kg). For heavier and older children, external fixation and locked lateral entry nails are viable options.

A common complication of elastic stable intramedullary nailing is pain and soft tissue irritation caused by the extraosseous portion of the nail tip at the insertion site. End caps provide increased stability during posterior-anterior bending tests but offer no significant advantages over the classical elastic nail configuration for other aspects, such as anterior-posterior bending or rotational control.

In general, external fixation has several advantages over elastic stable intramedullary nailing. These include a shorter operative time, reduced fluoroscopic exposure, a quicker time to partial weight-bearing, and lower malalignment rates. However, elastic stable intramedullary nailing is

© The Author(s), under exclusive license to Springer Nature Switzerland AG 2026

F. Canavese, *Advances in Pediatric Extremity Fracture Management*,
https://doi.org/10.1007/978-3-032-33306-3_15

associated with less skin irritation and a higher malalignment rate than external fixation. For this reason, more rigid fixation systems are preferred for older, heavier patients weighing more than 110 pounds (50 kg).

Traditionally, surgical techniques have recommended removing nails after fracture healing, typically within a few months to a year after surgery. However, there is some debate about whether hardware should always be removed. Studies have found that over 70% of patients do not require nail removal due to pain or irritation. While some patients reported persistent discomfort, it did not significantly interfere with daily activities. These results suggest that retaining flexible intramedullary nails could be a viable alternative to routine removal, thus avoiding the complications and inconvenience of a second surgery.

15.1 Machine Generated Summaries

Disclaimer: The summaries in this chapter were generated from Springer Nature publications using abstractive AI auto-summarization: An abstraction-based summarizer creates new text based on deep learning. New phrases are created to summarize the content. As the constituted sentences are machine selected, they may not fully reflect the body of the work, so we strongly advise that the original content is read and cited. The auto-generated summaries were curated by the author(s) to meet Springer Nature publication standards.

External Fixator Versus Elastic Stable Intramedullary Nail for Treatment of Metaphyseal-Diaphyseal Junction Fractures of the Pediatric Distal Femur: A Case-Control Study [32]

This is a machine-generated summary of:

Wen, Yuwei; Wang, Qiang; Song, Baojian; Feng, Wei; Zhu, Danjiang External fixator versus elastic stable intramedullary nail for treatment of metaphyseal-diaphyseal junction fractures of the pediatric distal femur: a case-control study [32]
Published in: BMC Musculoskeletal Disorders (2024)
Link to original: https://doi.org/10.1186/s12891-024-07469-z
Copyright of the summarized publication:
The Author(s) 2024
License: OpenAccess CC BY + CC0 4.0

This article is licensed under a Creative Commons Attribution 4.0 International License, which permits use, sharing, adaptation, distribution and reproduction in

any medium or format, as long as you give appropriate credit to the original author(s) and the source, provide a link to the Creative Commons licence, and indicate if changes were made. The images or other third party material in this article are included in the article's Creative Commons licence, unless indicated otherwise in a credit line to the material. If material is not included in the article's Creative Commons licence and your intended use is not permitted by statutory regulation or exceeds the permitted use, you will need to obtain permission directly from the copyright holder. To view a copy of this licence, visit http://creativecommons.org/licenses/by/4.0/. The Creative Commons Public Domain Dedication waiver (http://creativecommons.org/publicdomain/zero/1.0/) applies to the data made available in this article, unless otherwise stated in a credit line to the data.

If you want to cite the papers, please refer to the original.

For technical reasons we could not place the page where the original quote is coming from.

Research Highlights

Femoral fractures are a common pediatric injury, but distal femoral fractures are relatively rare, accounting for a small percentage of these cases. These injuries often occur due to sports activities or motor vehicle accidents, with a higher incidence in males. Treatment options for pediatric femoral fractures vary, with elastic stable intramedullary nailing (ESIN) and external fixation (EF) being two common methods. However, there is ongoing debate about the optimal treatment approach, particularly for proximal and distal femoral fractures. Now, a new study by Yuwei Wen and colleagues compares the clinical outcomes of EF and ESIN techniques in treating metaphyseal-diaphyseal junction (MDJ) fractures of the distal femur in children.

The study retrospectively analyzed medical records of children treated for femoral fractures at a hospital from January 2010 to January 2020. The researchers included patients whose fracture line was located on the MDJ and who were treated with either EF or ESIN. The study collected data on demographics, fracture characteristics, surgical details, and follow-up outcomes such as time to weight-bearing and fracture healing. In the EF group, Schanz pins were used for fixation, while ESIN involved retrograde insertion of pre-bent nails. Postoperative care varied between groups, with EF allowing earlier weight-bearing compared to ESIN. Statistical analyses were conducted to compare outcomes between the two groups.

The study found that both EF and ESIN are effective treatments for distal MDJ femoral fractures in children. However, EF demonstrated advantages over ESIN in terms of shorter operative time, reduced fluoroscopic exposure, quicker time to partial weight-bearing, and lower incidence of malalignment. While ESIN was associated with less skin irritation, it had a higher rate of malalignment compared to EF. The authors suggest that EF may be preferable in clinical scenarios where both treatment options are viable due to its benefits in reducing complications and avoiding implant removal surgery. Future studies could focus on prospective designs to further validate these findings and explore long-term outcomes in larger patient populations.

Improving Stability of Elastic Stable Intramedullary Nailing in a Transverse Midshaft Femur Fracture Model: Biomechanical Analysis of Using End Caps or a Third Nail [33]

This is a machine-generated summary of:

Rapp, Marion; Gros, Nina; Zachert, Gregor; Schulze-Hessing, Maaike; Stratmann, Christina; Wendlandt, Robert; Kaiser, Martin Michael Improving stability of elastic stable intramedullary nailing in a transverse midshaft femur fracture model: biomechanical analysis of using end caps or a third nail [33]
Published in: Journal of Orthopaedic Surgery and Research (2015)
Link to original: https://doi.org/10.1186/s13018-015-0239-z
Copyright of the summarized publication:
Rapp et al. 2015
License: OpenAccess CC BY + CC0 4.0

This article is distributed under the terms of the Creative Commons Attribution 4.0 International License (http://creativecommons.org/licenses/by/4.0), which permits unrestricted use, distribution, and reproduction in any medium, provided you give appropriate credit to the original author(s) and the source, provide a link to the Creative Commons license, and indicate if changes were made. The Creative Commons Public Domain Dedication waiver (http://creativecommons.org/publicdomain/zero/1.0/) applies to the data made available in this article, unless otherwise stated.

If you want to cite the papers, please refer to the original.

For technical reasons we could not place the page where the original quote is coming from.

Research Highlights

Fractures of the femoral diaphysis are common in children, particularly those over 6 years old, and are often treated with elastic stable intramedullary nailing (ESIN) to promote rapid recovery. However, complications such as instability have been reported, especially in complex fractures and older children. Now, a new study by Marion Rapp and colleagues investigates modifications to the ESIN technique to enhance stability in transverse femoral fractures by examining the use of end caps and a third nail.

The study employed a biomechanical approach using synthetic adolescent-sized composite femoral models to simulate transverse femoral fractures. The researchers divided the models into three groups: a control group with standard ESIN, a group with end caps added to the nails, and a group with an additional third nail. The models underwent various mechanical tests, including four-point bending, torsional testing, and shifting tests, using a Zwick universal testing machine. The results indicated that adding a third nail significantly increased stiffness across multiple stress planes compared to both the classical configuration and the modification with end caps. In contrast, the use of end caps did not enhance stability compared to the standard two-nail configuration.

The study advances our understanding of ESIN modifications by demonstrating that incorporating a third nail can improve stability in transverse femoral fractures without significant technical challenges. This finding suggests that clinical practice could benefit from adopting this modification to reduce complications associated with insufficient stability. Future study could focus on translating these biomechanical findings into clinical settings to assess long-term outcomes and potential impacts on recovery times in pediatric patients. Additionally, further research might explore other fracture types or configurations to optimize treatment strategies for pediatric femoral fractures.

Biomechanical Analysis of a Synthetic Femoral Spiral Fracture Model: Do End Caps Improve Retrograde Flexible Intramedullary Nail Fixation? [34]

This is a machine-generated summary of:

Kaiser, Martin M; Zachert, Gregor; Wendlandt, Robert; Rapp, Marion; Eggert, Rebecca; Stratmann, Christine; Wessel, Lucas M; Schulz, Arndt P; Kienast, Benjamin J Biomechanical analysis of a synthetic femoral spiral fracture model: Do end caps improve retrograde flexible intramedullary nail fixation? [34]
Published in: Journal of Orthopaedic Surgery and Research (2011)
Link to original: https://doi.org/10.1186/1749-799x-6-46
Copyright of the summarized publication:
Kaiser et al.; licensee BioMed Central Ltd. 2011
License: OpenAccess CC BY 2.0

This article is published under license to BioMed Central Ltd. This is an Open Access article distributed under the terms of the Creative Commons Attribution License (http://creativecommons.org/licenses/by/2.0), which permits unrestricted use, distribution, and reproduction in any medium, provided the original work is properly cited.

If you want to cite the papers, please refer to the original.

For technical reasons we could not place the page where the original quote is coming from.

Research Highlights

Femoral shaft fractures in children and adolescents have traditionally been managed with various treatment options, including casting and external fixation devices. However, in recent years, the approach for older children has shifted towards surgical interventions like elastic stable intramedullary nailing (ESIN) due to quicker recovery times and reduced immobilization complications. Despite its popularity, ESIN is not without issues, such as skin irritation and malalignment. Now, a new study by Martin M. Kaiser and colleagues explores whether the addition of End Caps to ESIN can enhance stability in treating spiral femoral fractures in synthetic bone models.

The study utilized synthetic adolescent-sized composite femoral models to simulate spiral fractures and assess the biomechanical stability of ESIN with and without End Caps. The researchers created identical spiral fractures on these models and performed retrograde intramedullary fixation using titanium nails, with some models also receiving cylindric hollow-threaded End Caps. The specimens underwent a series of mechanical tests, including bending, torsional, and compression tests, to evaluate the stability of the different configurations. Data were analyzed using statistical methods to determine any significant differences in stability between the two setups.

The findings revealed that while the use of End Caps provided increased stability during posterior-anterior bending tests, it did not offer significant advantages over the classical ESIN configuration in other aspects such as anterior-posterior bending or rotational control. The study highlights that adding End Caps did not significantly enhance overall fixation stability for spiral midshaft fractures in this synthetic model. Future studies could focus on further biomechanical research to refine this osteosynthesis technique and explore its applicability across various fracture types, including transverse and oblique fractures.

Retention of Flexible Intramedullary Nails Following Treatment of Pediatric Femur Fractures [35]

This is a machine-generated summary of:

Morshed, Saam; Humphrey, Marcie; Corrales, Luis A.; Millett, Meredith; Hoffinger, Scott A. Retention of flexible intramedullary nails following treatment of pediatric femur fractures [35]
Published in: Archives of Orthopaedic and Trauma Surgery (2007)
Link to original: https://doi.org/10.1007/s00402-007-0286-y
Copyright of the summarized publication:
Springer-Verlag 2007
All rights reserved.

If you want to cite the papers, please refer to the original.

For technical reasons we could not place the page where the original quote is coming from.

Research Highlights

Flexible intramedullary nailing is a widely used procedure for treating diaphyseal femur fractures in children, often yielding excellent outcomes. However, a common complication is pain and soft tissue irritation caused by the extraosseous portion of the nail tip at the insertion site. Traditionally, surgical techniques have recommended nail removal after fracture healing, typically within months to a year post-surgery. Now, a new study by Saam Morshed and colleagues investigates the safety of retaining these nails without routine removal, aiming to provide early follow-up data on symptoms and functional limitations in children treated with this approach.

The study was conducted as a retrospective review at a tertiary pediatric referral center, focusing on children with closed diaphyseal femur fractures treated with flexible intramedullary nails. Excluding those with underlying conditions or insufficient follow-up, 24 children were included in the analysis. The surgeries were performed using Synthes flexible titanium nails, cut to lie flush against the femoral cortex to minimize irritation. Post-operative management involved physical therapy and regular clinical assessments until full recovery. Follow-up interviews were conducted with 22 patients to assess pain levels and any need for further surgery. Statistical analyses were performed to evaluate associations between nail retention and various factors.

The study found that over 70% of patients did not require nail removal due to pain or irritation at an average follow-up of nearly 3 years. While some patients reported persistent discomfort, it did not significantly interfere with daily activities. The findings suggest that retaining flexible intramedullary nails could be a viable alternative to routine removal, potentially avoiding the complications and inconvenience of a second surgery. Future studies could focus on long-term outcomes and cost-effectiveness to further validate this approach as a standard treatment option for pediatric femur fractures.

Conclusion

Treatment options for pediatric femoral fractures depend on the patient's age and weight. Infants are usually treated conservatively, while older children are typically treated with elastic stable intramedullary nailing. Older children and individuals weighing over 110 pounds (50 kg) or over 50% of their ideal body weight may require more rigid fixation systems, such as external fixators and locked lateral entry nails. Though fractures at the junction of the distal diaphysis and metaphysis are rare, they account for 50% of fractures in non-walking children caused by abuse.

Bibliography

1. Heyworth BE, Hedequist DJ, Nasreddine AY, et al. Distal femoral valgus deformity following plate fixation of pediatric femoral shaft fractures. J Bone Joint Surg Am. 2013;95(6):526–33.
2. Li J, Rai S, Ze R, et al. Distal third femoral shaft fractures in school-aged children: a comparative study of elastic stable intramedullary nail and external fixator. Medicine. 2020;99(27):e21053.
3. Korobeinikov A, Popkov D. Use of external fixation for juxta-articular fractures in children. Injury. 2019;50(Suppl 1):S87–94.
4. Baghdadi S, Mahmoud MAH, Flynn JJM, et al. Unplanned return to the operating room (UpROR) after pediatric diaphyseal femoral fractures. J Pediatr Orthop. 2022;42(2):e120–5.
5. Ricci WM, Bellabarba C, Lewis R, et al. Angular malalignment after intramedullary nailing of femoral shaft fractures. J Orthop Trauma. 2001;15(2):90–5.
6. Khan HN, Ali M, Rashid RH, et al. Frequency of angular malalignment after intramedullary nailing for femur shaft fractures—a cross-sectional study. J Pak Med Assoc. 2021;71(Suppl 5 8):S4–7.

7. Li J, Guo X, Wang HQ, et al. Locking plate versus external fixation in the treatment of displaced femoral supracondylar fracture in children. J Orthop Surg Res. 2020;15(1):233. Published 2020 Jun 23.
8. Métaizeau JP. Stable elastic intramedullary nailing for fractures of the femur in children. J Bone Joint Surg. 2004;86 B:954–7.
9. Poolman RW, Kocher MS, Bhandari M. Pediatric femoral fractures: a systematic review of 2422 cases. J Orthop Trauma. 2006;20:648–54.
10. AWMF-Leitlinie Femurschaftfraktur. German Guidelines of the AWMF Study Group. 2014. http://www.awmf.org/leitlinien/detail/ll/006-016.html. Accessed 28 Dec 2014.
11. Rapp M, Albers K, Kaiser MM. Korrektureingriffe nach Operationen bei Femurschaftfrakturen im Kindesalter [Corrective procedures after operation of femoral shaft fractures in children.]. Chir Praxis. 2011;73:499–512.
12. Moroz LA, Launay F, Kocher MS, Newton PO, Frick SL, Sponseller PD, et al. Titanium elastic nailing of fractures of the femur in children. Predictors of complications and poor outcome. J Bone Joint Surg. 2006;88:1361–6.
13. Lazar-Antman MA, Leet AI. Effects of obesity on pediatric fracture care and management. J Bone Joint Surg Am. 2012;94:855–61.
14. Weiss JM, Choi P, Ghatan C, Skaggs DL, Kay RM. Complications with flexible nailing of femur fractures more than double with child obesity and weight >50 kg. J Child Orthop. 2009;3:53–8.
15. Kaiser MM, Wessel LM, Zachert G, Stratmann C, Eggert R, Gros N, et al. Biomechanical analysis of a synthetic femur spiral fracture model: influence of different materials on the stiffness in flexible intramedullary nailing. Clin Biomech. 2011;26:592–7.
16. Kaiser MM, Zachert G, Wendlandt R, Rapp M, Eggert C, Stratmann C, et al. Biomechanical analysis of a synthetic femoral spiral fracture model: do end caps improve retrograde flexible intramedullary nail fixation? J Orthop Surg Res. 2011;6:46.
17. Tschegg EK, Herndler S, Weninger P, Jamek M, Stanzl-Tschegg S, Redl H. Stiffness analysis of tibia-implant system under cyclic loading. Mater Sci Eng. 2008;C28:1203–8.
18. Kaiser MM, Zachert G, Wendlandt R, Eggert R, Stratmann C, Gros N, et al. Increasing stability by pre-bending the nails in elastic stable intramedullary nailing: a biomechanical analysis of a synthetic femoral spiral fracture model. J Bone Joint Surg. 2012;94:713–8.
19. Benz G, Kallieris S, Blume U. Biomechanik des experimentell gesetzten Biege- und Torsionsbruchs vor und nach Versorgung mit Nancy-Nägeln. Zentralbl Kinderchir. 2000;9:104–9.
20. Mahar AT, Lee SS, Lalonde FD, Impelluso T, Newton PO. Biomechanical comparison of stainless steel and titanium nails for fixation of simulated femoral fractures. J Pediatr Orthop. 2004;24:638–41.
21. Kaiser MM, Stratmann C, Zachert G, Schulze-Hessing M, Gros N, Eggert R, et al. Modification of elastic stable intramedullary nailing with a 3rd nail in a femoral spiral fracture model—results of biomechanical testing and a prospective clinical study. BMC Musculoskelet Disord. 2014;15:3.
22. Slongo T, Audigé L, Hunter JB, Berger SM. Clinical evaluation of end caps in elastic stable intramedullary nailing of femoral and tibial shaft fractures in children. Eur J Trauma Emerg Surg. 2011;37:305–12.
23. Domb BG, Sponseller PD, Ain M, Miller NH. Comparison of dynamic versus static external fixation for pediatric femur fractures. J Pediatr Orthop. 2002;22:428–30.
24. Probe R, Lindsey RW, Hadley NA, Barnes DA. Refracture of adolescent femoral shaft fractures: a complication of external fixation. A report of two cases. J Pediatr Orthop. 1993;13:102–5. https://doi.org/10.1097/01241398-199301000-00021.
25. Guidelines of the AWMF: Guideline of the german association of pediatric surgeons: Femur shaft fractures. 2008. http://www.awmf.org/leitlinien/detail/ll/006-016.html.
26. Narayanan UG, Hyman JE, Wainwright AM, Rang M, Alman BA. Complications of elastic stable intramedullary nail fixation of pediatric femoral fractures, and how to avoid them. J Pediatr Orthop. 2004;24:363–9. https://doi.org/10.1097/01241398-200407000-00004.

27. Ho CA, Skaggs DL, Tang CW, Kay RM. Use of flexible intramedullary nails in pediatric femur fractures. J Pediatr Orthop. 2006;26:497–504. https://doi.org/10.1097/01.bpo.0000226280.93577.c1.
28. Leet AI, Pichard CP, Ain MC. Surgical treatment of femoral fractures in obese children: does excessive body weight increase the rate of complications? J Bone Joint Surg Am. 2005;87:2609–13. https://doi.org/10.2106/JBJS.D.02019.
29. Flynn JM, Hresko T, Reynolds RA, Blasier RD, Davidson R, Kasser J. Titanium elastic nails for pediatric femur fractures: a multicenter study of early results with analysis of complications. J Pediatr Orthop. 2001;21(1):4–8.
30. Flynn JM, Luedtke L, Ganley TJ, Pill SG. Titanium elastic nails for pediatric femur fractures: lessons from the learning curve. Am J Orthop. 2002;31(2):71–4.
31. Bostman OM. Metallic or absorbable fracture fixation devices. A cost minimization analysis. Clin Orthop Relat Res. 1996;329:233–9.
32. Wen Y, Wang Q, Song B, Feng W, Zhu D. External fixator versus elastic stable intramedullary nail for treatment of metaphyseal-diaphyseal junction fractures of the pediatric distal femur: a case-control study. BMC Musculoskelet Disord. 2024;25:389. https://doi.org/10.1186/s12891-024-07469-z.
33. Rapp M, Gros N, Zachert G, Schulze-Hessing M, Stratmann C, Wendlandt R, Kaiser MM. Improving stability of elastic stable intramedullary nailing in a transverse midshaft femur fracture model: biomechanical analysis of using end caps or a third nail. J Orthop Surg Res. 2015;10:96. https://doi.org/10.1186/s13018-015-0239-z.
34. Kaiser MM, Zachert G, Wendlandt R, Rapp M, Eggert R, Stratmann C, Wessel LM, Schulz AP, Kienast BJ. Biomechanical analysis of a synthetic femoral spiral fracture model: do end caps improve retrograde flexible intramedullary nail fixation? J Orthop Surg Res. 2011;8:46. https://doi.org/10.1186/1749-799x-6-46.
35. Morshed S, Humphrey M, Corrales LA, Millett M, Hoffinger SA. Retention of flexible intramedullary nails following treatment of pediatric femur fractures. Arch Orthop Trauma Surg. 2007;127:509–14. https://doi.org/10.1007/s00402-007-0286-y.

Proximal and Distal Metaphyseal Tibia Fracture

16

Introduction by the Author

Fractures of the proximal tibial metaphysis are rare, with an estimated incidence of approximately six per 100,000 children per year. Non-displaced fractures are usually treated conservatively, while displaced fractures generally require surgical treatment and osteosynthesis.

Although trampoline use among children has become increasingly popular in recent decades, it has also been accompanied by a significant increase in related injuries, including proximal metaphyseal fractures. However, these fractures can be subtle and challenging to diagnose, especially for radiologists unfamiliar with their patterns. Convolutional neural networks, a type of machine learning, have been developed to improve detection of proximal and distal tibial metaphyseal lesions, including cases of suspected infant abuse.

Depending on whether they are displaced, proximal metaphyseal tibial fractures can be treated conservatively or surgically. A common complication following treatment is progressive valgus deformity, which has been observed after both conservative and surgical management.

Fractures of the distal tibial metaphysis are uncommon in children. The reported incidence of such injuries varies between 0.35% and 0.45% of all pediatric fractures.

Due to children's rapid bone healing and remodeling capabilities, these injuries can be treated non-operatively, especially when they are undisplaced. However, displaced fractures may necessitate surgical intervention. These fractures are typically managed through percutaneous pinning, elastic stable

© The Author(s), under exclusive license to Springer Nature Switzerland AG 2026
F. Canavese, *Advances in Pediatric Extremity Fracture Management*,
https://doi.org/10.1007/978-3-032-33306-3_16

intramedullary nailing, or external fixation. All three options have been shown to effectively treat these injuries. Nevertheless, the question of whether to fix the fibula in both bone fractures remains debated. Further investigation is needed to optimize treatment strategies for these complex injuries.

16.1 Machine Generated Summaries

Disclaimer: The summaries in this chapter were generated from Springer Nature publications using abstractive AI auto-summarization: An abstraction-based summarizer creates new text based on deep learning. New phrases are created to summarize the content. As the constituted sentences are machine selected, they may not fully reflect the body of the work, so we strongly advise that the original content is read and cited. The auto-generated summaries were curated by the author(s) to meet Springer Nature publication standards.

Trampoline Related Injuries in Children: Risk Factors and Radiographic Findings [17]

This is a machine-generated summary of:

Klimek, Peter Michael; Juen, David; Stranzinger, Enno; Wolf, Rainer; Slongo, Theddy Trampoline related injuries in children: risk factors and radiographic findings [17]
Published in: World Journal of Pediatrics (2013)
Link to original: https://doi.org/10.1007/s12519-013-0416-2
Copyright of the summarized publication:
Children's Hospital, Zhejiang University School of Medicine and Springer-Verlag Berlin Heidelberg 2013
All rights reserved.

If you want to cite the papers, please refer to the original.

For technical reasons we could not place the page where the original quote is coming from.

Research Highlights

Trampoline use among children has become increasingly popular, yet it is accompanied by a significant rise in related injuries over the past decades. Despite safety recommendations emphasizing adult supervision and limiting the number of jumpers, injuries continue to occur frequently. Now, a new study by Peter Michael Klimek and colleagues from the University of Bern, Switzerland, investigates the correlation between questionnaire data from parents and radiographic findings to identify children at risk for trampoline-related fractures.

The study was conducted at the Inselspital, University Hospital Bern, where all children with backyard trampoline injuries between 2005 and 2010 were included. Researchers reviewed patient records and radiographs while parents completed questionnaires detailing accident circumstances. The data collected included demographic information, accident details, and parental supervision levels. Radiographs were analyzed for fracture types and chronic changes by a pediatric radiologist blinded to questionnaire results. The study found that most injuries occurred when multiple children were jumping simultaneously, with proximal tibia fractures being particularly common in younger children during springtime. These fractures often resulted from axial forces leading to compression fractures with anterior angulation.

The findings highlight the need for enhanced safety measures and awareness regarding trampoline use among children. While parental supervision was evident in only a quarter of cases, it remains crucial in preventing injuries. The study suggests that neither safety nets nor larger trampolines significantly reduce injury severity, as most fractures occurred on net-secured trampolines. Future studies could focus on developing more effective safety guidelines and educational materials for parents to mitigate risks associated with trampoline use. Additionally, understanding seasonal variations in injury rates may help tailor prevention strategies more effectively.

Buckle Fracture of the Proximal Tibia in Children and Frequency of Association with Trampoline and Inflatable Bouncer Use [18]

This is a machine-generated summary of:

Saade-Lemus, Sandra; Nguyen, Jie Chen; Francavilla, Michael L.; Martin-Saavedra, Juan Sebastian; Ho-Fung, Victor M.; Kaplan, Summer L. Buckle fracture of the proximal tibia in children and frequency of association with trampoline and inflatable bouncer use [18]
Published in: Pediatric Radiology (2019)
Link to original: https://doi.org/10.1007/s00247-019-04450-0
Copyright of the summarized publication:
Springer-Verlag GmbH Germany, part of Springer Nature 2019
All rights reserved.

If you want to cite the papers, please refer to the original.

For technical reasons we could not place the page where the original quote is coming from.

Research Highlights

Hyperextension fractures of the lower extremity in children are less well understood compared to the more common "fall on outstretched hand" injuries of the upper extremity. These lower extremity injuries, particularly buckle fractures of the proximal tibia, often occur in young children and are associated with activities like trampoline use. However, these fractures can be subtle and challenging to diagnose, especially for radiologists unfamiliar with their patterns. Now, a new study by Sandra Saade-Lemus and colleagues investigates the appearance, etiology, and demographics of proximal tibial buckle fractures to improve diagnostic accuracy.

The study involved a retrospective review of radiograph reports from children under 10 years old who sustained proximal tibial buckle fractures. The researchers categorized the mechanisms of injury into bouncing (e.g., trampolines), falls, and other causes. Two experienced pediatric radiologists conducted a consensus image review to establish consistent descriptive terms for fracture patterns before independently reviewing the exams to assess interobserver agreement. The study found that bouncing mechanisms were the most common cause of these fractures, with trampolines being a significant contributor. Fracture patterns varied with age; younger children typically exhibited tibial buckling, while older children showed oblique fractures extending toward the physis.

The study advances our understanding of proximal tibial buckle fractures by highlighting age-related changes in fracture patterns and emphasizing the role of bouncing mechanisms like trampoline use. Future studies could explore interventions to reduce these injuries or investigate other factors influencing fracture patterns. The findings underscore the importance of training radiologists to recognize these subtle fracture patterns and suggest that clinicians should consider knee radiographs when evaluating leg pain in children with a history of axial loading activities. This research provides valuable insights into pediatric fracture diagnosis and prevention strategies as recreational activities involving trampolines become increasingly popular.

Greenstick Fractures of the Proximal Metaphyseal Tibia: A Retrospective Multicenter Study on the Outcome After Non-surgical or Surgical Treatment and the Occurrence of Posttraumatic Tibia Valga [19]

This is a machine-generated summary of:

Weigert, Annabelle; Lieber, Justus; Buergener, Daniel; Grosser, Kay; Strohm, Peter; Schmittenbecher, Peter P.; Zwingmann, Joern Greenstick fractures of the proximal metaphyseal tibia: a retrospective multicenter study on the outcome after non-surgical or surgical treatment and the occurrence of posttraumatic tibia valga [19]

Published in: European Journal of Trauma and Emergency Surgery (2022)
Link to original: https://doi.org/10.1007/s00068-022-02181-w
Copyright of the summarized publication:
The Author(s) 2022
License: OpenAccess CC BY 4.0

This article is licensed under a Creative Commons Attribution 4.0 International License, which permits use, sharing, adaptation, distribution and reproduction in any medium or format, as long as you give appropriate credit to the original author(s) and the source, provide a link to the Creative Commons licence, and indicate if changes were made. The images or other third party material in this article are included in the article's Creative Commons licence, unless indicated otherwise in a credit line to the material. If material is not included in the article's Creative Commons licence and your intended use is not permitted by statutory regulation or exceeds the permitted use, you will need to obtain permission directly from the copyright holder. To view a copy of this licence, visit http://creativecommons.org/licenses/by/4.0/.

If you want to cite the papers, please refer to the original.

For technical reasons we could not place the page where the original quote is coming from.

Research Highlights

Proximal metaphyseal tibia fractures, first described by Cozen et al., are rare injuries in children, with a low incidence rate. These fractures can be treated conservatively or surgically, depending on whether they are displaced. A common complication following treatment is the development of progressive valgus deformity, which has been observed after both conservative and surgical management. The pathogenesis of this deformity is not well understood, with several hypotheses proposed, including periosteal invagination and hypervascularity of the growth plate. Now, a new study by Annabelle Weigert and colleagues investigates whether the treatment method for greenstick fractures of the proximal metaphyseal tibia influences the occurrence and progression of valgus deformity.

The study involved collecting data from institutions with members of the SKT on patients treated for proximal tibia fractures within a specified period. Only greenstick fractures were included in the analysis, focusing on patients aged between specific age groups with available X-rays at trauma and follow-up. The medial proximal tibia angle (MPTA) was measured on radiographs to assess valgus deformity progression. Patients were divided into non-surgical and surgical treatment groups, with follow-up timelines defined for both short-term and long-term assessments. Statistical analyses compared MPTA values across different treatment methods and age groups. The results indicated that progressive valgus deformity occurred in both non-surgically and surgically treated patients, with significant increases in MPTA observed during follow-up.

The study highlights that progressive valgus deformity can occur regardless of treatment method for greenstick fractures of the proximal metaphyseal tibia. Surgical intervention did not prevent valgus progression and may only be beneficial in selected cases. The authors suggest that future studies should focus on long-term outcomes to better understand spontaneous correction mechanisms and refine surgical indications based on patient age and fracture characteristics. Further research is needed to elucidate the underlying mechanisms contributing to valgus deformity development post-treatment.

Machine Learning to Identify Distal Tibial Classic Metaphyseal Lesions of Infant Abuse: A Pilot Study [20]

This is a machine-generated summary of:

Tsai, Andy; Kleinman, Paul K. Machine learning to identify distal tibial classic metaphyseal lesions of infant abuse: a pilot study [20]
Published in: Pediatric Radiology (2022)
Link to original: https://doi.org/10.1007/s00247-022-05287-w
Copyright of the summarized publication:
The Author(s), under exclusive licence to Springer-Verlag GmbH Germany, part of Springer Nature 2022
All rights reserved.

If you want to cite the papers, please refer to the original.

For technical reasons we could not place the page where the original quote is coming from.

Research Highlights

The classic metaphyseal lesion (CML) is a specific injury often associated with inflicted trauma in infants, posing significant diagnostic challenges due to its subtle radiographic features. Despite the American College of Radiology's guidelines emphasizing high-detail techniques for detecting CMLs, these injuries can be easily overlooked, leading to profound clinical implications. Now, a new study by Andy Tsai and colleagues explores the potential of machine learning, specifically convolutional neural networks (CNNs), to improve the detection of distal tibial CMLs in suspected cases of infant abuse.

In this pilot study, the researchers developed a binary classification algorithm using a residual neural network (ResNet) to differentiate between normal and abnormal distal tibial radiographs. The study involved a retrospective review of skeletal surveys from a large children's hospital, identifying two cohorts: normal and CML-affected distal tibias. The radiographs were carefully curated and preprocessed to focus on the distal tibia, ensuring consistent image quality and alignment. The ResNet model was trained using cross-entropy loss with class weighting to address data imbalance and evaluated through fivefold cross-validation. This approach allowed for robust performance assessment despite the modest dataset size.

The study demonstrated promising results, achieving sensitivity and specificity ranges of 80–90% and 85–95%, respectively, with an overall accuracy range of 85–95% and a Kappa statistic indicating substantial agreement. These findings suggest that machine learning could serve as an effective tool for flagging potentially abnormal radiographs for further review by radiologists. Future studies should aim to include larger cohorts and incorporate other distal tibial pathologies to enhance the algorithm's robustness. Additionally, integrating automated object localization could streamline the process, making it more applicable in clinical settings. This research lays the groundwork for developing machine learning tools that complement traditional radiologic assessments in detecting high-specificity indicators of abuse like CMLs.

Outcome of Displaced Distal Tibial Metaphyseal Fractures in Children Between 6 and 15 Years of Age Treated by Elastic Stable Intramedullary Nails [21]

This is a machine-generated summary of:

Cravino, Mattia; Canavese, Federico; De Rosa, Vincenzo; Marengo, Lorenza; Samba, Antoine; Rousset, Marie; Mansour Khamallah, Mounira; Andreacchio, Antonio Outcome of displaced distal tibial metaphyseal fractures in children between 6 and 15 years of age treated by elastic stable intramedullary nails [21]
Published in: European Journal of Orthopaedic Surgery & Traumatology (2014)
Link to original: https://doi.org/10.1007/s00590-013-1402-z
Copyright of the summarized publication:
Springer-Verlag France 2014
All rights reserved.

If you want to cite the papers, please refer to the original.

For technical reasons we could not place the page where the original quote is coming from.

Research Highlights

Fractures of the distal tibial metaphysis in children are rare, accounting for a small percentage of all pediatric fractures. These injuries are often treated non-operatively due to children's rapid bone healing and remodeling capabilities. However, displaced fractures may necessitate surgical intervention, typically managed through percutaneous pinning or external fixation. Despite the established use of elastic stable intramedullary nailing (ESIN) for diaphyseal or metaphyseal fractures in children, there is a lack of clinical studies specifically addressing its application for distal tibial metaphysis fractures. Now, a new study by Mattia Cravino and colleagues retrospectively evaluates the clinical and radiographic outcomes of displaced distal tibia metaphyseal fractures in children treated with ESIN.

The study involved children aged 5–15 years who were treated at three pediatric orthopedic centers between June and August. All patients had displaced distal tibia metaphyseal fractures, with or without associated fibula fractures, and were managed using the ESIN technique as described by Métaizeau. The inclusion criteria required closed fractures with visible growth plates and no neurovascular injury. Surgical procedures involved closed reduction under general anesthesia, followed by stabilization with two intramedullary nails inserted through small incisions. Post-surgery, patients were immobilized in a below-knee cast for 6 weeks, with progressive weight-bearing allowed after cast removal. Follow-up assessments included clinical evaluations and radiographic examinations to monitor fracture healing and alignment.

The study demonstrated favorable outcomes for children treated with ESIN for displaced distal tibia metaphyseal fractures. Most patients returned to their daily activities without complications or limitations in movement. The findings suggest that ESIN is an effective treatment option, offering advantages such as reduced surgical time and lower infection rates compared to other methods. Future studies could explore long-term outcomes and potential growth plate disturbances due to the short follow-up period in this study. Additionally, the management of concomitant fibula fractures remains an area for further investigation to optimize treatment strategies for these complex injuries.

Conclusion

Fractures of the proximal or distal metaphyseal tibia are relatively uncommon. Depending on whether they are displaced, proximal metaphyseal tibial fractures can be treated either conservatively or surgically. A common complication following treatment is progressive valgus deformity, also known as Cozen's phenomenon.

Displaced distal metaphyseal fractures require fixation with percutaneous pinning or elastic stable intramedullary nailing. Whether to fix the fibula in both bone fractures remains debated.

Bibliography

1. Swischuk LE, John SD, Tschoepe EJ. Upper tibial hyperextension fractures in infants: another occult toddler's fracture. Pediatr Radiol. 1999;29:6–9.
2. Swischuk LE. Jumped off the trampoline: fell on knee: pain. Pediatr Emerg Care. 2009;25:366–7.
3. Dunbar JS, Owen HF, Nogrady MB, McLeese R. Obscure tibial fracture of infants—the toddler's fracture. J Can Assoc Radiol. 1964;15:136–44.
4. John SD, Moorthy CS, Swischuk LE. Expanding the concept of the toddler's fracture. Radiographics. 1997;17:367–76.
5. Skak SV, Jensen TT, Poulsen TD. Fracture of the proximal metaphysis of the tibia in children. Injury. 1987;18:149–56.
6. Kakel R. Trampoline fracture of the proximal tibial metaphysis in children may not progress into valgus: a report of seven cases and a brief review. Orthop Traumatol Surg Res. 2012;98:446–9.
7. Woodward GA, Furnival R, Schunk JE. Trampolines revisited: a review of 114 pediatric recreational trampoline injuries. Pediatrics. 1992;89:849–54.
8. American College of Radiology. ACR–SPR practice parameters for the performance and interpretation of skeletal surveys in children (Res. 10). In: American college of radiology (ACR) standards. Reston: American College of Radiology; 2016. p. 1–9.
9. Ciresan D, Meier U, Masci J, Schmidhuber J. Multi-column deep neural network for traffic sign classification. Neural Netw. 2012;32:333–8.

10. Liu X, Deng Z, Yang Y. Recent progress in semantic image segmentation. Artif Intell Rev. 2019;52:1–18.
11. Kingma DP, Ba J. Adam: a method for stochastic optimization. International Conference on Learning Representations (ICLR). 2015. https://dblp.org/rec/journals/corr/KingmaB14.html. Accessed 3 Feb 2022.
12. Métaizeau JP. Ostéosynthèse chez l'enfant: embrochage centromédullaire élastique, stable edition. Montpellier: Sauramps Médical; 1988.
13. Ligier JN, Métaizeau JP, Prévot J. Closed flexible medullary nailing in pediatric traumatololgy. Chir Pediatr. 1983;24:383–5.
14. Domzalski M, Lipton GE, Lee D, Guille JT. Fractures of the distal tibia metaphysis in children. Patterns of injury and results of treatment. J Pediatr Orthop. 2006;26:171–6.
15. Muller ME, Nazarian S, Koch P, Schatzker J. The comprehensive classification of fractures of long bones. Heidelberg: Springer; 1990.
16. Hansen BA, Greiff J, Bergmann F. Fractures of the tibia in children. Acta Orthop Scand. 1976;47:448–53.
17. Klimek PM, Juen D, Stranzinger E, Wolf R, Slongo T. Trampoline related injuries in children: risk factors and radiographic findings. World J Pediatr. 2013;9:169–74. https://doi.org/10.1007/s12519-013-0416-2.
18. Saade-Lemus S, Nguyen JC, Francavilla ML, Martin-Saavedra JS, Ho-Fung VM, Kaplan SL. Buckle fracture of the proximal tibia in children and frequency of association with trampoline and inflatable bouncer use. Pediatr Radiol. 2019;49:1327–34. https://doi.org/10.1007/s00247-019-04450-0.
19. Weigert A, Lieber J, Buergener D, Grosser K, Strohm P, Schmittenbecher PP, Zwingmann J. Greenstick fractures of the proximal metaphyseal tibia: a retrospective multicenter study on the outcome after non-surgical or surgical treatment and the occurrence of posttraumatic tibia valga. Eur J Trauma Emerg Surg. 2022;49:1459–65. https://doi.org/10.1007/s00068-022-02181-w.
20. Tsai A, Kleinman PK. Machine learning to identify distal tibial classic metaphyseal lesions of infant abuse: a pilot study. Pediatr Radiol. 2022;52:1095–103. https://doi.org/10.1007/s00247-022-05287-w.
21. Cravino M, Canavese F, De Rosa V, Marengo L, Samba A, Rousset M, Mansour Khamallah M, Andreacchio A. Outcome of displaced distal tibial metaphyseal fractures in children between 6 and 15 years of age treated by elastic stable intramedullary nails. Eur J Orthop Surg Traumatol. 2014;24:1603–8. https://doi.org/10.1007/s00590-013-1402-z.

17 Fractures of the Tibial Spine and Anterior Tibial Tuberosity

Introduction by the Author

Tibial spine fractures, which are avulsion fractures of the intercondylar eminence, are often associated with anterior cruciate ligament injuries. They are generally considered analogous to anterior cruciate ligament ruptures in adults. They typically occur in children between 8 and 14 years of age, predominantly affecting those who participate in competitive sports or who fall from a bicycle or motorcycle.

In growing patients, the tensile strength of the intercondylar eminence is lower than that of the anterior cruciate ligament. This leads to fractures when there is too much tension. Although the incidence of meniscal injuries in children with tibial eminence fractures is lower than in adults with anterior cruciate ligament ruptures, pediatric meniscal tears and entrapments need to be systematically evaluated. Magnetic resonance imaging is beneficial for assessing concomitant injuries before treatment in nonsurgical cases. However, it may not be valuable for detecting entrapments if arthroscopy is planned.

The most common classification system for these fractures was described by Meyers and McKeever and modified by Zariczny. There are four types of fractures, which are classified according to the amount of displacement: no or minimally displaced (type 1); displaced with posterior hinge (type 2); avulsion (type 3); and comminuted (type 4).

Types 1 and 2 fractures are generally treated conservatively with a long-leg cast in extension.

There is agreement that surgical treatment for displaced and comminuted fractures can lead to satisfactory clinical outcomes, though there is no consensus on the optimal treatment. Some advocate conservative management, while others recommend open or arthroscopic surgery.

© The Author(s), under exclusive license to Springer Nature Switzerland AG 2026
F. Canavese, *Advances in Pediatric Extremity Fracture Management*,
https://doi.org/10.1007/978-3-032-33306-3_17

Patients regain a full range of motion and return to their pre-injury activity levels without experiencing any instability. Although patients develop residual knee laxity, which is detected instrumentally, this does not result in subjective instability or functional limitations.

Acute tibial tuberosity fractures are also rare and often occur in athletic adolescent males nearing skeletal maturity. These fractures account for a small percentage of all proximal tibial and physeal injuries, with an incidence ranging from 0.4% to 2.7%. The Watson-Jones classification system categorizes fractures based on the extent to which the proximal tibial epiphysis is involved and displaced. In type I, a small fragment of the tubercle is avulsed and displaced slightly anteriorly. In type II, the secondary ossification center of the tubercle has coalesced with the proximal tibial epiphysis, resulting in avulsion of the entire tubercle. In type III, the fracture line extends into the articular surface.

Despite their rarity, tibial tuberosity fractures can significantly impact the extensor mechanism of the knee. In severe cases, the proximal tibia may evolve into recurvatum due to anterior growth arrest. Careful management and long-term follow-up are necessary to detect growth arrest.

17.1 Machine Generated Summaries

Disclaimer: The summaries in this chapter were generated from Springer Nature publications using abstractive AI auto-summarization: An abstraction-based summarizer creates new text based on deep learning. New phrases are created to summarize the content. As the constituted sentences are machine selected, they may not fully reflect the body of the work, so we strongly advise that the original content is read and cited. The auto-generated summaries were curated by the author(s) to meet Springer Nature publication standards.

Meniscal Injuries in Skeletally Immature Children with Tibial Eminence Fractures. Systematic Review of Literature [39]

This is a machine-generated summary of:

Severyns, Mathieu; Odri, Guillaume Anthony; Vendeuvre, Tanguy; Marchand, Jean-Baptiste; Germaneau, Arnaud; Dramé, Moustapha Meniscal injuries in skeletally immature children with tibial eminence fractures. Systematic review of literature [39]

Published in: International Orthopaedics (2023)

Link to original: https://doi.org/10.1007/s00264-023-05787-w

Copyright of the summarized publication:
The Author(s) under exclusive licence to SICOT aisbl 2023
Copyright comment: Springer Nature or its licensor (e.g. a society or other partner) holds exclusive rights to this article under a publishing agreement with the author(s) or other rightsholder(s); author self-archiving of the accepted manuscript version of this article is solely governed by the terms of such publishing agreement and applicable law.
All rights reserved.

If you want to cite the papers, please refer to the original.

For technical reasons we could not place the page where the original quote is coming from.

Research Highlights

Tibial eminence fractures (TEFs), also known as tibial spine fractures, are avulsions of the anterior cruciate ligament (ACL) from its tibial insertion site, predominantly affecting children aged eight to 14. In this age group, the ACL is biomechanically stronger than its tibial attachment, leading to these fractures. While adult studies have extensively documented meniscal lesions associated with ACL ruptures, there is limited understanding of such injuries in children with TEFs. Now, a new study by Mathieu Severyns and colleagues systematically reviews the literature to determine the frequency of meniscal lesions in skeletally immature patients with TEFs, using MRI and arthroscopy as diagnostic tools.

The study conducted a comprehensive literature search across PubMed, Scopus, and Embase databases up to May 2023. Articles were selected based on predefined criteria, focusing on observational studies that reported data on intercondylar tibial fractures. The researchers extracted data on study design, sample size, age, sex ratio, fracture classification, treatment techniques, and diagnostic methods for meniscal lesions. Statistical analyses were performed to compare proportions of lesions identified by different diagnostic methods. The review included 26 studies with a total of 1032 patients. Findings indicated that while MRI is useful for identifying concomitant injuries like meniscal tears before treatment, it does not significantly enhance detection of entrapments compared to arthroscopy.

The study advances our understanding of TEFs by highlighting a significant rate of associated meniscal tears and entrapments in children. It suggests that while MRI is beneficial for pre-treatment assessment of concomitant injuries in non-surgical cases, it may not add value for detecting entrapments if arthroscopy is planned. Future study could focus on refining MRI techniques to improve detection of soft tissue entrapments and further explore the correlation between fracture severity and associated injuries. This could lead to optimized treatment protocols and better prognostic outcomes for pediatric patients with TEFs.

Cartilaginous Avulsion Fracture of the Tibial Spine in a 5-Year-Old Girl [40]

This is a machine-generated summary of:

Kim, Jung Ryul; Song, Ji Hun; Lee, Ju Hong; Lee, Sang Yong; Yoo, Wan Hee
Cartilaginous avulsion fracture of the tibial spine in a 5-year-old girl [40]
Published in: Skeletal Radiology (2008)
Link to original: https://doi.org/10.1007/s00256-007-0428-x
Copyright of the summarized publication:
ISS 2007
All rights reserved.

If you want to cite the papers, please refer to the original.

For technical reasons we could not place the page where the original quote is coming from.

Research Highlights

The anterior tibial spine serves as the distal attachment site for the anterior cruciate ligament (ACL), and in children, this area is cartilaginous before the proximal tibia fully ossifies. When excessive stress is applied to the ACL, it can lead to a fracture through the cancellous bone beneath the tibial spine, particularly in children, where such fractures are more common than ACL tears seen in adults. However, tibial spine fractures have not been reported in children below a certain age. Now, a new study by Jung Ryul Kim and colleagues reports the first case of a purely cartilaginous avulsion fracture of the tibial spine in a 3-year-old female patient, which was not visible on radiographs.

The study details a case where a young girl presented with knee pain after slipping on a trampoline. Initial radiographs showed no bony lesions, but further investigation with magnetic resonance imaging (MRI) revealed an avulsion injury of the articular cartilage attached to the ACL at the tibial eminence and a large effusion. Diagnostic arthroscopy confirmed that the anterior portion of the avulsed fragment had a posterior hinge and was classified as a type II tibial eminence fracture according to Meyers and McKeever. The patient underwent arthroscopic reduction and fixation using pull-out sutures, achieving anatomical reduction. Post-surgery, she was placed in a long-leg cast for 6 weeks before beginning range of motion and strengthening exercises.

At one-year follow-up, the patient exhibited full range of motion and excellent knee stability without pain. This case highlights that while tibial eminence avulsion injuries are common in older children, they can also occur in younger patients with purely cartilaginous structures. The study suggests that MRI can be crucial for diagnosing such occult injuries when radiographs fail to reveal them. Future study could explore differential injury patterns in skeletally immature knees under various loading conditions to better understand these injuries' mechanisms and improve diagnostic protocols.

Clinical and Radiological Results of Arthroscopically Treated Tibial Spine Fractures in Childhood [41]

This is a machine-generated summary of:

Perugia, D.; Basiglini, L.; Vadalà, A.; Ferretti, A. Clinical and radiological results of arthroscopically treated tibial spine fractures in childhood [41]
Published in: International Orthopaedics (2008)
Link to original: https://doi.org/10.1007/s00264-008-0697-6
Copyright of the summarized publication:
Springer-Verlag 2008
All rights reserved.

If you want to cite the papers, please refer to the original.
For technical reasons we could not place the page where the original quote is coming from.

Research Highlights

Tibial eminence fractures, commonly occurring in children aged eight to twelve, are often compared to anterior cruciate ligament (ACL) ruptures in adults due to similar injury mechanisms. These fractures typically result from falls during activities like cycling or motorcycling. The prevailing belief is that the tibial eminence's fragility, combined with the high elasticity of childhood ligaments, contributes to these injuries. However, there is a lack of consensus on the optimal treatment for type II fractures, with some advocating for conservative management and others recommending surgical intervention. Now, a new study by D. Perugia and colleagues investigates the clinical and radiological outcomes of patients who underwent arthroscopic reduction for anterior tibial eminence fractures.

The study involved ten patients treated surgically at a single institution between November and October. The participants, with an average age of 11.5 years, sustained injuries primarily during sports activities or falls from motorcycles. All patients with type II and III fractures underwent arthroscopic reduction using reabsorbable polydioxanone sutures for fixation. The surgical procedure included arthroscopic debridement and careful evaluation for associated chondral or meniscal lesions. Post-operative care involved immobilization in full extension and a structured rehabilitation protocol to restore range of motion (ROM) and muscle strength. Clinical assessments were conducted using international knee evaluation scales, while radiological evaluations ensured proper fracture consolidation.

The study's findings indicate that surgical treatment can lead to satisfactory clinical outcomes, with all patients regaining full ROM and returning to pre-injury activity levels without reported instability. Despite some residual knee laxity detected instrumentally, it did not translate into subjective instability or functional limitations for the patients. Future studies could explore the presence of rotational knee laxity observed in some cases, potentially linked to undetected peripheral knee injuries. Additionally, further research might investigate long-term outcomes across different fracture types to refine treatment strategies and improve patient care.

Arthroscopic Percutaneous Pullout Suture Transverse Tunnel Technique Repair for Tibial Spine Fractures in Skeletally Immature Patients [42]

This is a machine-generated summary of:

Zhou, Yi; Deng, Guozhen; She, Hongjiang; Zhou, Yangyang; Xiang, Bingyan; Bai, Fan Arthroscopic percutaneous pullout suture transverse tunnel technique repair for tibial spine fractures in skeletally immature patients [42]
Published in: International Orthopaedics (2023)
Link to original: https://doi.org/10.1007/s00264-023-05756-3
Copyright of the summarized publication:
The Author(s) under exclusive licence to SICOT aisbl 2023
Copyright comment: Springer Nature or its licensor (e.g. a society or other partner) holds exclusive rights to this article under a publishing agreement with the author(s) or other rightsholder(s); author self-archiving of the accepted manuscript version of this article is solely governed by the terms of such publishing agreement and applicable law.
All rights reserved.

If you want to cite the papers, please refer to the original.

For technical reasons we could not place the page where the original quote is coming from.

Research Highlights

Tibial spine fractures (TSF) are avulsion fractures of the intercondylar eminence often associated with anterior cruciate ligament (ACL) injuries, predominantly affecting children and adolescents engaged in competitive sports. In skeletally immature patients, the tensile strength of the intercondylar eminence is lower than that of the ACL, leading to fractures under excessive tensile load. Traditionally, surgical anatomic reduction is recommended for type II, III, and IV fractures due to complications from conservative treatment. Now, a new study by Yi Zhou and colleagues introduces a percutaneous pullout suture transverse tunnel (PP-STT) technique aimed at providing epiphyseal protection during TSF repair in skeletally immature patients (SIPs).

The study compared the clinical and radiological outcomes of the PP-STT technique with the traditional transtibial pullout suture (TS-PLS) technique. The researchers reviewed medical data from SIPs with type II, III, or IV TSF treated between February and November. Patients were divided into two groups based on the surgical technique used. The PP-STT technique involved creating soft tissue tunnels and a transverse bone tunnel below the tibial tuberosity to pass sutures through, avoiding direct drilling through the tibial epiphyseal plate. In contrast, the TS-PLS technique used transtibial bone tunnels through the epiphyseal plate. Both techniques aimed for anatomical reduction of displaced fragments under arthroscopic visualization.

The study found that both surgical techniques resulted in satisfactory clinical and radiological outcomes without significant differences between them. However, the PP-STT technique offers an advantage by minimizing potential iatrogenic injury to the tibial epiphyseal plate, which is crucial for bone growth in SIPs. Future study could focus on long-term outcomes and further refine techniques to enhance safety and efficacy in pediatric orthopedic surgery. Despite limitations such as short follow-up time and small sample size, this study provides valuable insights into safer surgical options for treating TSF in young patients.

MRI Evaluation of Pediatric Tibial Eminence Fractures: Comparison Between Conventional and "CT-Like" Ultrashort Echo Time (UTE) Images [43]

This is a machine-generated summary of:

Nguyen, Jie C.; Guariento, Andressa; Williams, Brendan A.; Lawrence, J. Todd R.; Ganley, Theodore J.; Venkatesh, Tanvi P.; Sze, Raymond W. MRI evaluation of pediatric tibial eminence fractures: comparison between conventional and "CT-like" ultrashort echo time (UTE) images [43]
Published in: Skeletal Radiology (2022)
Link to original: https://doi.org/10.1007/s00256-022-04000-0
Copyright of the summarized publication:
ISS 2022
All rights reserved.

If you want to cite the papers, please refer to the original.

For technical reasons we could not place the page where the original quote is coming from.

Research Highlights

Tibial eminence avulsion fractures, occurring at the insertion of the anterior cruciate ligament (ACL), are rare but significant injuries in pediatric patients, often resulting from sports-related activities or accidents. These fractures can lead to knee instability and long-term dysfunction if not properly diagnosed and treated. The Meyers and McKeever classification system is commonly used to guide treatment decisions based on fracture displacement, with imaging playing a crucial role in assessing these injuries. However, conventional MRI sequences have limitations in visualizing bone structures due to longer echo times. Now, a new study by Jie C. Nguyen and colleagues explores the use of ultrashort echo time (UTE) MRI sequences to improve the detection and characterization of tibial eminence fractures in children.

The study was conducted at a tertiary children's hospital, where researchers retrospectively reviewed MRI examinations of pediatric knees, focusing on those with UTE images. The study included children with tibial eminence fractures and an age-matched reference group without fractures. Using a 3-Tesla MRI scanner, both conventional and UTE sequences were acquired, with images reviewed by radiologists and surgeons blinded to clinical outcomes. The study aimed to compare the diagnostic accuracy and inter-reader agreement between conventional MRI and UTE-enhanced images for fracture detection and characterization. Statistical analyses were performed to assess sensitivity, specificity, and inter-reader reliability.

The addition of UTE images did not significantly impact the already high diagnostic accuracy for fracture detection but improved inter-reader agreement on fracture characterization. This enhanced agreement led to changes in management decisions in some cases, highlighting the potential of UTE sequences to provide more precise information on fracture displacement and morphology. Future studies could focus on validating these findings with larger sample sizes and surgical correlations, as well as exploring the application of UTE imaging for other anatomical sites in both pediatric and adult populations. The integration of UTE into routine clinical practice could enhance treatment decision-making by offering comprehensive osseous and soft tissue assessment within a single imaging session.

Type III Fractures of the Anterior Tibial Tuberosity in Adolescents: Two Case Reports [44]

This is a machine-generated summary of:

Ares-Rodriguez, Oscar; Seijas, Roberto; Núñez-Pereira, Susana; Aguirre-Canyadell, Marius Type III fractures of the anterior tibial tuberosity in adolescents: two case reports [44]

Published in: European Journal of Orthopaedic Surgery & Traumatology (2008)
Link to original: https://doi.org/10.1007/s00590-008-0322-9
Copyright of the summarized publication:
Springer-Verlag 2008
All rights reserved.

If you want to cite the papers, please refer to the original.

For technical reasons we could not place the page where the original quote is coming from.

Research Highlights

Acute tibial tubercle avulsion fractures are rare injuries, often occurring in athletic adolescent males nearing skeletal maturity. These fractures account for a small percentage of all proximal tibial and physeal injuries, with an incidence between 0.4% and 2.7% of all epiphyseal injuries. Despite their rarity, these injuries can significantly impact the extensor mechanism of the knee, necessitating careful management. Now, a new study by Oscar Ares-Rodriguez and colleagues presents two cases of displaced intra-articular fractures of the tibial tuberosity, providing insights into surgical treatment approaches and outcomes.

The study details two cases involving adolescent males who sustained tibial tuberosity fractures during sports activities—one from a basketball jump and the other from a soccer-related impact. Both patients underwent open reduction and internal fixation using cannulated cancellous bone screws to restore the extensor mechanism and ensure articular congruency. The surgical approach included medial arthrotomy for visualization and precise reduction of fracture fragments. Postoperative care involved immobilization followed by a structured rehabilitation program focusing on progressive quadriceps strengthening. At 6 weeks post-surgery, both patients began active rehabilitation exercises, ultimately resuming sports activities within 12 weeks post-injury.

The study highlights successful surgical outcomes with full restoration of joint motion and no complications in both cases. The authors emphasize the importance of anatomical reduction and stable fixation to prevent long-term sequelae such as genu recurvatum or growth disturbances. Future study could explore long-term follow-up to assess potential growth alterations or late-onset complications. Additionally, further research might investigate optimal rehabilitation protocols to enhance recovery timelines while minimizing risks associated with early return to sports activities. This study contributes valuable clinical insights into managing this uncommon but impactful injury in adolescent athletes.

Conclusion

Tibial spine fractures, which are avulsion fractures of the intercondylar eminence, are often associated with anterior cruciate ligament injuries. The optimal treatment for displaced fractures remains debated: open surgery versus arthroscopy. Acute tibial tuberosity fractures account for a small percentage of all proximal tibial and physeal injuries. Despite correct diagnosis and treatment, these injuries carry a high risk of growth arrest (procurvatum).

Bibliography

1. Shimberg JL, Aoyama JT, Leska TM, et al. Tibial spine fractures: how much are we missing without pretreatment advanced imaging? A multicenter study. Am J Sports Med. 2020;48:3208–13.
2. Rhodes JT, Cannamela PC, Cruz AI, et al. Incidence of meniscal entrapment and associated knee injuries in tibial spine avulsions. J Pediatr Orthop. 2018;38:e38–42.
3. Johnson AC, Wyatt JD, Treme G, et al. Incidence of associated knee injury in pediatric tibial eminence fractures. J Knee Surg. 2014;27:215–9.
4. Kocher MS, Micheli LJ, Gerbino P, et al. Tibial eminence fractures in children: prevalence of meniscal entrapment. Am J Sports Med. 2003;31:404–7.
5. Burstein DB, Viola A, Fulkerson JP. Entrapment of the medial meniscus in a fracture of the tibial eminence. Arthroscopy. 1988;4:47–50.

6. Falstie-Jensen S, Sondergard Petersen PE. Incarceration of the meniscus in fractures of the intercondylar eminence of the tibia in children. Injury. 1984;15:236–8.
7. Chandler JT, Miller TK. Tibial eminence fracture with meniscal entrapment. Arthroscopy. 1995;11:499–502.
8. Mah JY, Adili A, Otsuka NY, et al. Follow-up study of arthroscopic reduction and fixation of type III tibial-eminence fractures. J Pediatr Orthop. 1998;18:475–7.
9. Feucht MJ, Brucker PU, Camathias C, et al. Meniscal injuries in children and adolescents undergoing surgical treatment for tibial eminence fractures. Knee Surg Sports Traumatol Arthrosc. 2017;25:445–53.
10. Shea KG, Grimm NL, Laor T, et al. Bone bruises and meniscal tears on mri in skeletally immature children with tibial eminence fractures. J Pediatr Orthop. 2011;31:150–2.
11. Lewis E, Zionts MD. Fractures around the knee in children. J Am Acad Orthop Surg. 2002;10:345–55.
12. William K, Accousti MD, Baxter R, Willis MD. Tibial eminence fractures. Orthop Clin N Am. 2003;34:365–75.
13. Noyes FR, Delucas JL, Torvik PJ. Biomechanics of ACL failure: an analysis of strain-rate sensitivity and mechanism of failure in primates. J Bone Joint Surg. 1974;56-A:236–53.
14. Woo SL, Hollis JM, Adams DJ, et al. Tensile properties of the human femur-anterior cruciate ligament-tibia complex. The effects of specimen age and orientation. Am J Sports Med. 1991;19:217–25.
15. Baxter MP, Willey JJ. Fractures of the tibial spine in children. An evaluation of knee stability. J Bone Joint Surg. 1988;70-B:228–30.
16. Mulhall KJ, Dowdall J, Grannell M, et al. Tibial spine fractures. An analysis of outcome in surgically treated type III injuries. Injury. 1999;30:289–92.
17. Smith JB. Knee instability after fractures of the intercondylar eminence of the tibia. J Pediatr Orthop. 1984;4:462–4.
18. Grönkvist H, Hirsch G, Johansson L. Fracture of the anterior tibial spine in children. J Pediatr Orthop. 1984;4:465–8.
19. Meyers MH, McKeever FM. Fracture of the intercondylar eminence of the tibia. J Bone Joint Surg Am. 1959;41-A:209–22.
20. Meyers MH, McKeever FM. Fracture of the intercondylar eminence of the tibia. J Bone Joint Surg Am. 1970;52:1677–84.
21. Canale ST. Fractures and dislocation in children. In: Campbell's operative orthopaedics. 9th ed. Philadelphia: Mosby; 1998. p. 2488–90.
22. Lubowitz JH, Elson WS, Guttmann D. Part II: arthroscopic treatment of tibial plateau fractures: intercondylar eminence fractures. Arthroscopy. 2005;21:86–92.
23. Hunter RE, Willis JA. Arthroscopic fixation of avulsion fractures of the tibial eminence: technique and outcome. Arthroscopy. 2004;20:113–21.
24. Baxter MP, Wiley JJ. Fractures of the tibial spine in children. An evaluation of knee stability. J Bone Joint Surg Br. 1988;70:228–30.
25. Willis RB, Blokker C, Stoll TM, et al. Long-term follow-up of anterior tibial eminence fractures. J Pediatr Orthop. 1993;13:361–4.
26. Tuca M, Bernal N, Luderowski E, Green DW. Tibial spine avulsion fractures. Curr Opin Pediatr. 2019;31(1):103–11. https://doi.org/10.1097/MOP.0000000000000719.
27. Wiegand N, Naumov I, Vamhidy L, et al. Arthroscopic treatment of tibial spine fracture in children with a cannulated Herbert screw. Knee. 2014;21:481–5.
28. Su W, Wang P, Wang H, Lin C. A simple, modified arthroscopic suture fixation of avulsion fracture of the tibial intercondylar eminence in children. J Pediatr Orthop B. 2011;20(1):17–21. https://doi.org/10.1097/BPB.0b013e32832d8452.
29. Havlas V, Kautzner J, Trč T, Kaplan A. Arthroscopic technique using crossed K-wires for avulsion fractures of intercondylar eminence in children. Acta Chir Orthop Traumatol Cechoslov. 2011;78(4):343–7.

30. Kristinsson J, Elsoe R, Jensen HP, et al. Satisfactory outcome following arthroscopic fixation of tibial intercondylar eminence fractures in children and adolescents using bioabsorbable nails. Arch Orthop Trauma Surg. 2021;141:1945–51.
31. Kocher MS, Foreman ES, Micheli LJ. Laxity and functional outcome after arthroscopic reduction and internal fixation of displaced tibial spine fractures in children. Arthroscopy. 2003;19:1085–90.
32. Edmonds EW, Fornari ED, Dashe J, Roocroft JH, King MM, Pennock AT. Results of displaced pediatric tibial spine fractures. J Pediatr Orthop. 2015;35(7):651–6. https://doi.org/10.1097/BPO.0000000000000356.
33. Zhao C, Bi Q, Bi M. Management of a type two avulsion fracture of the tibial intercondylar eminence in children: arthroscopic suture fixation versus conservative immobilization. Int Orthop. 2018;42(6):1363–9. https://doi.org/10.1007/s00264-018-3855-5.
34. Green D, Tuca M, Luderowski E, Gausden E, Goodbody C, Konin G. A new, MRI-based classification system for tibial spine fractures changes clinical treatment recommendations when compared to Myers and Mckeever. Knee Surg Sports Traumatol Arthrosc. 2019;27(1):86–92.
35. Chotel F, Raux S, Accadbled F, et al. Cartilaginous tibial eminence fractures in children: which recommendations for management of this new entity? Knee Surg Sports Traumatol Arthrosc. 2016;24:688–96.
36. Ehrenborg G. The Osgood–Schlatter lesion. A clinical and experimental study. Acta Chir Scand Suppl. 1962;288:1–36.
37. Bolesta MJ, Fitch RD. Tibial tubercle avulsions. J Pediatr Orthop. 1986;6(2):186–92.
38. McKoy BE, Stanitski CL. Acute tibial tubercle avulsion fractures. Orthop Clin North Am. 2003;34:397–403.
39. Severyns M, Odri GA, Vendeuvre T, Marchand J-B, Germaneau A, Dramé M. Meniscal injuries in skeletally immature children with tibial eminence fractures. Systematic review of literature. Int Orthop. 2023;47:2439–48. https://doi.org/10.1007/s00264-023-05787-w.
40. Kim JR, Song JH, Lee JH, Lee SY, Yoo WH. Cartilaginous avulsion fracture of the tibial spine in a 5-year-old girl. Skeletal Radiol. 2008;37:343–5. https://doi.org/10.1007/s00256-007-0428-x.
41. Perugia D, Basiglini L, Vadalà A, Ferretti A. Clinical and radiological results of arthroscopically treated tibial spine fractures in childhood. Int Orthop. 2008;33:243–8. https://doi.org/10.1007/s00264-008-0697-6.
42. Zhou Y, Deng G, She H, Zhou Y, Xiang B, Bai F. Arthroscopic percutaneous pullout suture transverse tunnel technique repair for tibial spine fractures in skeletally immature patients. Int Orthop. 2023;47:1353–60. https://doi.org/10.1007/s00264-023-05756-3.
43. Nguyen JC, Guariento A, Williams BA, Lawrence JTR, Ganley TJ, Venkatesh TP, Sze RW. MRI evaluation of pediatric tibial eminence fractures: comparison between conventional and "CT-like" ultrashort echo time (UTE) images. Skeletal Radiol. 2022;51:1603–10. https://doi.org/10.1007/s00256-022-04000-0.
44. Ares-Rodriguez O, Seijas R, Núñez-Pereira S, Aguirre-Canyadell M. Type III fractures of the anterior tibial tuberosity in adolescents: two case reports. Eur J Orthop Surg Traumatol. 2008;18:399–403. https://doi.org/10.1007/s00590-008-0322-9.

Diaphyseal Tibia and Fibula Fracture 18

Introduction by the Author

Tibia diaphyseal fractures are the second most common type of fracture in hospitalized children, accounting for 15% of all fractures in children. Forty percent of tibia fractures occur in the mid diaphysis. These fractures are often the result of high- or low-energy trauma and often require surgical intervention when significantly displaced to prevent complications such as shortening or rotation.

Traditionally, they are treated with closed reduction and immobilization in a long-leg cast. While this method is generally effective, it has limitations, particularly in cases of polytrauma or fracture instability. Closed reduction and immobilization are still recommended for diaphyseal fractures of the tibia and fibula in children under 5 years of age who weigh less than 25 kg.

Elastic stable intramedullary nailing has emerged as an alternative treatment option, offering benefits such as rapid recovery and low infection rates. This technique provides stable fixation and good rotational stability with minimal invasiveness and low rates of postoperative complications, even in children weighing up to 110 pounds (50 kg). The most common complications are residual malalignment or skin irritation. Major complications are rare, occurring in fewer than 5% of cases and more frequently in open fractures. Additionally, elastic stable intramedullary nailing is preferred to external fixation for treating open tibial fractures, including Gustilo types II and IIIA. It yields comparable outcomes to an external fixator with fewer complications, such as pin tract infections.

In diaphyseal tibial and fibular fractures, the fibula is generally not fixed because it heals spontaneously in almost all cases.

Due to their distance from active growth plates, diaphyseal tibial and fibular fractures have limited remodeling potential, especially in children over 8 years of age.

© The Author(s), under exclusive license to Springer Nature Switzerland AG 2026
F. Canavese, *Advances in Pediatric Extremity Fracture Management*,
https://doi.org/10.1007/978-3-032-33306-3_18

18.1 Machine Generated Summaries

Disclaimer: The summaries in this chapter were generated from Springer Nature publications using abstractive AI auto-summarization: An abstraction-based summarizer creates new text based on deep learning. New phrases are created to summarize the content. As the constituted sentences are machine selected, they may not fully reflect the body of the work, so we strongly advise that the original content is read and cited. The auto-generated summaries were curated by the author(s) to meet Springer Nature publication standards.

Epidemiology of Paediatric Lower Extremity Fractures in a Tertiary Care Center in Switzerland [61]

This is a machine-generated summary of:

Chaibi, Emmélie; Zambelli, Pierre-Yves; Merckaert, Sophie Epidemiology of paediatric lower extremity fractures in a tertiary care center in Switzerland [61]
Published in: European Journal of Trauma and Emergency Surgery (2020)
Link to original: https://doi.org/10.1007/s00068-020-01400-6
Copyright of the summarized publication:
Springer-Verlag GmbH Germany, part of Springer Nature 2020
All rights reserved.

If you want to cite the papers, please refer to the original.
For technical reasons we could not place the page where the original quote is coming from.

Research Highlights

Pediatric fractures are a significant concern, accounting for a substantial percentage of injuries in children and leading to emergency consultations. In Switzerland, traumatic injuries are the leading cause of hospital admissions for children, with lower extremity fractures being particularly prevalent. Despite the high incidence of these injuries, there is limited epidemiological data specific to the Swiss pediatric population, especially concerning the correlation between board sports and lower extremity fractures. Now, a new study by Emmélie Chaibi and colleagues investigates the epidemiology and injury patterns of lower extremity fractures in children consulting a tertiary referral hospital in Switzerland.

The study conducted by Chaibi et al. involved a monocentric retrospective analysis of pediatric traumatic injuries at the Children's University Hospital of Lausanne over a 1-year period. The researchers collected data on patients up to 16 years old who presented with lower extremity fractures. Radiographic and clinical data were meticulously recorded and verified by medical professionals. The study classified fractures using established systems and analyzed variables such as age, gender, season, mechanism of injury, and treatment methods. Descriptive statistics were employed to tabulate the findings, revealing that boys had a higher risk ratio for traumatic injuries compared to girls. The study also found that tibia fractures were most common during winter months, often linked to board sports.

The findings from this study provide valuable insights into the epidemiology of pediatric fractures in Switzerland, highlighting the significant role of seasonal activities like skiing in fracture prevalence. The research underscores the importance of training junior residents in managing pediatric trauma cases effectively. Future studies could expand on these findings by incorporating multi-centric data over extended periods to enhance understanding and improve prevention strategies. The retrospective nature and short-term follow-up are limitations that future research could address to provide more comprehensive clinical outcome analyses.

Displaced Tibia Shaft Fractures in Children Treated by Elastic Stable Intramedullary Nailing: Results and Complications in Children Weighing 50 kg (110 lb) or More [26]

This is a machine-generated summary of:

Marengo, Lorenza; Paonessa, Matteo; Andreacchio, Antonio; Dimeglio, Alain; Potenza, Alberto; Canavese, Federico Displaced tibia shaft fractures in children treated by elastic stable intramedullary nailing: results and complications in children weighing 50 kg (110 lb) or more [26]

Published in: European Journal of Orthopaedic Surgery & Traumatology (2015)
Link to original: https://doi.org/10.1007/s00590-015-1729-8

Copyright of the summarized publication:
Springer-Verlag France 2015
All rights reserved.

If you want to cite the papers, please refer to the original.

For technical reasons we could not place the page where the original quote is coming from.

Research Highlights

The elastic stable intramedullary nailing (ESIN) technique is a well-established method for stabilizing long bone fractures, particularly in pediatric orthopedic surgery. It offers stable fixation and good rotational stability with minimal invasiveness and low postoperative complications. Despite its widespread use, especially for displaced tibia shaft fractures in children under 50 kg, there is limited research on its effectiveness in heavier children. Now, a new study by Lorenza Marengo and colleagues addresses this gap by evaluating the clinical and radiographic outcomes of ESIN in children weighing 50 kg or more.

The study retrospectively analyzed 106 children treated for displaced tibia shaft fractures using ESIN from September 2010 to May 2020 at two institutions. The inclusion criteria required patients to have closed displaced tibia shaft fractures, weigh at least 50 kg, and have no associated neurovascular injuries. The researchers collected demographic data, fracture characteristics, and surgical details from medical records. Radiographic evaluations were performed to classify fracture types and assess angulation and translation. The surgical technique involved closed manipulations under fluoroscopic control followed by the insertion of pre-contoured titanium elastic nails. Patients were followed up clinically and radiographically for at least 1 year post-surgery to monitor fracture healing and complications.

The study found that ESIN is a viable option for treating displaced tibia shaft fractures in children weighing 50 kg or more, with an overall complication rate lower than previously reported studies. The only major complication was anterior compartment syndrome in one patient. The authors noted no significant correlation between nail size/medullary canal diameter ratio and complication rates, suggesting that weight exceeding 50 kg is the primary factor influencing outcomes. Future studies could further explore the role of body mass index and refine guidelines for nail sizing to optimize treatment outcomes in this patient population. Despite some limitations, such as its retrospective nature and limited sample size, the study provides valuable insights into the use of ESIN in heavier pediatric patients.

Outcomes and Complications Following Flexible Intramedullary Nailing for the Treatment of Tibial Fractures in Children: A Meta-Analysis [62]

This is a machine-generated summary of:

Fanelli, Daniele; Perrotta, Gerardo; Stocco, Fabio; Agilinko, Joshua; Castioni, Davide; Mercurio, Michele; Gasparini, Giorgio; Barker, Simon Outcomes and complications following flexible intramedullary nailing for the treatment of tibial fractures in children: a meta-analysis [62]

Published in: Archives of Orthopaedic and Trauma Surgery (2021)

Link to original: https://doi.org/10.1007/s00402-021-03839-7

Copyright of the summarized publication:

The Author(s), under exclusive licence to Springer-Verlag GmbH, DE part of Springer Nature 2021

All rights reserved.

If you want to cite the papers, please refer to the original.

For technical reasons we could not place the page where the original quote is coming from.

Research Highlights

Tibia shaft fractures are the second most common fractures in hospitalized children, often resulting from both high and low energy trauma. Traditional treatment involves closed reduction and immobilization in a long leg cast, which is generally effective but has limitations, especially in cases of polytrauma or fracture instability. Flexible intramedullary nailing (FIN) has emerged as an alternative, offering benefits such as rapid recovery and low infection rates. However, there remains a need for clarity on the comparative clinical and cost-effectiveness of different treatment options for pediatric tibial fractures. Now, a new study by Daniele Fanelli and colleagues evaluates the surgical outcomes and complications of FIN in pediatric tibia shaft fractures through a systematic review and meta-analysis.

The study followed the Preferred Reporting Items for Systematic Reviews and Meta-Analyses guidelines, conducting comprehensive searches across PubMed/MedLine, Scopus, and Cochrane Central databases. The authors included studies that reported clinical outcomes of FIN for pediatric tibia fractures with at least 6 months of follow-up. Data extraction focused on demographics, fracture characteristics, surgical outcomes, and complications. The meta-analysis used fixed or random effect models based on heterogeneity to estimate complication rates and compare outcomes between open and closed fractures. The analysis included 13 studies with varying levels of evidence, assessing both qualitative and quantitative data to provide insights into the nature and rate of complications associated with FIN.

The study found that while almost one-third of patients undergoing FIN experienced complications, most were minor, such as residual malalignment or skin irritation. Major complications were rare, occurring in less than 5% of cases. Open fractures had a higher complication rate compared to closed ones. The findings suggest that FIN is an effective treatment option for unstable tibia shaft fractures in children, with satisfactory time to union and return to physical activity. Future study could focus on direct comparative analyses with other treatment methods to establish clearer guidelines for managing pediatric tibial fractures. Additionally, standardizing definitions for outcomes like malunion and non-union could enhance consistency across future research.

Application of Unilateral External Fixation by the "Joystick Technique" in the Treatment of Pediatric Tibia Shaft Fractures: Technical Note [63]

This is a machine-generated summary of:

Wang, Xinhui; Zhang, Zhe; Hou, Xizhi; Wang, Bao; Li, Yongdong; Zhang, Tao
Application of unilateral external fixation by the "joystick technique" in the treatment of pediatric tibia shaft fractures: technical note [63]
Published in: Journal of Orthopaedic Surgery and Research (2021)
Link to original: https://doi.org/10.1186/s13018-021-02625-w
Copyright of the summarized publication:
The Author(s) 2021
License: OpenAccess CC BY + CC0 4.0

This article is licensed under a Creative Commons Attribution 4.0 International License, which permits use, sharing, adaptation, distribution and reproduction in any medium or format, as long as you give appropriate credit to the original author(s) and the source, provide a link to the Creative Commons licence, and indicate if changes were made. The images or other third party material in this article are included in the article's Creative Commons licence, unless indicated otherwise in a credit line to the material. If material is not included in the article's Creative Commons licence and your intended use is not permitted by statutory regulation or exceeds the permitted use, you will need to obtain permission directly from the copyright holder. To view a copy of this licence, visit http://creativecommons.org/licenses/by/4.0/. The Creative Commons Public Domain Dedication waiver (http://creativecommons.org/publicdomain/zero/1.0/) applies to the data made available in this article, unless otherwise stated in a credit line to the data.

If you want to cite the papers, please refer to the original.

For technical reasons we could not place the page where the original quote is coming from.

Research Highlights

Tibia fractures are a prevalent injury among children, often requiring surgical intervention when significantly displaced to prevent complications such as shortening or rotation. Traditional surgical methods like open reduction and internal fixation, while effective, pose risks including trauma and infection. Minimally invasive techniques are thus sought after to mitigate these issues. Now, a new study by Xinhui Wang and colleagues explores the use of a unilateral external fixator combined with a joystick technique for fracture reduction in pediatric tibia shaft fractures, aiming to enhance clinical outcomes while minimizing surgical trauma.

The study retrospectively analyzed children with tibia shaft fractures treated at the Third Hospital of Hebei Medical University. Patients included had closed or Gustilo I type fractures with significant displacement. The surgical procedure involved external fixation under general anesthesia, using half-pins strategically placed following the "near-near, far-far" principle to optimize fixation strength. For older children, an additional external fixator was applied for increased stability. Postoperative care included elevation of the limb, antibiotic treatment, and guided weight-bearing exercises. The study reported successful fracture healing in all patients without major complications, highlighting the effectiveness of this minimally invasive approach.

The findings suggest that unilateral external fixation combined with joystick reduction offers a promising alternative for treating pediatric tibia shaft fractures, providing benefits such as reduced trauma and early functional recovery. Future study could focus on larger sample sizes and randomized controlled trials to further validate these results. Additionally, addressing challenges like fixation strength and pin-tract infection remains crucial for optimizing this technique's application in clinical settings. This approach may represent a significant advancement in pediatric orthopedic surgery by offering a less invasive yet effective treatment option for complex fractures.

External Fixation Versus Elastic Stable Intramedullary Nailing in the Treatment of Open Tibial Shaft Fractures in Children [64]

This is a machine-generated summary of:

Hong, Pan; Rai, Saroj; Tang, Xin; Liu, Ruikang; Li, Jin External fixation versus elastic stable intramedullary nailing in the treatment of open tibial shaft fractures in children [64]
Published in: Journal of Orthopaedic Surgery and Research (2021)
Link to original: https://doi.org/10.1186/s13018-021-02679-w
Copyright of the summarized publication:
The Author(s) 2021
License: OpenAccess CC BY + CC0 4.0

This article is licensed under a Creative Commons Attribution 4.0 International License, which permits use, sharing, adaptation, distribution and reproduction in any medium or format, as long as you give appropriate credit to the original author(s) and the source, provide a link to the Creative Commons licence, and indicate if changes were made. The images or other third party material in this article are included in the article's Creative Commons licence, unless indicated otherwise in a credit line to the material. If material is not included in the article's Creative Commons licence and your intended use is not permitted by statutory regulation or exceeds the permitted use, you will need to obtain permission directly from the copyright holder. To view a copy of this licence, visit http://creativecommons.org/licenses/by/4.0/. The Creative Commons Public Domain Dedication waiver (http://creativecommons.org/publicdomain/zero/1.0/) applies to the data made available in this article, unless otherwise stated in a credit line to the data.

If you want to cite the papers, please refer to the original.

For technical reasons we could not place the page where the original quote is coming from.

Research Highlights

Tibial fractures are common injuries in children, often involving the diaphysis and distal metaphyseal region. While closed reduction and casting are standard treatments for closed tibial shaft fractures, surgical stabilization is necessary for more complex cases such as comminuted or unstable fractures, open fractures, and polytrauma. Despite the popularity of external fixators (EF) for open injuries, complications like pin tract infection and refracture are prevalent. Elastic stable intramedullary nailing (ESIN) has shown acceptable outcomes for open tibial fractures. Now, a new study by Pan Hong and colleagues compares the clinical outcomes of EF versus ESIN in treating open tibial shaft fractures in children.

The study retrospectively reviewed patients aged 3–15 years with open tibial shaft fractures treated at their institute from January 2010 to January 2020. Patients were categorized into EF and ESIN groups based on their surgical procedure, excluding those with GA grade I injuries, comminuted fractures, pathological fractures, neuromuscular disorders, metabolic diseases, previous tibial fractures or instrumentation, polytrauma, or body weight over 50 kg. The choice of surgical method depended on the surgeon's preference. Antimicrobial therapy was administered early with first-generation cephalosporins and linezolid as needed. Radiographic assessments were conducted to monitor limb length discrepancy (LLD), angulation, and union. Complications were classified as major or minor. Statistical analyses were performed using SPSS software.

The study found that ESIN provided satisfactory clinical outcomes with fewer complications compared to EF in selected patients with open tibial shaft fractures. Although ESIN required secondary surgery for hardware removal, it resulted in faster radiological union and fewer cases of refracture compared to EF. The incidence of implant prominence was higher in the ESIN group but manageable. Future studies could explore cost-effectiveness and address allocation bias due to surgeon preference in treatment choice. Overall, ESIN is a viable option for GA grade II and IIIA open tibial fractures with comparable outcomes to EF but fewer complications like pin tract infections.

Residual Angulation of Distal Tibial Diaphyseal Fractures in Children Younger than Ten Years [65]

This is a machine-generated summary of:

Jung, Sung Taek; Park, Hyuk; Lee, Ju-Hyung; Kim, Jung Ryul Residual angulation of distal tibial diaphyseal fractures in children younger than 10 years [65]
Published in: Journal of Orthopaedic Surgery and Research (2014)
Link to original: https://doi.org/10.1186/s13018-014-0084-5
Copyright of the summarized publication:
Jung et al.; licensee BioMed Central Ltd. 2014
Copyright comment: This article is published under license to BioMed Central Ltd. This is an Open Access article distributed under the terms of the Creative Commons Attribution License (http://creativecommons.org/licenses/by/4.0), which permits unrestricted use, distribution, and reproduction in any medium, provided the original work is properly credited. The Creative Commons Public Domain Dedication waiver (http://creativecommons.org/publicdomain/zero/1.0/) applies to the data made available in this article, unless otherwise stated.

If you want to cite the papers, please refer to the original.
For technical reasons we could not place the page where the original quote is coming from.

Research Highlights

The normal process of bone remodeling in children allows for the realignment of initially malunited bone fragments, making anatomic reduction less critical in pediatric fractures compared to adults. Children's bones adapt to stresses from body weight, muscle action, and joint forces, often correcting residual angulation spontaneously. However, tibial angular deformities, particularly distal tibial fractures, pose challenges due to muscle activity and reduced growth potential in the distal tibia. Now a new study by Sung Taek Jung and colleagues from Chonbuk National University investigates residual angulation and factors influencing it after pediatric distal tibial fractures.

The study retrospectively analyzed children under 10 years old with distal tibial fractures treated at two tertiary centers. Excluding certain fracture types and cases with inadequate follow-up, the researchers included 51 fractures in their analysis. They assessed radiographic angulation changes from immediate postoperative to final follow-up images. Treatment methods varied based on fracture stability, including casting, elastic stable intramedullary nailing (ESIN), or external fixation (EF). Statistical analyses identified factors associated with residual deformities, revealing that initial angulations greater than 10° and treatment methods other than casting were linked to persistent valgus deformities.

The study highlights that spontaneous remodeling of distal tibial fractures in children is often incomplete, particularly for valgus deformities. While varus angulations showed improvement over time, valgus deformities persisted or worsened. The authors suggest that stabilizing fibular fractures might prevent valgus progression and recommend further research to explore this possibility. The findings underscore the importance of precise reduction in treating pediatric distal tibial fractures to minimize long-term deformities and suggest that a small amount of varus reduction may be preferable to an acceptable range of valgus angulation.

Conclusion

Diaphyseal fractures of the tibia and fibula are common. Elastic stable intramedullary nailing is the preferred treatment for displaced fractures in children over 5 years old. For younger children, closed reduction and long-leg cast immobilization may be more appropriate.

Bibliography

1. Landin LA. Fracture patterns in children. Analysis of 8,682 fractures with special reference to incidence, etiology and secular changes in a Swedish urban population 1950–1979. Acta Orthop Scand Suppl. 1983;202:1–109.
2. Lyons RA, Delahunty AM, Kraus D, et al. Children's fractures: a population based study. Inj Prev. 1999;5:129–32.
3. Joeris A, Lutz N, Wicki B, Slongo T, Audigé L. An epidemiological evaluation of pediatric long bone fractures—a retrospective cohort study of 2716 patients from two Swiss tertiary pediatric hospitals. BMC Pediatr. 2014;20(14):314.
4. Cooper C, et al. Epidemiology of childhood fractures in Britain: a study using the general practice research database. J Bone Miner Res. 2004;19(12):1976–81.
5. Rennie L, et al. The epidemiology of fractures in children. Injury. 2007;38(8):913–22.

6. Song HR, Oh CW, Shin HD, Kim SJ, Kyung HS, Baek SH, Park BC, Ihn JC. Treatment of femoral shaft fractures in young children: comparison between conservative treatment and retrograde flexible nailing. J Pediatr Orthop B. 2004;13(4):275–80. https://doi.org/10.1097/01.bpb.0000111023.13276.43.
7. Ramseier LE, Janicki JA, Weir S, Narayanan UG. Femoral fractures in adolescents: a comparison of four methods of fixation. J Bone Joint Surg Am. 2010;92:1122–9.
8. Lascombes P, Nespola A, Poircuitte JM, Popkov D, de Gheldere A, Haumont T, Journeau P. Early complications with flexible intramedullary nailing in childhood fractures: 100 cases managed with precurved tip and shaft nails. Orthop Traumatol Surg Res. 2012;98:369–75.
9. Flynn JM, Hresko T, Reynolds RA, Blasier RD, Davidson R, Kasser J. Titanium elastic nails for pediatric femur fractures: a multicenter study of early results with analysis of complications. J Pediatr Orthop. 2001;21:4–8.
10. Luhmann SJ, Schootman M, Schoenecker PL, Dobbs MB, Gordon JE. Complications of titanium elastic nails for pediatric femoral shaft fractures. J Pediatr Orthop. 2003;23:443–7.
11. Weiss JM, Choi P, Ghatan C, Skaggs DL, Kay RM. Complications with flexible nailing of femur fractures more than double with child obesity and weight >50 kg. J Child Orthop. 2009;3:53–8.
12. Ho CA, Skaggs DL, Tang CW, Kay RM. Use of flexible intramedullary nails in pediatric femur fractures. J Pediatr Orthop. 2006;26:497–504. https://doi.org/10.1097/01.bpo.0000226280.93577.c1.
13. Ligier JN, Métaizeau JP, Prévot J. Closed flexible medullary nailing in pediatric traumatololgy. Chir Pediatr. 1983;24:383–5.
14. Ligier JN, Métaizeau JP, Prévot J, Lascombes P. Elastic stable intramedullary nailing of femoral shaft fractures in children. J Bone Joint Surg Br. 1988;70:74–7.
15. Goodwin RC, Gaynor T, Mahar A, Oka R, Lalond FD. Intramedullary flexible nail fixation of unstable pediatric tibial diaphyseal fractures. J Pediatr Orthop. 2005;25:570–6.
16. Srivastava AK, Mehlman CT, Wall EJ, Do TT. Elastic stable intramedullary nailing of tibial shaft fractures in children. J Pediatr Orthop. 2008;28:152–8.
17. Karladani AH, Granhed H, Edshage B, Jerre R, Styf J. Displaced tibial shaft fractures: a prospective randomized study of closed intramedullary nailing versus cast treatment in 53 patients. Acta Orthop Scand. 2000;71:160–7.
18. Canavese F, Botnari A, Andreacchio A, Marengo L, Samba A, Dimeglio A, Rousset M. Displaced tibial shaft fractures with intact fibula in children: nonoperative management versus operative treatment with elastic stable intramedullary nailing. J Pediatr Orthop. 2015; (Epub ahead of print).
19. Mark GS, Rajan RA. Elastic intramedullary nailing in unstable fractures of the paediatric tibial diaphysis: a systematic review. J Child Orthop. 2010;4:45–51.
20. Deakin DE, Winter H, Jain P, Bache CE. Malunion following flexible intramedullary nails for tibial and femoral fractures in adolescents. J Child Orthop. 2010;4:571–7.
21. Sankar WN, Jones KJ, Horn RD, Wells L. Titanium elastic nails for pediatric tibial shaft fractures. J Child Orthop. 2010;1:281–6.
22. Norman D, Peskin B, Ehrenraich A, et al. The use of external fixators in the immobilization of pediatric fractures. Arch Orthop Trauma Surg. 2002;122:379–82. https://doi.org/10.1007/s00402-001-0383-2.
23. Lascombes P, Haumont T, Journeau P. Use and abuse of flexible intramedullary nailing in children and adolescents. J Pediatr Orthop. 2006;26:827–34.
24. Kc KM, Acharya P, Sigdel A. Titanium Elastic Nailing System (TENS) for tibia fractures in children: functional outcomes and complications. J Nepal Med Assoc. 2016;55:55–60.
25. Lascombes P, Huber H, Fay R, et al. Flexible intramedullary nailing in children: nail to medullary canal diameters optimal ratio. J Pediatr Orthop. 2013;33:403–8. https://doi.org/10.1097/BPO.0b013e318285c54d.
26. Marengo L, Paonessa M, Andreacchio A, et al. Displaced tibia shaft fractures in children treated by elastic stable intramedullary nailing: results and complications in children weighing

50 kg (110 lb) or more. Eur J Orthop Surg Traumatol. 2016;26:311–7. https://doi.org/10.1007/s00590-015-1729-8.
27. Goodbody CM, Lee RJ, Flynn JM, Sankar WN. Titanium elastic nailing for pediatric tibia fractures: do older, heavier kids do worse? J Pediatr Orthop. 2016;36:472–7. https://doi.org/10.1097/BPO.0000000000000483.
28. Heo J, Oh C-W, Park K-H, et al. Elastic nailing of tibia shaft fractures in young children up to 10 years of age. Injury. 2016;47:832–6. https://doi.org/10.1016/j.injury.2015.10.024.
29. Kubiak EN, Egol KA, Scher D, Wasserman B, Feldman D, Kovac KJ. Operative treatment of tibial fractures in children: are elastic stable intramedullary nails an improvement over external fixation? J Bone Joint Surg Am. 2005;87:1761–8.
30. Pandya NK, Edmonds EW. Immediate intramedullary flexible nailing of open pediatric tibial shaft fractures. J Pediatr Orthop. 2012;32:770–6. https://doi.org/10.1097/BPO.0b013e318270468b.
31. Shen K, Cai H, Wang Z, Xu Y. Elastic stable intramedullary nailing for severely displaced distal tibial fractures in children. Medicine. 2016;95:e4980. https://doi.org/10.1097/MD.0000000000004980.
32. Canavese F, Botnari A, Andreacchio A, et al. Displaced tibial shaft fractures with intact fibula in children: nonoperative management versus operative treatment with elastic stable intramedullary nailing. J Pediatr Orthop. 2016;36:667–72. https://doi.org/10.1097/BPO.0000000000000528.
33. Gicquel P, Giacomelli M-C, Basic B, et al. Problems of operative and non-operative treatment and healing in tibial fractures. Injury. 2005;36(Suppl 1):A44–50. https://doi.org/10.1016/j.injury.2004.12.012.
34. Karaman I, Halici M, Kafadar IH, et al. Mid-term results of the elastic intramedullary nailing in paediatric long bone shaft fractures: a prospective study of 102 cases. J Pediatr Orthop Part B. 2014;23:212–20. https://doi.org/10.1097/01.bpb.0000444460.95927.05.
35. O'Brien T, Weisman DS, Ronchetti P, et al. Flexible titanium nailing for the treatment of the unstable pediatric tibial fracture. J Pediatr Orthop. 2004;24:601–9. https://doi.org/10.1097/00004694-200411000-00001.
36. Pennock AT, Bastrom TP, Upasani VV. Elastic intramedullary nailing versus open reduction internal fixation of pediatric tibial shaft fractures. J Pediatr Orthop. 2017;37:e403–8. https://doi.org/10.1097/BPO.0000000000001065.
37. Ozkul E, Gem M, Arslan H, et al. How safe is titanium elastic nail application in the surgical treatment of tibia fractures in children? Acta Orthop Belg. 2014;80:76–81.
38. Uludağ A, Tosun HB. Treatment of unstable pediatric tibial shaft fractures with titanium elastic nails. Medicina. 2019;55:266. https://doi.org/10.3390/medicina55060266.
39. Baldwin KD, Babatunde OM, Russell Huffman G, Hosalkar HS. Open fractures of the tibia in the pediatric population: a systematic review. J Child Orthop. 2009;3:199–208. https://doi.org/10.1007/s11832-009-0169-6.
40. Perry DC, Wright JG, Cooke S, et al. A consensus exercise identifying priorities for research into clinical effectiveness among children's orthopaedic surgeons in the United Kingdom. Bone Joint J. 2018;100-B:680–4. https://doi.org/10.1302/0301-620X.100B5.BJJ-2018-0051.
41. Palmu SA, Auro S, Lohman M, et al. Tibial fractures in children. A retrospective 27-year follow-up study. Acta Orthop. 2014;85:513–7. https://doi.org/10.3109/17453674.2014.916489.
42. Patel NK, Horstman J, Kuester V, Sambandam S, Mounasamy V. Pediatric tibial shaft fractures. Indian J Orthop. 2018;52:522–8.
43. Kleiner JE, Raducha JE, Cruz AI Jr. Increasing rates of surgical treatment for paediatric tibial shaft fractures: a national database study from between 2000 and 2012. J Child Orthop. 2019;13:213–9.
44. Cruz AI Jr, Raducha JE, Swarup I, Schachne JM, Fabricant PD. Evidence-based update on the surgical treatment of pediatric tibial shaft fractures. Curr Opin Pediatr. 2019;31:92–102.
45. Beltsios M, Savvidou O, Kovanis J, Alexandropoulos P, Papagelopoulos P. External fixation as a primary and definitive treatment for tibial diaphyseal fractures. Strateg Trauma Limb Reconstr. 2009;4:81–7.

46. Simon A-L, Apostolou N, Vidal C, et al. Paediatric tibial shaft fractures treated by open reduction and stabilization with monolateral external fixation. J Child Orthop. 2018;12:20–8. https://doi.org/10.1302/1863-2548.12.170056.
47. Kuyucu E, Kara A, Say F, Erdil M, Bülbül M, Gülenç B. Application of hybrid external fixation by the "joystick method" in bicondylar tibial plateau fractures: technical note. Ulus Travma Acil Cerrahi Derg. 2018;24:263–7.
48. Gordon JE, Schoenecker PL, Oda JE, Ortman MR, Szymanski DA, Dobbs MB, et al. A comparison of monolateral and circular external fixation of unstable diaphyseal tibial fractures in children. J Pediatr Orthop B. 2003;12:338–45.
49. Gordon JE, O'Donnell JC. Tibia fractures: what should be fixed? J Pediatr Orthop. 2012;32(Suppl 1):S52–61. https://doi.org/10.1097/BPO.0b013e318254c7be.
50. Charalambous CP, Alvi F, Siddique I, Zenios M, Hirst P, Marshall P. Casting versus surgical fixation for grade IIIA open tibial diaphysial fractures in children: effect on the rate of infection and the need for secondary surgical procedures to promote bone union. Int Orthop. 2005;29(6):392–5. https://doi.org/10.1007/s00264-005-0009-3.
51. Pandya NK. Flexible intramedullary nailing of unstable and/or open tibia shaft fractures in the pediatric population. J Pediatr Orthop. 2016;36(Suppl 1):S19–23. https://doi.org/10.1097/BPO.0000000000000754.
52. Nandra RS, Wu F, Gaffey A, Bache CE. The management of open tibial fractures in children: a retrospective case series of eight years' experience of 61 cases at a paediatric specialist Centre. Bone Joint J. 2017;99-B:544–53. https://doi.org/10.1302/0301-620X.99B4.37855.
53. Economedes DM, Abzug JM, Paryavi E, Herman MJ. Outcomes using titanium elastic nails for open and closed pediatric tibia fractures. Orthopedics. 2014;37(7):e619–24. https://doi.org/10.3928/01477447-20140626-52.
54. Gasco J, de Pablos J. Bone remodeling in malunited fractures in children. Is it reliable? J Pediatr Orthop B. 1997;6(2):126–32. https://doi.org/10.1097/01202412-199704000-00008.
55. Dwyer AJ, John B, Krishen M, Hora R. Remodeling of tibial fractures in children younger than 12 years. Orthopedics. 2007;30(5):393–6.
56. Cozen L. Fracture of the proximal portion of the tibia in children followed by valgus deformity. Surg Gynecol Obstet. 1953;97:183–8.
57. Ogden JA, et al. Tibia Valga after proximal metaphyseal fractures in childhood: a normal biologic response. J Pediatr Orthop. 1995;15(4):489–94.
58. Gustilo RB. Current concepts in the management of open fractures. Instr Course Lect. 1987;36:359–66.
59. Steinert V, Bennek J. Tibial fractures in children. Zentralbl Chir. 1966;91(38):1387–92.
60. Beaty JH, Kasser JR. Fractures in children. Philadelphia: Lippincott Williams & Wilkins; 2010.
61. Chaibi E, Zambelli PY, Merckaert S. Epidemiology of paediatric lower extremity fractures in a tertiary care center in Switzerland. Eur J Trauma Emerg Surg. 2020;8:3449–59. https://doi.org/10.1007/s00068-020-01400-6.
62. Fanelli D, Perrotta G, Stocco F, Agilinko J, Castioni D, Mercurio M, Gasparini G, Barker S. Outcomes and complications following flexible intramedullary nailing for the treatment of tibial fractures in children: a meta-analysis. Arch Orthop Trauma Surg. 2021;142:1469–82. https://doi.org/10.1007/s00402-021-03839-7.
63. Wang X, Zhang Z, Hou X, Wang B, Li Y, Zhang T. Application of unilateral external fixation by the "joystick technique" in the treatment of pediatric tibia shaft fractures: technical note. J Orthop Surg Res. 2021;16:493. https://doi.org/10.1186/s13018-021-02625-w.
64. Hong P, Rai S, Tang X, Liu R, Li J. External fixation versus elastic stable intramedullary nailing in the treatment of open tibial shaft fractures in children. J Orthop Surg Res. 2021;16:528. https://doi.org/10.1186/s13018-021-02679-w.
65. Jung ST, Park H, Lee JH, Kim JR. Residual angulation of distal tibial diaphyseal fractures in children younger than ten years. J Orthop Surg Res. 2014;9:84. https://doi.org/10.1186/s13018-014-0084-5.

Distal Tibial Epiphyseal Fractures: Salter-Harris, Tillaux and Triplane Fractures

19

Introduction by the Author

Physeal injuries of the distal tibia are the second most common type of injury after distal radius injuries and carry a high risk of complications. If distal tibial epiphyseal fractures, particularly transitional fractures such as Tillaux and triplane fractures, are not properly treated, complications such as growth arrest and angular deformities may result. Growth disturbance incidence varies between 2% and 40%, and it is believed to be influenced by several factors, including fracture type and initial displacement. Age is a critical factor in predicting growth disturbances following distal tibial physeal fractures, likely because younger children have greater growth potential. Additionally, Salter-Harris types 3 and 4 fractures are more prevalent in the growth disturbance group, indicating a higher risk associated with these fracture types. Furthermore, patients with concurrent fibula fractures have a higher incidence of growth disorders.

While these fractures can be suspected based on plain radiographs of the ankle, Computed Tomography scans are necessary for an accurate diagnosis and to guide appropriate management strategies for these complex fractures.

Based on ankle position, direction of force, and degree of closure of the distal tibial physis, pediatric physeal fractures tend to occur in a predictable pattern and are classified accordingly using the Dias-Tachdjian classification system, which is based on "mechanism of injury".

The most common ankle injury in children is a Salter-Harris type distal tibial physeal fracture. These fractures account for 32%–60% of ankle injuries in this age group. These fractures are not usually associated with growth disturbances because they occur in the hypertrophic zone, where issues with growth are less likely to occur. However, the incidence of premature physeal closure increases 3.5-fold in the presence of a residual gap. Open reduction and removal of the interposed periosteum are recommended to decrease this risk, which is higher if displacement exceeds 3 mm at the time of injury.

© The Author(s), under exclusive license to Springer Nature Switzerland AG 2026
F. Canavese, *Advances in Pediatric Extremity Fracture Management*,
https://doi.org/10.1007/978-3-032-33306-3_19

Triplane and Tillaux fractures result from supination, external rotation, and compression stress, resulting in unpredictable, multiplanar fracture patterns.

Tillaux fractures account for 3%–7% of distal tibial epiphyseal fractures. They involve the anterolateral quadrant of the distal tibial physis and can be classified as Salter-Harris type 3 with intraarticular involvement. These fractures often result from external rotation of the foot and can lead to premature physeal closure. Those with less than 2 mm of displacement can be treated conservatively, while those with greater displacement require surgical intervention to prevent joint incongruity and deformity.

Triplane fractures of the distal tibia are a type of Salter-Harris 4 fracture, representing approximately 10%–15% of pediatric ankle fractures. These complex injuries usually occur during the period of physeal closure, between 12 and 15 years of age, and involve a combination of coronal, transverse, and sagittal fractures, affecting the articular surface, the epiphysis, and the metaphysis. They often occur in adolescents due to the unique pattern of growth plate fusion that occurs during this developmental stage. Although triplane fractures are relatively common among distal tibial growth plate injuries, they can lead to serious complications, such as growth arrest or angular deformity, if not managed properly.

Anatomical reduction (closed or open) and fixation are crucial for successful outcomes in these complex fractures.

19.1 Machine Generated Summaries

Disclaimer: The summaries in this chapter were generated from Springer Nature publications using abstractive AI auto-summarization: An abstraction-based summarizer creates new text based on deep learning. New phrases are created to summarize the content. As the constituted sentences are machine selected, they may not fully reflect the body of the work, so we strongly advise that the original content is read and cited. The auto-generated summaries were curated by the author(s) to meet Springer Nature publication standards.

Pediatric Ankle Injuries: Utilizing the Dias-Tachdjian Classification [80]

This is a machine-generated summary of:

Pomeranz, Christy B.; Bartolotta, Roger J. Pediatric ankle injuries: utilizing the Dias-Tachdjian classification [80]
Published in: Skeletal Radiology (2019)

Link to original: https://doi.org/10.1007/s00256-019-03356-0
Copyright of the summarized publication:
ISS 2019
All rights reserved.

If you want to cite the papers, please refer to the original.

For technical reasons we could not place the page where the original quote is coming from.

Research Highlights

Physeal fractures of long bones are prevalent in the pediatric population, with a significant portion involving the distal tibia. These injuries pose a risk of permanent damage to the growth plate, potentially leading to growth arrest. Numerous classification systems exist to describe these fractures, but they often lack consideration for both the physis and the mechanism of injury. Now, a new study by Christy B. Pomeranz and colleagues reviews the Dias-Tachdjian classification system, which uniquely addresses both aspects, offering insights into radiographic interpretation and management implications.

The study delves into the Dias-Tachdjian classification system, which categorizes pediatric ankle fractures based on both the mechanism of injury and physeal involvement. This system is particularly relevant for young children with open physes and includes four primary injury mechanisms: supination-inversion, supination-plantar flexion, pronation-eversion external rotation (PEER), and supination-external rotation (SER). The authors conducted a retrospective analysis of pediatric ankle fractures, highlighting that supination injuries are more common than pronation injuries. They provide detailed descriptions of each fracture pattern and their respective treatments, ranging from conservative casting to surgical interventions like open reduction and internal fixation. The study also emphasizes the importance of understanding fracture patterns as children approach skeletal maturity, where changes in physeal closure can alter fracture characteristics.

The main advancement presented by Pomeranz et al. is the application of a simplified algorithm for using the Dias-Tachdjian classification in clinical practice. This approach aids in identifying associated fractures and planning appropriate management strategies. The study underscores the importance of recognizing specific fracture patterns that may lead to complications such as primary physeal closure and angular deformities. Future study could focus on refining this classification system further or exploring its application in diverse clinical settings to enhance pediatric fracture management outcomes.

Incidence of Growth Disturbance After Distal Tibia Physeal Fracture in Children [81]

This is a machine-generated summary of:

Chen, Hui; Chen, Zhao; Chen, Peisheng; Zheng, Zibing; Lin, Jinrun Incidence of growth disturbance after distal tibia physeal fracture in children [81]
Published in: Journal of Orthopaedic Surgery and Research (2022)
Link to original: https://doi.org/10.1186/s13018-022-03427-4
Copyright of the summarized publication:
The Author(s) 2022
License: OpenAccess CC BY + CC0 4.0

This article is licensed under a Creative Commons Attribution 4.0 International License, which permits use, sharing, adaptation, distribution and reproduction in any medium or format, as long as you give appropriate credit to the original author(s) and the source, provide a link to the Creative Commons licence, and indicate if changes were made. The images or other third party material in this article are included in the article's Creative Commons licence, unless indicated otherwise in a credit line to the material. If material is not included in the article's Creative Commons licence and your intended use is not permitted by statutory regulation or exceeds the permitted use, you will need to obtain permission directly from the copyright holder. To view a copy of this licence, visit http://creativecommons.org/licenses/by/4.0/. The Creative Commons Public Domain Dedication waiver (http://creativecommons.org/publicdomain/zero/1.0/) applies to the data made available in this article, unless otherwise stated in a credit line to the data.

If you want to cite the papers, please refer to the original.

For technical reasons we could not place the page where the original quote is coming from.

Research Highlights

Distal tibia physeal fractures are a common injury in children, second only to distal radius physis injuries. These fractures can lead to growth disturbances, such as angular deformities and leg length discrepancies, due to the vulnerability of the physis. The incidence of growth disturbances varies widely, and multiple factors are thought to contribute, including fracture type and initial displacement. However, the specific factors influencing growth disturbances remain unclear. Now, a new study by Hui Chen and colleagues aims to assess the factors related to growth disturbance after distal tibia physeal fractures in children.

The study was conducted at Fuzhou Second Hospital Affiliated with Xiamen University and involved a retrospective review of patient data from September 2010 to September 2020. Children with distal tibia physeal fractures were categorized into two groups: those with growth disturbances and those without. The researchers collected data on various factors, including age, gender, fracture classification, displacement, and surgical details. Patients were further divided into early and delayed operation groups based on the time from injury to surgery. Statistical analyses were performed using SPSS software to identify significant differences between the groups. The study found that younger age was significantly associated with growth disturbances, as was the presence of Salter–Harris types III and IV fractures.

The findings suggest that age is a critical factor in predicting growth disturbances following distal tibia physeal fractures, likely due to the greater growth potential in younger children. Additionally, Salter–Harris types III and IV fractures were more prevalent in the growth disturbance group, indicating a higher risk associated with these fracture types. The study also noted that patients with concurrent fibula fractures had a higher incidence of growth disorders. Future studies could focus on long-term follow-up to better understand the progression of growth disturbances over time and explore interventions that might mitigate these risks in younger patients or those with complex fracture types.

Growth Plate Fractures of the Distal Tibia: Is CT Imaging Necessary? [82]

This is a machine-generated summary of:

Lemburg, Stefan P.; Lilienthal, Eggert; Heyer, Christoph M. Growth plate fractures of the distal tibia: is CT imaging necessary? [82]
Published in: Archives of Orthopaedic and Trauma Surgery (2010)
Link to original: https://doi.org/10.1007/s00402-010-1140-1
Copyright of the summarized publication:
Springer-Verlag 2010
All rights reserved.

If you want to cite the papers, please refer to the original.

For technical reasons we could not place the page where the original quote is coming from.

Research Highlights

Growth plate fractures of the distal tibia are among the most common fractures in children, second only to other growth plate injuries. These fractures can lead to significant complications, such as posttraumatic arthrosis and bone deformation, due to their potential to disrupt normal bone growth. The classification and treatment of these fractures are complex, with various imaging modalities available for evaluation. However, there is a lack of systematic comparisons between conventional radiography (CR) and computed tomography (CT) in assessing these injuries. Now, a new study by Stefan P. Lemburg and colleagues aims to address this gap by comparing CR and CT in evaluating distal tibial growth plate fractures to determine the incremental diagnostic benefit of CT.

The study retrospectively analyzed cases of children under 18 years with distal tibial growth plate injuries treated at their institution. The researchers included patients who had undergone both CR and CT imaging within 24 hours of injury. Two experienced radiologists independently evaluated the images without knowledge of the patients' clinical histories or outcomes. The study assessed the accuracy of CR compared to CT in identifying fracture characteristics such as metaphyseal involvement, articular surface dehiscence, and ridge formation. Statistical analyses were conducted to evaluate sensitivity, specificity, and overall accuracy for each imaging modality.

The findings revealed that CR had a significantly lower accuracy than CT in detecting certain fracture characteristics, particularly for complex fracture types like triplane fractures. While CR was adequate for classifying Salter-Harris (SH) type I and II fractures, it often misclassified SH type III and IV fractures compared to CT results. The study suggests that CT should be considered when precise fracture classification is crucial for determining treatment options, especially in complex cases where surgical intervention may be necessary. Future studies could explore the impact of these imaging differences on clinical outcomes and therapeutic decisions, potentially guiding more effective management strategies for pediatric patients with distal tibial growth plate fractures.

Growth Arrest Lines and Intra-Epiphyseal Silhouettes: A Case Series [83]

This is a machine-generated summary of:

Kennedy, Ian W; Irwin, Greg J; Huntley, James S Growth arrest lines and intra-epiphyseal silhouettes: a case series [83]
Published in: BMC Research Notes (2014)
Link to original: https://doi.org/10.1186/1756-0500-7-27
Copyright of the summarized publication:
Kennedy et al.; licensee BioMed Central Ltd. 2014
License: OpenAccess CC BY 2

This article is published under license to BioMed Central Ltd. This is an Open Access article is distributed under the terms of the Creative Commons Attribution License (https://creativecommons.org/licenses/by/2.0), which permits unrestricted use, distribution, and reproduction in any medium, provided the original work is properly credited. The Creative Commons Public Domain Dedication waiver (https://creativecommons.org/publicdomain/zero/1.0/) applies to the data made available in this article, unless otherwise stated.

Copyright comment This article is published under license to BioMed Central Ltd. This is an Open Access article distributed under the terms of the Creative Commons Attribution License (http://creativecommons.org/licenses/by/2.0), which permits unrestricted use, distribution, and reproduction in any medium, provided the original work is properly cited. The Creative Commons Public Domain

Dedication waiver (http://creativecommons.org/publicdomain/zero/1.0/) applies to the data made available in this article, unless otherwise stated.

If you want to cite the papers, please refer to the original.

For technical reasons we could not place the page where the original quote is coming from.

Research Highlights

Growth arrest lines, also known as Harris lines, are transverse metaphyseal lines visible on radiographs that indicate a temporary cessation of bone growth. These lines have been used as markers of disease in various fields, including paleontology, and can arise from systemic illnesses like septicaemia or localized trauma such as fractures. Despite their clinical significance, the precise etiology and implications of growth arrest lines remain incompletely understood. Now, a new study by Ian W. Kennedy and colleagues explores the occurrence and clinical significance of growth arrest lines in three pediatric patients who experienced trauma.

The study presents a case series involving three young girls who sustained different types of traumatic injuries leading to the formation of growth arrest lines. The first case involved a knee hyperflexion injury with ligament avulsions, managed surgically, resulting in both metaphyseal and intra-epiphyseal arrest lines visible on post-operative radiographs. The second case described a displaced tibial spine fracture requiring surgical intervention, with similar radiographic findings. The third case involved a comminuted distal tibial fracture near the growth plate, where serial radiographs showed the migration of arrest lines away from the physis over time. These cases highlight the formation of intra-epiphyseal silhouettes, which are rarely reported in literature, suggesting that articular trauma rather than impaired blood supply may contribute to their development.

The study advances our understanding of growth arrest lines by documenting rare intra-epiphyseal silhouettes secondary to trauma and emphasizing their potential role in assessing growth plate damage. Future study could focus on further elucidating the mechanisms behind these formations and their long-term implications for bone development. Additionally, understanding the relationship between Harris lines and articular surfaces could provide insights into predicting bone deformities following physeal injuries. This research underscores the importance of recognizing growth arrest lines as indicators of past stressors and their utility in clinical assessments post-trauma.

Open Reduction and Internal Fixation for Displaced Salter-Harris Type II Fractures of the Distal Tibia: A Retrospective Study of Sixty-Five Cases in Children [84]

This is a machine-generated summary of:

Yuan, Quanwen; Zhen, Yunfang; Guo, Zhixiong; Zhang, Fuyong; Fang, Jianfeng; Zhu, Zhenhua; Zhu, Lunqing; Shen, Xiaofang; Yin, Chunhua; Liu, Yao; Yao, Feng; Wu, Lin; Wang, Xiaodong Open reduction and internal fixation for dis-

placed Salter-Harris type II fractures of the distal tibia: a retrospective study of sixty-five cases in children [84]
Published in: Journal of Orthopaedic Surgery and Research (2021)
Link to original: https://doi.org/10.1186/s13018-021-02359-9
Copyright of the summarized publication:
The Author(s) 2021
License: OpenAccess CC BY + CC0 4.0

This article is licensed under a Creative Commons Attribution 4.0 International License, which permits use, sharing, adaptation, distribution and reproduction in any medium or format, as long as you give appropriate credit to the original author(s) and the source, provide a link to the Creative Commons licence, and indicate if changes were made. The images or other third party material in this article are included in the article's Creative Commons licence, unless indicated otherwise in a credit line to the material. If material is not included in the article's Creative Commons licence and your intended use is not permitted by statutory regulation or exceeds the permitted use, you will need to obtain permission directly from the copyright holder. To view a copy of this licence, visit http://creativecommons.org/licenses/by/4.0/. The Creative Commons Public Domain Dedication waiver (http://creativecommons.org/publicdomain/zero/1.0/) applies to the data made available in this article, unless otherwise stated in a credit line to the data.

If you want to cite the papers, please refer to the original.

For technical reasons we could not place the page where the original quote is coming from.

Research Highlights

Salter-Harris type II distal tibia physeal fractures are the most common ankle injuries in children, typically associated with a lower risk of growth disturbances due to the fracture line's location in the hypertrophic zone. However, recent studies have reported a higher incidence of premature physeal closure (PPC) than previously thought, particularly in S-H II fractures compared to S-H III and IV fractures. The optimal treatment for displaced S-H II distal tibia fractures remains controversial, with differing opinions on whether open reduction and internal fixation (ORIF) can reduce PPC incidence. Now, a new study by Quanwen Yuan and colleagues reviews the outcomes of ORIF in treating S-H II distal tibia fractures with displacement greater than 3 mm, focusing on the rate of PPC.

In this retrospective study, medical records and radiographs of patients treated for S-H II distal tibia fractures at a single institution were analyzed. The study included patients with more than 3 mm initial displacement who underwent ORIF to remove interposed periosteum and achieve anatomical reduction. The researchers recorded various parameters such as age, sex, injury mechanism, and follow-up duration. Surgical procedures involved open reduction under general anesthesia using an anterolateral approach to remove soft tissue interposition before fixation with Kirschner wires or screws. The study found that all patients had residual displacement greater than 3 mm after closed reduction but achieved less than 2 mm displacement following

ORIF. Despite successful anatomical reduction, 19 out of 65 patients developed PPC, with concomitant fibular fracture significantly associated with increased PPC risk.

The study highlights that while ORIF is effective in achieving anatomical reduction for displaced S-H II distal tibia fractures, PPC remains a common complication. The presence of a concomitant fibular fracture was identified as a significant predictor of PPC, suggesting that more severe initial displacement may lead to greater physeal damage. Future studies should explore long-term outcomes and consider follow-up until skeletal maturity to better understand PPC development. Additionally, further research is needed to determine whether nonoperative treatments could yield similar results without the complications associated with surgical intervention.

Displaced Juvenile Tillaux Fractures [85]

This is a machine-generated summary of:

Tiefenboeck, Thomas M.; Binder, Harald; Joestl, Julian; Tiefenboeck, Michael M.; Boesmueller, Sandra; Krestan, Christian; Schurz, Mark Displaced juvenile Tillaux fractures [85]
Published in: Wiener klinische Wochenschrift (2016)
Link to original: https://doi.org/10.1007/s00508-016-1059-9
Copyright of the summarized publication:
The Author(s) 2016
License: OpenAccess CC BY 4.0

This article is distributed under the terms of the Creative Commons Attribution 4.0 International License (http://creativecommons.org/licenses/by/4.0/), which permits unrestricted use, distribution, and reproduction in any medium, provided you give appropriate credit to the original author(s) and the source, provide a link to the Creative Commons license, and indicate if changes were made.

If you want to cite the papers, please refer to the original.

For technical reasons we could not place the page where the original quote is coming from.

Research Highlights

Juvenile Tillaux fractures, first described by Paul Jules Tillaux, are avulsion fractures of the distal tibial physis that occur predominantly in adolescents. These fractures are significant due to their involvement of the weight-bearing articular surface and the potential for posttraumatic ankle arthritis if not properly treated. Despite their clinical importance, treatment protocols for these fractures vary widely in the literature, with recommendations ranging from immobilization for nondisplaced fractures to surgical intervention for those with significant displacement. Now, a new study by Thomas M. Tiefenboeck and colleagues presents one of the largest single-center reports on displaced juvenile Tillaux fractures, focusing on clinical-functional and radiographic outcomes.

The study retrospectively evaluated patients treated for physeal injuries of the distal tibia at a single institution between 2000 and 2010. Seven patients met the inclusion criteria, with data available for five patients at a mean long-term follow-up of 42 months. Diagnosis was confirmed through clinical examination and imaging, including X-rays and CT scans. Most patients underwent open reduction and internal fixation (ORIF) followed by plaster cast immobilization. The study utilized a standardized treatment protocol, with non-weight-bearing mobilization recommended for at least 6 weeks post-surgery. Outcomes were assessed using the Foot and Ankle Score, which showed significant improvement over time.

The findings suggest that ORIF combined with postoperative plaster cast immobilization leads to excellent outcomes in displaced Tillaux fractures. All patients achieved full recovery without complications, except one who experienced temporary joint stiffness resolved through physical therapy. The study highlights the importance of anatomical reduction in achieving favorable results and minimizing long-term complications. Future studies could explore alternative methods such as arthroscopic-assisted reduction, which allows direct visualization of fracture fragments and associated chondral injuries. However, this study's retrospective design and small sample size limit its generalizability, underscoring the need for further research to establish standardized treatment guidelines for juvenile Tillaux fractures.

Closed Reduction and Internal Fixation for Tillaux Fractures, Based on Pre-Operative Three-Dimensional Computed Tomography [86]

This is a machine-generated summary of:

Lee, Jong Wha; Cho, Jae Ho; Song, Hyung Keun; Chung, Jun Young; Park, Young Uk; Kim, Tae Hun Closed reduction and internal fixation for tillaux fractures, based on pre-operative three-dimensional computed tomography [86]

Published in: European Journal of Orthopaedic Surgery & Traumatology (2024)
Link to original: https://doi.org/10.1007/s00590-024-03910-0

Copyright of the summarized publication:
The Author(s), under exclusive licence to Springer-Verlag France SAS, part of Springer Nature 2024

Copyright comment: Springer Nature or its licensor (e.g. a society or other partner) holds exclusive rights to this article under a publishing agreement with the author(s) or other rightsholder(s); author self-archiving of the accepted manuscript version of this article is solely governed by the terms of such publishing agreement and applicable law.

All rights reserved.

If you want to cite the papers, please refer to the original.

For technical reasons we could not place the page where the original quote is coming from.

Research Highlights

Tillaux fractures, a type of Salter-Harris physeal fracture, involve the avulsion of the anterolateral distal tibial epiphysis and are common in adolescents, often resulting from sports-related trauma. These fractures occur due to the unique closure pattern of the distal tibial physis, making the lateral portion more susceptible to avulsion forces. While fractures with less than 2 mm displacement can be treated conservatively, those with greater displacement require surgical intervention to prevent joint incongruity and deformity. Now, a new study by Jong Wha Lee and colleagues explores a detailed closed reduction technique for treating Tillaux fractures using pre-operative three-dimensional computed tomography (3D-CT) analysis to identify fracture patterns and guide surgical intervention.

The study involved 42 patients with Tillaux fractures who underwent surgical treatment at a single institution between 2010 and 2020. The researchers used pre-operative 3D-CT scans to analyze fracture fragment displacement patterns, focusing on varus tilt and external rotation. Patients with more than a 2 mm fracture gap after initial closed reduction attempts underwent surgery. The surgical technique involved reducing the fracture fragment through a small skin incision using mosquito forceps under image intensifier guidance. The reduction force was applied in specific directions to counteract varus tilt and external rotation, followed by fixation with a cannulated screw. Post-operative management included non-weight bearing for 4 weeks and evaluation of bone union through radiographs.

The study's findings highlight the importance of understanding anatomical fracture patterns for successful closed reduction in Tillaux fractures. The consistent pattern of varus tilt and external rotation informed the direction of reduction forces, leading to satisfactory outcomes in most cases. Future studies could focus on multicenter trials to validate these findings further and explore post-operative CT comparisons for precise anatomical assessments. The research underscores the potential for improved clinical outcomes through enhanced anatomical understanding and tailored surgical techniques, although challenges remain in cases with significant initial displacement or periosteal impingement.

Concurrent Ipsilateral Tillaux Fracture and Medial Malleolar Fracture in Adolescents: Management and Outcome [87]

This is a machine-generated summary of:

Yuan, Quanwen; Guo, Zhixiong; Wang, Xiaodong; Dai, Jin; Zhang, Fuyong; Fang, Jianfeng; Yin, Chunhua; Yu, Wentao; Zhen, Yunfang Concurrent ipsilateral Tillaux fracture and medial malleolar fracture in adolescents: management and outcome [87]
Published in: Journal of Orthopaedic Surgery and Research (2020)
Link to original: https://doi.org/10.1186/s13018-020-01961-7
Copyright of the summarized publication:
The Author(s) 2020
License: OpenAccess CC BY + CC0 4.0

This article is licensed under a Creative Commons Attribution 4.0 International License, which permits use, sharing, adaptation, distribution and reproduction in any medium or format, as long as you give appropriate credit to the original author(s) and the source, provide a link to the Creative Commons licence, and indicate if changes were made. The images or other third party material in this article are included in the article's Creative Commons licence, unless indicated otherwise in a credit line to the material. If material is not included in the article's Creative Commons licence and your intended use is not permitted by statutory regulation or exceeds the permitted use, you will need to obtain permission directly from the copyright holder. To view a copy of this licence, visit http://creativecommons.org/licenses/by/4.0/. The Creative Commons Public Domain Dedication waiver (http://creativecommons.org/publicdomain/zero/1.0/) applies to the data made available in this article, unless otherwise stated in a credit line to the data.

If you want to cite the papers, please refer to the original.

For technical reasons we could not place the page where the original quote is coming from.

Research Highlights

Physeal injuries of the distal tibia are common in adolescents and carry a significant risk of complications, particularly Tillaux fractures, which involve the anterolateral quadrant of the distal tibial physis. These fractures often result from external rotation of the foot and can lead to premature physeal closure. While medial malleolar fractures (MMF) have been less frequently studied due to their lower rate of growth disturbance, they play a crucial role in ankle stability. Now, a new study by Quanwen Yuan and colleagues at the Children's Hospital of Soochow University explores the rare combination of Tillaux fracture and MMF in adolescents, aiming to understand their mechanism, diagnosis, and treatment options.

The study retrospectively reviewed six cases of Tillaux fracture associated with MMF treated between January and December. The patients, aged around 14 years on average, were evaluated using lateral plain radiographs and computerized tomography (CT) scans to assess fracture displacement and associated injuries. The researchers classified MMFs using Salter-Harris criteria when the physis was involved or Herscovici classification otherwise. Treatment involved open reduction and internal fixation (ORIF) with Kirschner wires for Tillaux fractures, while MMFs were managed with closed reduction or ORIF depending on the fracture type. Postoperative care included immobilization with a short-leg cast and non-weight-bearing instructions for 4–6 weeks. Functional outcomes were assessed using the American Orthopedic Foot and Ankle Society (AOFAS) scores.

The study highlights that anatomical reduction and fixation are crucial for successful outcomes in these complex fracture cases. Despite some instances of nonunion in MMFs due to lack of internal fixation, most fractures healed within 8–12 weeks without significant complications like premature physeal closure or leg length discrepancy. Future study could focus on larger sample sizes and longer follow-up periods to better understand injury mechanisms and refine treatment protocols for these rare fracture combinations in adolescents. The findings suggest that internal fixation may be more effective for MMFs in this age group, emphasizing the need for tailored approaches based on specific fracture characteristics.

Triplane Fractures: Do We Need Cross-Sectional Imaging? [88]

This is a machine-generated summary of:

Schneidmueller, D.; Sander, A. L.; Wertenbroek, M.; Wutzler, S.; Kraus, R.; Marzi, I.; Laurer, H. Triplane fractures: do we need cross-sectional imaging? [88]
Published in: European Journal of Trauma and Emergency Surgery (2013)
Link to original: https://doi.org/10.1007/s00068-013-0338-7
Copyright of the summarized publication:
Springer-Verlag Berlin Heidelberg 2013
All rights reserved.

If you want to cite the papers, please refer to the original.
For technical reasons we could not place the page where the original quote is coming from.

Research Highlights

The Triplane fracture, a transitional fracture of the ankle, is a topic of interest in pediatric traumatology due to its occurrence during a specific period of adolescence when the epiphyseal plate is closing. This fracture type extends into three planes, allowing for further stratification into Triplane I and II fractures. Traditionally, classification and treatment decisions have been based on plain radiographs. However, with the increased availability of cross-sectional imaging, there is debate over its necessity in diagnosing these fractures. Now, a new study by D. Schneidmueller and colleagues investigates whether cross-sectional imaging impacts the classification and treatment of Triplane fractures.

In this retrospective study conducted at the University of Frankfurt's Trauma Department, researchers analyzed pediatric ankle fracture cases with both plain radiographs and cross-sectional imaging. The study involved 30 cases, including 15 Triplane fractures. Observers with varying levels of experience reviewed the images to classify fractures and suggest treatments. The study found that cross-sectional imaging significantly improved the correct classification of Triplane fractures compared to conventional radiographs alone. For non-specialized observers, correct classification increased from 60% with X-rays to 80% with additional imaging. Specialized observers also showed improved accuracy with cross-sectional imaging, aligning more closely with expert consensus on treatment recommendations.

The study highlights that while conventional X-rays remain essential for initial fracture detection, cross-sectional imaging provides valuable additional information for classifying transitional fractures like Triplane I and II. This enhanced accuracy supports more precise treatment strategies, particularly for experienced pediatric trauma surgeons. Future studies could focus on comparing outcomes between operative and conservative treatments to establish clearer guidelines. Despite the small sample size limiting definitive conclusions on treatment outcomes, this research underscores the potential benefits of incorporating cross-sectional imaging into standard diagnostic protocols for complex pediatric ankle fractures.

The Incidence and Treatment Outcome of Atypical Triplane Fractures in Adolescents [89]

This is a machine-generated summary of:

Kang, Hyunseong; Kang, Taehan; Lim, Chaemoon The Incidence and Treatment Outcome of Atypical Triplane Fractures in Adolescents [89]
Published in: Indian Journal of Orthopaedics (2022)
Link to original: https://doi.org/10.1007/s43465-022-00679-4
Copyright of the summarized publication:
Indian Orthopaedics Association 2022
All rights reserved.

If you want to cite the papers, please refer to the original.

For technical reasons we could not place the page where the original quote is coming from.

Research Highlights

Triplane fractures, which occur in the sagittal, coronal, and axial planes, account for a small percentage of pediatric ankle fractures and typically affect children between 10 and 15 years of age due to physeal closure. These fractures are complex and can be misclassified using traditional systems like Salter-Harris. Atypical triplane fractures (ATFs) have been described in case reports but lack consensus on optimal treatment strategies. Now, a new study by Hyunseong Kang and colleagues investigates the incidence, fracture patterns, injury mechanisms, treatment outcomes, and proposes treatment recommendations for ATFs.

The study was conducted retrospectively on patients under 18 years treated for triplane fractures over a decade. Classical triplane fractures were excluded, focusing on ATFs with follow-up until skeletal maturity. Fractures were classified using a modified system by Yung et al., and all underwent initial closed reduction under sedation. Satisfactory reductions were immobilized with short leg casts; otherwise, open reduction with internal fixation was performed. Radiographic evaluations included plain radiography and CT scans to assess fracture displacement and configuration. Clinical outcomes were measured using the American Orthopedic Foot and Ankle Society score for the ankle-hindfoot, alongside pain assessments and range of motion evaluations.

The study found that both operative and non-operative treatments yielded good clinical outcomes for ATFs. Non-operative management with closed reduction and cast immobilization was effective for extra-articular ATFs with displacement less than 2 mm. The authors suggest that broader indications for non-operative treatment could be beneficial in children with extra-articular triplane fractures to avoid complications associated with surgery. Future studies should focus on larger sample sizes and randomized controlled trials to confirm these findings and further refine treatment protocols for ATFs. The study highlights the importance of accurate diagnosis using CT scans to guide appropriate management strategies for these complex fractures.

Extra-Articular Triplane Fracture of the Distal Tibia: A Case Report [90]

This is a machine-generated summary of:

O'Connor, D. K.; Mulligan, Michael E. Extra-articular triplane fracture of the distal tibia: a case report [90]
Published in: Pediatric Radiology (1998)
Link to original: https://doi.org/10.1007/s002470050367
Copyright of the summarized publication:
Springer-Verlag Berlin Heidelberg 1998
All rights reserved.

If you want to cite the papers, please refer to the original.

For technical reasons we could not place the page where the original quote is coming from.

Research Highlights

Triplane fractures of the distal tibia are complex injuries typically involving a combination of coronal, transverse, and sagittal fractures. These fractures often occur in adolescents due to the unique pattern of growth plate fusion during this developmental stage. While triplane fractures are relatively common among distal tibial growth plate injuries, they can lead to serious complications such as growth arrest or angular deformity if not properly managed. Now, a new study by D. K. O'Connor and colleagues reports an unusual variation of the triplane fracture that includes an extra-articular epiphyseal component, a variation not previously described in radiologic literature.

In this study, the authors present a case involving a young boy who sustained an ankle injury after landing awkwardly from a jump. Initial radiographs revealed a coronal metaphyseal fracture with widening of the anterior physis and associated soft-tissue swelling. A CT scan provided further clarity, demonstrating the coronal nature of the metaphyseal fracture and a sagittal fracture extending into the medial malleolus while sparing the tibiotalar joint. This detailed imaging allowed for accurate classification of the fracture as extra-articular, which significantly influenced the treatment approach. The patient was successfully managed with closed reduction and casting, avoiding more invasive procedures like open reduction and internal fixation.

The main advance highlighted by this study is the identification of an extra-articular variant of triplane fractures, which has important implications for treatment decisions. Recognizing this variant can help orthopedic surgeons opt for less invasive management strategies when appropriate, reducing potential complications associated with surgical intervention. Future study could focus on further characterizing these fracture variants and developing guidelines for their management to improve outcomes in pediatric patients with similar injuries. Additionally, increased use of CT imaging in evaluating suspected triplane fractures may lead to better identification and understanding of these complex injuries.

Triplane Fracture of the Distal Fibula [91]

This is a machine-generated summary of:

Ruffing, Thomas; Muhm, Markus; Winkler, Hartmut Triplane Fracture of the Distal Fibula [91]
Published in: European Journal of Trauma and Emergency Surgery (2009)
Link to original: https://doi.org/10.1007/s00068-009-9030-3
Copyright of the summarized publication:
Urban & Vogel München 2010
All rights reserved.

If you want to cite the papers, please refer to the original.

For technical reasons we could not place the page where the original quote is coming from.

Research Highlights

Triplane fractures are complex injuries that typically occur in the distal tibia of adolescents due to the unique pattern of growth plate closure during this developmental stage. These fractures involve three planes: the articular surface, the epiphysis, and the metaphysis. However, triplane fractures in locations other than the distal tibia are rare and not well-documented. Now, a new study by Thomas Ruffing and colleagues from the Department of Trauma and Reconstructive Surgery at Westpfalz-Klinikum GmbH in Kaiserslautern, Germany, reports a unique case of a triplane fracture in the distal fibula of a 14-year-old girl.

The study details the diagnostic and surgical approach taken to address this unusual fracture. Initially, an X-ray revealed a flake in the joint space between the talus and distal fibula. A computed tomography (CT) scan was then performed, which showed a fracture starting at the metaphyseal articular face, crossing the physis, and ending at the epiphyseal articular face of the distal fibula. Despite an open growth plate lateral to the fracture zone, there was no subdivision into metaphyseal and epiphyseal fragments. The surgical intervention involved open reduction via lateral incision after antiedematous therapy. The intraoperative findings confirmed that the flake was part of both the medial metaphysis and epiphysis of the distal fibula. The fracture was stabilized using K-wires for epiphysiolysis and a transarticular PDS suture for the flake.

This case represents a significant advancement in understanding transitional fractures outside typical locations like the distal tibia. The successful treatment highlights potential strategies for managing similar injuries in rare anatomical sites. Future study could focus on further elucidating the physiological course of physeal closure in various bones to better predict and treat such fractures. Additionally, MRI investigations might be necessary to verify hypotheses regarding epiphyseodesis patterns in less commonly affected areas like the distal fibula.

Comparison of Surgical Outcomes Between Bioabsorbable and Metal Screw Fixation for Distal Tibial Physeal Fracture in Children and Adolescent [92]

This is a machine-generated summary of:

Kim, Woo Sub; Oh, Min Joon; Park, Moon Seok; Sung, Ki Hyuk Comparison of surgical outcomes between bioabsorbable and metal screw fixation for distal tibial physeal fracture in children and adolescent [92]

Published in: International Orthopaedics (2024)
Link to original: https://doi.org/10.1007/s00264-024-06284-4

Copyright of the summarized publication:
The Author(s) under exclusive licence to SICOT aisbl 2024

Copyright comment: Springer Nature or its licensor (e.g. a society or other partner) holds exclusive rights to this article under a publishing agreement with the author(s) or other rightsholder(s); author self-archiving of the accepted manuscript version of this article is solely governed by the terms of such publishing agreement and applicable law.

All rights reserved.

If you want to cite the papers, please refer to the original.

For technical reasons we could not place the page where the original quote is coming from.

Research Highlights

Ankle fractures are a common type of pediatric fracture, with distal tibial fractures accounting for a significant portion of growth plate injuries in children and adolescents. These fractures, particularly transitional ones like Tillaux and triplane fractures, can lead to complications such as growth arrest and angular deformities if not properly treated. Traditional treatment often involves metal screw fixation, which necessitates a second surgery for screw removal, posing additional risks and costs.

Now, a new study by Woo Sub Kim and colleagues explores the use of bioabsorbable screws as an alternative to metal screws for the fixation of distal tibial physeal fractures in children, aiming to reduce the need for secondary surgeries.

The study was conducted retrospectively at a single institution and included patients aged 18 years or younger who underwent open reduction and internal fixation (ORIF) using either metal or bioabsorbable screws. The researchers collected demographic data, radiographic measurements, and clinical outcomes from medical records. Patients were divided into two groups based on the type of screw used. The surgical procedures were performed under general anesthesia, with bioabsorbable screws being implemented from March 2018 onwards. Radiographic assessments included measurements of limb length discrepancy (LLD) and lateral distal tibial angle (LDTA), while clinical outcomes were evaluated using the Oxford Ankle and Foot Questionnaire. Statistical analyses compared variables such as hospital stay duration, medical costs, and surgical outcomes between the two groups.

The study found no significant differences in radiographic or clinical outcomes between the metal and bioabsorbable screw groups. However, patients treated with bioabsorbable screws experienced shorter hospital stays due to the elimination of the need for implant removal surgery. Despite higher initial costs associated with bioabsorbable implants, these findings suggest potential benefits in terms of patient satisfaction and reduced exposure to general anesthesia. Future studies with larger cohorts and longer follow-up periods are needed to confirm these results and assess long-term complications associated with bioabsorbable implants. The use of bioabsorbable screws may offer a promising alternative for treating pediatric distal tibia physeal fractures by avoiding secondary surgeries while maintaining effective clinical outcomes.

Epiphyseal Hyperplasia Caused by an Ectopic Ossification Center of the Distal Tibia: Presentation of a Pediatric Case with 13 Years of Radiological Surveillance [93]

This is a machine-generated summary of:

Scheipl, Susanne; Tauber, Stefan; Bergovec, Marko; Leithner, Andreas; Ranner, Gerhard Epiphyseal hyperplasia caused by an ectopic ossification center of the distal tibia: presentation of a pediatric case with 13 years of radiological surveillance [93]
Published in: Skeletal Radiology (2018)
Link to original: https://doi.org/10.1007/s00256-018-2894-8
Copyright of the summarized publication:
ISS 2018
All rights reserved.

If you want to cite the papers, please refer to the original.

For technical reasons we could not place the page where the original quote is coming from.

Research Highlights

Several authors have described ossification variabilities and the extension of growth plate cartilage into the metaphysis as signs of healing fractures. However, these descriptions do not match the clinical and radiographic presentation of a unique case reported in this study. A 7-year-old boy presented with a cortical lytic lesion in his distal tibial metaphysis, initially suggestive of a malignant process. Further imaging revealed that the lesion was due to hyperplastic epiphyseal cartilage, likely from an ectopic ossification center. Now, a new study by Susanne Scheipl and colleagues documents this unprecedented case, highlighting the importance of distinguishing self-limiting conditions from diseases requiring invasive diagnosis or therapy.

The study involved a comprehensive clinical and radiological evaluation of the patient over several years. Initial radiographs showed a cortical lytic lesion with indistinct borders, raising suspicion of malignancy. However, MRI and CT scans revealed a tongue-shaped cartilaginous lesion extending from the epiphyseal plate into the metaphysis, with no signs of aggressive disease such as bone marrow edema or soft-tissue infiltration. The interdisciplinary team decided against an immediate biopsy, opting instead for long-term monitoring through clinical examinations and MRI scans. Over time, the lesion acquired an eccentric shape and gradually ossified in parallel with physiological physeal fusion. By the time the boy's epiphyseal plates fused, the cartilaginous lesion had fully mineralized without affecting leg length or function.

The long-term follow-up supports the diagnosis of a self-limiting benign cartilaginous process, likely representing a developmental variant such as an ectopic ossification center extending into the metaphysis. This case underscores the need for awareness of such conditions to avoid unnecessary invasive procedures. Future study could focus on identifying similar cases to better understand their natural history and potential implications for pediatric orthopedic practice. The findings contribute to existing literature by documenting a unique presentation that challenges current understanding and highlights variability in pediatric bone development.

Classic Metaphyseal Lesion of Distal Tibia Following Footling Breech Delivery [94]

This is a machine-generated summary of:

Lee, Gloria S.; Methratta, Sosamma T.; Frasier, Lori D. Classic metaphyseal lesion of distal tibia following footling breech delivery [94]
Published in: Pediatric Radiology (2019)
Link to original: https://doi.org/10.1007/s00247-019-04490-6
Copyright of the summarized publication:
Springer-Verlag GmbH Germany, part of Springer Nature 2019
All rights reserved.

If you want to cite the papers, please refer to the original.

For technical reasons we could not place the page where the original quote is coming from.

Research Highlights

Classic metaphyseal lesions (CMLs) are fractures highly indicative of child abuse, particularly in infants under 1 year old. These fractures, often found in fatal abuse cases, are characterized by their "corner" or "bucket handle" appearance on radiographs and typically occur at the proximal tibia, distal tibia, distal femur, and proximal humerus. However, CMLs have also been reported in rare instances of birth trauma during cesarean sections and breech extractions. Despite these reports, a CML of the distal tibia associated with birth trauma had not been documented until now. A new study by Gloria S. Lee and colleagues presents a unique case of a distal tibial CML following an emergent cesarean section with a double footling presentation.

In this study, the authors describe the case of an infant delivered at 36 weeks' gestation due to severe pre-eclampsia in the mother. The delivery was complicated by a footling breech position, requiring significant traction forces on the infant's legs during extraction. Post-delivery examination revealed multiple bruises and decreased movement in the extremities. Radiographs taken on the first day showed a CML of the right distal tibial metaphysis, with follow-up imaging indicating healing. The authors emphasize that distinguishing this CML from one caused by child abuse was straightforward due to the absence of manipulations like external cephalic version prior to delivery and the clear obstetric history indicating traumatic delivery forces.

This case highlights that while CMLs are typically associated with non-accidental trauma, they can also occur due to significant birth trauma under specific circumstances. The study underscores the importance of thorough obstetric and delivery history reviews when assessing neonatal fractures to differentiate between accidental and non-accidental causes. Future study could focus on further characterizing the conditions under which CMLs might arise from birth trauma to improve diagnostic accuracy and prevent misinterpretation as abuse.

Conclusion

Complications are common with distal tibial epiphyseal fractures. The most common complication is growth arrest of the distal tibial growth plate, which can result in angular deformities and shortening. Anatomic reduction and surgical fixation are recommended for fractures with more than 2 mm of displacement.

Bibliography

1. Dias LS, Tachdjian MO. Physeal injuries of the ankle in children: classification. Clin Orthop Relat Res. 1978;136:230–3.
2. Kärrholm J, Hansson LI, Laurin S. Pronation injuries of the ankle in children. Retrospective study of radiographical classification and treatment. Acta Orthop Scand. 1983;54(1):1–17.

3. Kärrholm J, Hansson LI, Laurin S. Supination-adduction injuries of the ankle in children-radiographical classification and treatment. Arch Orthop Trauma Surg. 1983;101(3):193–200.
4. Blackburn EW, Aronsson DD, Rubright JH, Lisle JW. Ankle fractures in children. J Bone Joint Surg Am. 2012;94(13):1234–44.
5. D'Angelo F, Solarino G, Tanas D, Zani A, Cherubino P, Moretti B. Outcome of distal tibia physeal fractures: a review of cases as related to risk factors. Injury. 2017;48(Suppl 3):S7–S11.
6. Kraus R, Kaiser M. Growth disturbances of the distal tibia after physeal separation—what do we know, what do we believe we know? A review of current literature. Eur J Pediatr Surg. 2008;18:295–9.
7. Spiegel PG, Cooperman DR, Laros GS. Epiphyseal fractures of the distal ends of the tibia and fibula. A retrospective study of two hundred and thirty-seven cases in children. J Bone Joint Surg Am. 1978;60(8):1046–50.
8. Kling TJ, Bright RW, Hensinger RN. Distal tibial physeal fractures in children that may require open reduction. J Bone Joint Surg Am. 1984;66:647–57.
9. Basener CJ, Mehlman CT, Dipasquale TG. Growth disturbance after distal femoral growth plate fractures in children: a meta-analysis. J Orthop Trauma. 2009;23:663–7.
10. Rohmiller MT, Gaynor TP, Pawelek J, et al. Salter-Harris I and II fractures of the distal tibia: does mechanism of injury relate to premature physeal closure? J Pediatr Orthop. 2006;26:322–8.
11. Leary JT, Handling M, Talerico M, et al. Physeal fractures of the distal tibia: predictive factors of premature physeal closure and growth arrest. J Pediatr Orthop. 2009;29:356–61.
12. Russo F, Moor MA, Mubarak SJ, et al. Salter-Harris II fractures of the distal tibia: does surgical management reduce the risk of premature physeal closure? J Pediatr Orthop. 2013;33:524–9.
13. Rang M. Injuries of the epiphysis, growth plate and perichondral ring. In: Rang M, editor. Children's fracture. Philadelphia: Lippincott; 1983. p. 10.
14. Salter R. Epiphyseal plate injuries. In: Letts R, editor. Management of pediatric fracture. New York: Churchill Livingstone; 1994. p. 10.
15. Dugan G, Herndon WA, Mcguire R. Distal tibial physeal injuries in children: a different treatment concept. J Orthop Trauma. 1987;1:63–7.
16. Pacicca D, Cramer K, Tornetta P. Is anatomic reduction necessary for displaced physeal fractures of the distal tibia? In: Programs and abstracts of the American Academy of Orthopaedic Surgeons 68th annual meeting. 2001. p. 131.
17. Mac Nealy GA, Rogers LF, Hernandez R, Poznanski AK. Injuries of the distal tibial epiphysis: systematic radiographic evaluation. AJR Am J Roentgenol. 1982;138:683–9.
18. Pesl T, Havranek P. Rare injuries to the distal tibiofibular joint in children. Eur J Pediatr Surg. 2006;16:255–9.
19. Brown SD, Kasser JR, Zurakowski D, Jaramillo D. Analysis of 51 tibial triplane fractures using CT with multiplanar reconstruction. AJR Am J Roentgenol. 2004;183:1489–95.
20. Ogden JA. Growth slowdown and arrest lines. J Paediatr Orthop. 1984;4:409–15. https://doi.org/10.1097/01241398-198408000-00003.
21. Harris HA. The growth of the long bones in childhood with special reference to certain bony striations of the metaphysis and the role of vitamins. Arch Intern Med. 1926;38:785–93. https://doi.org/10.1001/archinte.1926.00120300102009.
22. Nowak O, Piontek J. The frequency of appearance of transverse (Harris) lines in the tibia in relationship to age at death. Ann Hum Biol. 2002;29:314–25. https://doi.org/10.1080/03014460110086105.
23. Abraham A, Macnicol MF. Growth arrest lines and recurrent patellar dislocation: a new sign. Knee. 2001;8:163–5. https://doi.org/10.1016/S0968-0160(00)00074-0.
24. Ogden JA. Chondro-osseous development and growth. In: Urist MR, editor. Fundamental and clinical bone physiology. Philadelphia: Lippincott; 1981.
25. Peterson HA. Epiphyseal growth plate fractures. Heidelberg: Springer; 2007.
26. Barmada A, Gaynor T, Mubarak SJ. Premature physeal closure following distal tibia physeal fractures: a new radiographic predictor. J Pediatr Orthop. 2003;23:733–9.

27. Koury SI, Stone CK, Harrell G, La Charite DD. Recognition and management of Tillaux fractures in adolescents. Pediatr Emerg Care. 1999;15(1):37–9.
28. Horn BD, Crisci K, Krug M, Pizzutillo PD, MacEwen GD. Radiologic evaluation of juvenile Tillaux fractures of the distal tibia. J Pediatr Orthop. 2001;21(2):162–4.
29. Stefanich RJ, Lozman J. The juvenile fracture of Tillaux. Clin Orthop Relat Res. 1986;210:219–27.
30. Kaya A, Altay T, Ozturk H, Karapinar L. Open reduction and internal fixation in displaced juvenile Tillaux fractures. Injury. 2007;38(2):201–5.
31. Choudhry IK, Wall EJ, Eismann EA, Crawford AH, Wilson L. Functional outcome analysis of triplane and Tillaux fractures after closed reduction and percutaneous fixation. J Pediatr Orthop. 2014;34:139–43. https://doi.org/10.1097/bpo.0000000000000085.
32. Crawford AH. Triplane and Tillaux fractures: is a 2 mm residual gap acceptable? J Pediatr Orthop. 2012;32(Suppl 1):S69–73.
33. Kennedy MA, Sama AE, Padavan S. The Tillaux fracture: a case report. J Emerg Med. 1998;16(4):603–6.
34. Mizuta T, Benson WM, Foster BK, Paterson DC, Morris LL. Statistical analysis of the incidence of physeal injuries. J Pediatr Orthop. 1987;7:518–23.
35. Duchesneau S, Fallat LM. The Tillaux fracture. J Foot Ankle Surg. 1996;35(2):127–33.
36. Wuerz TH, Gurd DP. Pediatric physeal ankle fracture. J Am Acad Orthop Surg. 2013;21(4):234–44. https://doi.org/10.5435/JAAOS-21-04-234.
37. Tanaka M, Shibano K, Tagawa Y, Kawai H, Hamada M. Juvenile Tillaux fracture with disrupted anteroinferior tibiofibular ligament: a case report. Knee Surg Sports Traumatol Arthrosc. 2009;17(10):1239–42.
38. Ayas MS, Köse A, Terzi E, Dincer R, Topal M, Uymur EY, Şahin A. Surgical management of displaced adolescent Tillaux fractures with the mini-open technique. Ulus Travma Acil Cerrahi Derg. 2021;27(1):109–14.
39. Schlesinger I, Wedge JH. Percutaneous reduction and fixation of displaced juvenile Tillaux fractures: a new surgical technique. J Pediatr Orthop. 1993;13(3):389–91.
40. Horn BD, Crisci K, Krug M, Pizzutillo PD, MacEwen GD. Radiologic evaluation of juvenile Tillaux fractures of the distal tibia. J Pediatr Orthop. 2001;21:162–4.
41. Seel EH, Noble S, Clarke NM, Uglow MG. Outcome of distal tibial physeal injuries. J Pediatr Orthop B. 2011;20(4):242–8.
42. Cass JR, Peterson HA. Salter-Harris type-IV injuries of the distal tibial epiphyseal growth plate, with emphasis on those involving the medial malleolus. J Bone Joint Surg Am. 1983;65(8):1059–70.
43. Cottalorda J, Beranger V, Louahem D, Camilleri JP, Launay F, Dimeglio A, et al. Salter-Harris type III and IV medial malleolar fractures: growth arrest: is it a fate? A retrospective study of 48 cases with open reduction. J Pediatr Orthop. 2008;28(6):652–5.
44. Petratos DV, Kokkinakis M, Ballas EG, Anastasopoulos JN. Prognostic factors for premature growth plate arrest as a complication of the surgical treatment of fractures of the medial malleolus in children. Bone Joint J. 2013;95-B(3):419–23.
45. Herscovici D Jr, Scaduto JM, Infante A. Conservative treatment of isolated fractures of the medial malleolus. J Bone Joint Surg Br. 2007;89 B(1):89–93.
46. Petit P, Panuel M, Faure F, et al. Acute fracture of the distal tibial physis: role of gradient-echo MR imaging versus plain film examination. Am J Roentgenol. 1996;166:1203–6.
47. Kay RM, Matthys GA. Paediatric ankle fractures: evaluation and treatment. J Am Acad Orthop Surg. 2001;9:268–78.
48. von Laer L. Classification, diagnosis, and treatment of transitional fractures of the distal part of the tibia. J Bone Joint Surg Am. 1985;67(5):687–98.
49. Jarvis JG, Miyanji F. The complex triplane fracture: ipsilateral tibial shaft and distal triplane fracture. J Trauma. 2001;51:714–6.
50. Lohman M, Kivisaari A, Kallio P, et al. Acute paediatric ankle trauma: MRI versus plain radiography. Skel Radiol. 2001;30:504–11.
51. Rogers L. The ankle. Philadelphia: Churchill Livingstone; 2002.

52. Clement DA, Worlock PH. Triplane fracture of the distal tibia. A variant in cases with an open growth plate. J Bone Joint Surg Br. 1987;69:412–5.
53. Cone RO III, Nguyen V, Flournoy JG, et al. Triplane fracture of the distal tibial epiphysis: radiographic and CT studies. Radiology. 1984;153:763–7.
54. Jones S, Phillips N, Ali F, Fernandes JA, Flowers MJ, Smith TW. Triplane fractures of the distal tibia requiring open reduction and internal fixation. Pre-operative planning using computed tomography. Injury. 2003;34:293–8.
55. Spiegel PG, Mast JW, Cooperman DR, Laros GS. Triplane fractures of the distal tibial epiphysis. Clin Orthop Relat Res. 1984;188:74–89.
56. Spiegel PG, et al. Triplane fractures of the distal tibial epiphysis. Clin Orthop Relat Res. 1984;188:74–89.
57. Yung CS, Kuong EE, Chow W. A previously unreported type of extra-articular triplane fracture: a revised classification system. J Orthop Surg (Hong Kong). 2019;27(1):2309499019828500.
58. Thawrani D, et al. Reliability and necessity of computerized tomography in distal tibial physeal injuries. J Pediatr Orthop. 2011;31(7):745–50.
59. Schnetzler KA, Hoernschemeyer D. The pediatric triplane ankle fracture. J Am Acad Orthop Surg. 2007;15(12):738–47.
60. O'Connor DK, Mulligan ME. Extra-articular triplane fracture of the distal tibia: a case report. Pediatr Radiol. 1998;28:332–3.
61. Fenelon C, Murphy EP, Galbraith JG, Kearns SR. The burden of hardware removal in ankle fractures: how common is it, why do we do it and what is the cost? A ten-year review. Foot Ankle Surg. 2019;25(4):546–9.
62. Naumann MG, Sigurdsen U, Utvåg SE, Stavem K. Incidence and risk factors for removal of an internal fixation following surgery for ankle fracture: a retrospective cohort study of 997 patients. Injury. 2016;47(8):1783–8.
63. Bostman O, Pihlajamaki H. Routine implant removal after fracture surgery: a potentially reducible consumer of hospital resources in trauma units. J Trauma. 1996;41(5):846–9.
64. Kasai T, Matsumoto T, Iga T, Tanaka S. Complications of implant removal in ankle fractures. J Orthop. 2019;16(3):191–4.
65. Gogolewski S. Resorbable polymers for internal fixation. Clin Mater. 1992;10(1–2):13–20.
66. Juutilainen T, Pätiälä H, Ruuskanen M, Rokkanen P. Comparison of costs in ankle fractures treated with absorbable or metallic fixation devices. Arch Orthop Trauma Surg. 1997;116(4):204–8.
67. Ojeda-Thies C, Bonsfills N, Albinana J. Solitary epiphyseal enchondroma of the proximal femur in a 23-month-old girl. J Pediatr Orthop. 2008;28(5):565–8.
68. Henderson ER, Pohlmann RA, Hollowell ML, Gebhardt MC. Epiphyseal lesion of the humerus in a child. Solitary epiphyseal enchondroma of the humeral greater tuberosity. Skeletal Radiol. 2013;42(7):1001–2; 1021–3.
69. Jones KB, Buckwalter JA, Frassica FJ, McCarthy EF. Intracortical chondroma: a report of two cases. Skeletal Radiol. 2006;35(5):298–301.
70. Niethard M, Rogalski M, Deja M, Zacher J. Partial physeal growth arrest with increasing genu varum deformity caused by a cortical enchondroma—a case report. Z Orthop Unfall. 2008;146(6):725–9.
71. Kleinman PK, Marks SC Jr, Spevak MR, Belanger PL, Richmond JM. Extension of growth-plate cartilage into the metaphysis: a sign of healing fracture in abused infants. AJR Am J Roentgenol. 1991;156(4):775–9.
72. Laor T, Hartman AL, Jaramillo D. Local physeal widening on MR imaging: an incidental finding suggesting prior metaphyseal insult. Pediatr Radiol. 1997;27(8):654–62.
73. Jans LB, Jaremko JL, Ditchfield M, Verstraete KL. Evolution of femoral condylar ossification at MR imaging: frequency and patient age distribution. Radiology. 2011;258(3):880–8.
74. O'Connell A, Donoghue VB. Can classic metaphyseal lesions follow uncomplicated caesarean section? Pediatr Radiol. 2007;37:488–91.
75. Lysack JT, Soboleski D. Classic metaphyseal lesion following external cephalic version and cesarean section. Pediatr Radiol. 2003;33:422–4.

76. Morris S, Cassidy N, Stephens M, et al. Birth-associated femoral fractures: incidence and outcome. J Pediatr Orthop. 2002;22:27–30.
77. Grayev AM, Boal DK, Wallach DM, Segal LS. Metaphyseal fractures mimicking abuse during treatment for clubfoot. Pediatr Radiol. 2001;31:559–63.
78. Della Grotta LM, Marine MB, Harris TL, Karmazyn B. Classic metaphyseal lesion acquired during physical therapy. Clin Imaging. 2019;54:100–2.
79. Burrell T, Opfer E, Berglund L, et al. A witnessed case of a classic metaphyseal fracture caused during IV line placement in a child: insight into mechanism of injury. J Forensic Leg Med. 2015;35:51–3.
80. Pomeranz CB, Bartolotta RJ. Pediatric ankle injuries: utilizing the Dias-Tachdjian classification. Skeletal Radiol. 2020;49:521–30. https://doi.org/10.1007/s00256-019-03356-0.
81. Chen H, Chen Z, Chen P, Zheng Z, Lin J. Incidence of growth disturbance after distal tibia physeal fracture in children. J Orthop Surg Res. 2022;17(1):529. https://doi.org/10.1186/s13018-022-03427-4.
82. Lemburg SP, Lilienthal E, Heyer CM. Growth plate fractures of the distal tibia: is CT imaging necessary? Arch Orthop Trauma Surg. 2010;130:1411–7. https://doi.org/10.1007/s00402-010-1140-1.
83. Kennedy IW, Irwin GJ, Huntley JS. Growth arrest lines and intra-epiphyseal silhouettes: a case series. BMC Res Notes. 2014;7:27. https://doi.org/10.1186/1756-0500-7-27.
84. Yuan Q, Zhen Y, Guo Z, Zhang F, Fang J, Zhu Z, Zhu L, Shen X, Yin C, Liu Y, Yao F, Wu L, Wang X. Open reduction and internal fixation for displaced Salter-Harris type II fractures of the distal tibia: a retrospective study of sixty-five cases in children. J Orthop Surg Res. 2021;16:224. https://doi.org/10.1186/s13018-021-02359-9.
85. Tiefenboeck TM, Binder H, Joestl J, Tiefenboeck MM, Boesmueller S, Krestan C, Schurz M. Displaced juvenile Tillaux fractures. Wien Klin Wochenschr. 2017;129:169–75. https://doi.org/10.1007/s00508-016-1059-9.
86. Lee JW, Cho JH, Song HK, Chung JY, Park YU, Kim TH. Closed reduction and internal fixation for Tillaux fractures, based on pre-operative three-dimensional computed tomography. Eur J Orthop Surg Traumatol. 2024;34:2365–71. https://doi.org/10.1007/s00590-024-03910-0.
87. Yuan Q, Guo Z, Wang X, Dai J, Zhang F, Fang J, Yin C, Yu W, Zhen Y. Concurrent ipsilateral Tillaux fracture and medial malleolar fracture in adolescents: management and outcome. J Orthop Surg Res. 2020;15:423. https://doi.org/10.1186/s13018-020-01961-7.
88. Schneidmueller D, Sander AL, Wertenbroek M, Wutzler S, Kraus R, Marzi I, Laurer H. Triplane fractures: do we need cross-sectional imaging? Eur J Trauma Emerg Surg. 2013;40:37–43. https://doi.org/10.1007/s00068-013-0338-7.
89. Kang H, Kang T, Lim C. The incidence and treatment outcome of atypical triplane fractures in adolescents. Indian J Orthop. 2022;56:2133–40. https://doi.org/10.1007/s43465-022-00679-4.
90. O'Connor DK, Mulligan ME. Extra-articular triplane fracture of the distal tibia: a case report. Pediatr Radiol. 1998;28:332–3. https://doi.org/10.1007/s002470050367.
91. Ruffing T, Muhm M, Winkler H. Triplane fracture of the distal fibula. Eur J Trauma Emerg Surg. 2009;36:392–6. https://doi.org/10.1007/s00068-009-9030-3.
92. Kim WS, Oh MJ, Park MS, Sung KH. Comparison of surgical outcomes between bioabsorbable and metal screw fixation for distal tibial physeal fracture in children and adolescent. Int Orthop. 2024;48:2681–7. https://doi.org/10.1007/s00264-024-06284-4.
93. Scheipl S, Tauber S, Bergovec M, Leithner A, Ranner G. Epiphyseal hyperplasia caused by an ectopic ossification center of the distal tibia: presentation of a pediatric case with 13 years of radiological surveillance. Skeletal Radiol. 2018;47:1029–37. https://doi.org/10.1007/s00256-018-2894-8.
94. Lee GS, Methratta ST, Frasier LD. Classic metaphyseal lesion of distal tibia following footling breech delivery. Pediatr Radiol. 2019;49:1840–2. https://doi.org/10.1007/s00247-019-04490-6.

20 Pelvic Fractures

Introduction by the Author

Pelvic fractures are relatively common in adults. They account for approximately 4% of all fractures. However, they are rare in children. They comprise only 2% of all pediatric fractures. Up to 10% of pediatric pelvic fractures are unstable.

These fractures occur in the ilium, pubis, or ischium and are often associated with high-energy trauma. Due to the complex anatomy of the pelvis and the potential for associated severe injuries, they can result in significant mortality. Though less common than in adults, pelvic fractures in children are associated with significant morbidity and costly treatment. These injuries pose significant challenges due to the high risk of mortality from associated bleeding.

Due to the forceful nature of these accidents, additional injuries often accompany pelvic fractures. Extremity and genitourinary injuries are particularly common in pediatric cases. Unlike adult cases, vascular hemorrhaging is uncommon in pediatric pelvic fractures. Although pelvic fractures in children are uncommon, the associated mortality rate is reportedly as high as 25%. The leading cause of death in children with pelvic fractures is combined injury rather than the fracture itself.

The skeleton of an immature pediatric patient is more flexible, with greater joint laxity and abundant cartilage. These characteristics allow for superior shock absorption and increased remodeling potential. These characteristics make nonsurgical management an attractive option for pediatric patients. This approach includes bed rest, traction, pelvic slings, and hip spica casts. However, recent evidence suggests that this approach may lead to complications affecting quality of life. Therefore, surgical intervention is recommended

© The Author(s), under exclusive license to Springer Nature Switzerland AG 2026
F. Canavese, *Advances in Pediatric Extremity Fracture Management*,
https://doi.org/10.1007/978-3-032-33306-3_20

for unstable fracture patterns to prevent late complications such as low back pain, limb length discrepancy, early sacroiliac fusion, iliac wing undergrowth, and hemi-pelvis undergrowth. These complications have been reported in up to 30% of skeletally immature patients with pelvic fractures. Unlike adults, children with pelvic fractures typically die from associated central nervous system or abdominal organ injuries rather than pelvic hemorrhage.

Surgical strategies such as external fixation and pelvic angiography are also indicated for pediatric cases. While most pediatric patients with unstable pelvic fractures had favorable outcomes with external fixation, those aged 8 years or older with severely displaced fractures (Tile C) and immediate postoperative displacement of 10 mm or more experienced poorer outcomes.

20.1 Machine Generated Summaries

Disclaimer: The summaries in this chapter were generated from Springer Nature publications using abstractive AI auto-summarization: An abstraction-based summarizer creates new text based on deep learning. New phrases are created to summarize the content. As the constituted sentences are machine selected, they may not fully reflect the body of the work, so we strongly advise that the original content is read and cited. The auto-generated summaries were curated by the author(s) to meet Springer Nature publication standards.

Multicenter Epidemiological Analysis of Related Factors in 10,808 Hospitalized Children with Lower Limb and Pelvic Fractures in China [47]

This is a machine-generated summary of:

Qiu, Xin; Zhu, Tianfeng; Deng, Hansheng; Chen, Jianlin; Feng, Haoran; Huang, Zilong; Li, Jiahui; Wang, Xinyu; Liu, Shizhe; Wang, Shuaiyin; Gu, Zhenkun; Wu, Zhengyu; Yang, Qisong; Liu, Gen; Feng, Guoshuang; Sechi, Leonardo Antonio; Caggiari, Gianfilippo; You, Chao; Fu, Guibing Multicenter epidemiological analysis of related factors in 10,808 hospitalized children with lower limb and pelvic fractures in China [47]
Published in: Scientific Reports (2024)
Link to original: https://doi.org/10.1038/s41598-024-77970-x
Copyright of the summarized publication:
The Author(s) 2024
License: OpenAccess CC BY-NC-ND 4.0

This article is licensed under a Creative Commons Attribution-NonCommercial-NoDerivatives 4.0 International License, which permits any non-commercial use, sharing, distribution and reproduction in any medium or format, as long as you give appropriate credit to the original author(s) and the source, provide a link to the Creative Commons licence, and indicate if you modified the licensed material. You do not have permission under this licence to share adapted material derived from this article or parts of it. The images or other third party material in this article are included in the article's Creative Commons licence, unless indicated otherwise in a credit line to the material. If material is not included in the article's Creative Commons licence and your intended use is not permitted by statutory regulation or exceeds the permitted use, you will need to obtain permission directly from the copyright holder. To view a copy of this licence, visit http://creativecommons.org/licenses/by-nc-nd/4.0/.

If you want to cite the papers, please refer to the original.

For technical reasons we could not place the page where the original quote is coming from.

Research Highlights

Unintentional childhood injuries, particularly fractures, have emerged as a significant global public health issue, with fractures being the most common type of injury among children. These injuries vary based on local climate, culture, and activities, leading to diverse causative factors across different regions. In China, where children constitute a substantial portion of the population, there is limited research on the patterns and trends of lower limb and pelvic fractures in children. Now a new study by Xin Qiu and colleagues addresses this gap by conducting a retrospective analysis of epidemiological data from tertiary pediatric hospitals in China to better understand these fracture patterns and their associated injuries.

The study involved analyzing medical records of hospitalized children with lower limb and pelvic fractures from December 2015 to December 2020. Data were collected using the International Statistical Classification of Diseases and Related Health Problems coding system, focusing on age, sex, causes of injury, fracture sites, treatment modalities, and concomitant trauma to other systems. The researchers categorized patients into age groups—infants, preschool children, school children, and adolescents—and classified fracture sites anatomically. Statistical analyses were performed using SPSS software to identify significant differences in treatment approaches across age groups and fracture sites. The study found that preschool children had the highest incidence of fractures, with males more frequently affected than females across all age groups. The most common fracture sites were the tibia, femur, and fibula shafts.

The study advances our understanding of pediatric fractures in China by highlighting the prevalence of lower limb and pelvic fractures among preschool-aged children and identifying falling over as the leading cause of these injuries. It underscores the need for targeted preventive interventions tailored to specific age groups to reduce fracture incidence. Future study directions could include developing comprehensive intervention strategies involving health education for children, parents, communities, and schools to enhance safety awareness and reduce injury risks. Additionally, interdisciplinary collaboration is essential for managing high-energy trauma cases involving pelvic fractures and multi-system injuries in children.

Pelvic Angiography Is Effective for Emergency Pediatric Patients with Pelvic Fractures: A Propensity-Score-Matching Study with a Nationwide Trauma Registry in Japan [48]

This is a machine-generated summary of:

Katayama, Yusuke; Kitamura, Tetsuhisa; Hirose, Tomoya; Kiguchi, Takeyuki; Matsuyama, Tasuku; Takahashi, Hiroki; Kiyohara, Kosuke; Sado, Junya; Adachi, Shingo; Noda, Tomohiro; Izawa, Junichi; Nakagawa, Yuko; Shimazu, Takeshi Pelvic angiography is effective for emergency pediatric patients with pelvic fractures: a propensity-score-matching study with a nationwide trauma registry in Japan [48]
Published in: European Journal of Trauma and Emergency Surgery (2019)
Link to original: https://doi.org/10.1007/s00068-019-01154-w
Copyright of the summarized publication:
Springer-Verlag GmbH Germany, part of Springer Nature 2019
License: OpenAccess CC BY 4.0

This article is distributed under the terms of the Creative Commons Attribution 4.0 International License (http://creativecommons.org/licenses/by/4.0/), which permits unrestricted use, distribution, and reproduction in any medium, provided you give appropriate credit to the original author(s) and the source, provide a link to the Creative Commons license, and indicate if changes were made.

If you want to cite the papers, please refer to the original.

For technical reasons we could not place the page where the original quote is coming from.

Research Highlights

Pelvic fractures in children, though less common than in adults, pose significant challenges due to the high risk of mortality from associated bleeding. Traditional treatment strategies like external fixation and pelvic angiography (PA) are well-documented for adults but less so for pediatric cases. The Eastern Association for the Surgery of Trauma guidelines recommend emergency PA for adult patients with pelvic fractures who exhibit hemodynamic instability or signs of ongoing bleeding. However, the effectiveness of PA in pediatric patients remains underexplored. Now, a new study by Yusuke Katayama and colleagues investigates the association between PA implementation and outcomes in emergency pediatric patients with pelvic fractures using data from the Japanese Trauma Data Bank (JTDB).

The study utilized a retrospective observational design, analyzing data from the JTDB spanning several years. Pediatric patients aged 16 years or younger with pelvic fractures were included, excluding those with cardiopulmonary arrest upon hospital arrival or missing critical data. The researchers employed propensity-score matching to compare outcomes between patients who received PA and those who did not. The main endpoint was hospital mortality, and statistical analyses were conducted using logistic regression models to adjust for potential confounders such as age, injury severity, and shock status on arrival. The study found that among matched cohorts, hospital mortality was significantly lower in the PA group compared to the non-PA group, particularly among patients presenting with shock.

The findings suggest that implementing PA in pediatric patients with pelvic fractures can lead to improved survival rates, especially in those with hemodynamic instability. This study highlights the potential benefits of angiographic assessment and intervention in managing severe pediatric trauma cases. Future studies could focus on refining catheter selection for children and exploring non-invasive techniques like CT-guided surgery to enhance treatment efficacy further. Additionally, understanding the decision-making process behind PA implementation could provide insights into optimizing care protocols for pediatric trauma patients.

Prehospital Predictors of Risk for Pelvic Fractures in Pediatric Trauma Patients [49]

This is a machine-generated summary of:

Nabaweesi, Rosemary; Arnold, Meghan A.; Chang, David C.; Rossberg, Mark I.; Ziegfeld, Susan; Sawaya, David E.; Bathurst, Melinda A.; Colombani, Paul; Abdullah, Fizan Prehospital predictors of risk for pelvic fractures in pediatric trauma patients [49]

Published in: Pediatric Surgery International (2008)
Link to original: https://doi.org/10.1007/s00383-008-2195-8
Copyright of the summarized publication:
Springer-Verlag 2008
All rights reserved.

If you want to cite the papers, please refer to the original.

For technical reasons we could not place the page where the original quote is coming from.

Research Highlights

Pelvic fractures in children, though uncommon, are associated with significant morbidity and costly treatment. The American College of Surgeons Committee on Trauma recommends pelvic radiography for all patients with multisystem blunt traumatic injuries, but there is a need to refine criteria to reduce unnecessary imaging in pediatric cases. Now, a new study by Rosemary Nabaweesi and colleagues at The Johns Hopkins Children's Center investigates factors that may help identify pediatric trauma patients at the highest risk for pelvic fractures.

The study involved a retrospective analysis of data from the Johns Hopkins Children's Center pediatric trauma registry, focusing on patients younger than 18 years who sustained blunt injuries. Excluding those with penetrating or burn injuries, the researchers analyzed demographic, etiological, and clinical variables of 1000 patients to determine the presence of pelvic fractures via radiography. Statistical analyses, including Pearson's chi-square test and Mann–Whitney rank sum test, were used to compare children with and without pelvic fractures. The study found that older children, males, and Caucasians were at higher risk. Additionally, injuries occurring in streets or highways and mechanisms such as being struck as a pedestrian or involved in motor vehicle crashes significantly increased the likelihood of pelvic fractures.

The study advances understanding by identifying specific demographic and mechanistic factors that predict pelvic fracture risk in pediatric trauma patients. These findings suggest that targeted use of pelvic radiography based on these criteria could reduce unnecessary imaging. Future study could focus on developing a decision instrument incorporating these factors to guide clinical practice effectively. Such an instrument could minimize radiation exposure and resource use while maintaining diagnostic accuracy. Despite limitations like missing data on physical findings, this research provides a foundation for more precise imaging guidelines in pediatric trauma care.

The Clinical Characteristics and Management of Paediatric Pelvic Fractures: A Changing Landscape Based on Skeletal Maturity [50]

This is a machine-generated summary of:

Lu, Victor; Gowrishankar, Shrav; Arshad, Zaki; Thahir, Azeem; Lenihan, Jonathan; Mcdonald, Scott; Rawal, Jaikirty; Hull, Peter; Chou, Daud; Carrothers, Andrew The clinical characteristics and management of paediatric pelvic fractures: a changing landscape based on skeletal maturity [50]

Published in: European Journal of Trauma and Emergency Surgery (2022)
Link to original: https://doi.org/10.1007/s00068-022-02108-5
Copyright of the summarized publication:
The Author(s) 2022
License: OpenAccess CC BY 4.0

This article is licensed under a Creative Commons Attribution 4.0 International License, which permits use, sharing, adaptation, distribution and reproduction in any medium or format, as long as you give appropriate credit to the original author(s)

and the source, provide a link to the Creative Commons licence, and indicate if changes were made. The images or other third party material in this article are included in the article's Creative Commons licence, unless indicated otherwise in a credit line to the material. If material is not included in the article's Creative Commons licence and your intended use is not permitted by statutory regulation or exceeds the permitted use, you will need to obtain permission directly from the copyright holder. To view a copy of this licence, visit http://creativecommons.org/licenses/by/4.0/.

If you want to cite the papers, please refer to the original.

For technical reasons we could not place the page where the original quote is coming from.

Research Highlights

Paediatric pelvic fractures (PPFs) are rare, typically resulting from high-energy trauma such as motor vehicle accidents (MVAs). These injuries often accompany other traumas, with extremity injuries being common due to the elasticity of the paediatric pelvis. Despite the severity of these incidents, vascular hemorrhage is less frequent in children compared to adults. However, there is limited data specifically addressing mortality risks associated with PPFs. Now, a new study by Victor Lu and colleagues conducts a 10-year retrospective analysis of paediatric pelvic fracture cases at a level one trauma center, aiming to clarify factors such as fracture types, associated injuries, and mortality rates.

The study reviewed medical records and radiographs of children under 16 years who sustained pelvic fractures from blunt-force trauma. Excluding firearm injuries, data were categorized into epidemiological, radiographical, clinical, and associated injury details. The modified Torode classification was used to assess fracture types, while skeletal maturity was determined by triradiate cartilage status. Statistical analyses were performed to compare outcomes between skeletally mature and immature groups. The findings revealed that pedestrian MVAs were the most common mechanism of injury for skeletally immature patients. The study also noted that skeletally immature patients were more likely to sustain rami fractures and less likely to require surgical intervention for pelvic injuries compared to their mature counterparts.

The study advances understanding by highlighting the distinct characteristics and treatment needs of skeletally immature patients with PPFs. It suggests that those with closed triradiate cartilage can be managed similarly to adults due to comparable injury patterns and treatment requirements. Future studies could focus on long-term outcomes and health economics analyses to optimize paediatric pelvic trauma care. Additionally, establishing multicenter collaborations may enhance data collection for these rare cases, ultimately improving management strategies and patient outcomes in this vulnerable population.

Surgical Management of Paediatric Pelvic Fractures: A Prospective Case Series and Early Experience from a Level One Egyptian Trauma Centre [51]

This is a machine-generated summary of:

Arafa, Mohamed; Khalifa, Ahmed A.; Fergany, Ali; Abdelhafez, Mostafa A.; Mohamedean, Aly; Adam, Faisal Fahmy; Farouk, Osama Surgical management of paediatric pelvic fractures: a prospective case series and early experience from a level one Egyptian trauma centre [51]
Published in: International Orthopaedics (2022)
Link to original: https://doi.org/10.1007/s00264-022-05509-8
Copyright of the summarized publication:
The Author(s) 2022
License: OpenAccess CC BY 4.0

This article is licensed under a Creative Commons Attribution 4.0 International License, which permits use, sharing, adaptation, distribution and reproduction in any medium or format, as long as you give appropriate credit to the original author(s) and the source, provide a link to the Creative Commons licence, and indicate if changes were made. The images or other third party material in this article are included in the article's Creative Commons licence, unless indicated otherwise in a credit line to the material. If material is not included in the article's Creative Commons licence and your intended use is not permitted by statutory regulation or exceeds the permitted use, you will need to obtain permission directly from the copyright holder. To view a copy of this licence, visit http://creativecommons.org/licenses/by/4.0/.

If you want to cite the papers, please refer to the original.

For technical reasons we could not place the page where the original quote is coming from.

Research Highlights

Pediatric pelvic fractures (PPF) are a significant concern due to the unique characteristics of the pediatric skeleton, which includes inherent flexibility and a cartilaginous cover that acts as a shock absorber. These injuries differ from adult pelvic fractures and often result from significant trauma. Traditionally, nonsurgical management has been the standard approach for PPF, relying on the pediatric skeleton's ability to remodel. However, this approach has led to various long-term complications such as malunion, nonunion, scoliosis, and pelvic asymmetry. Now, a new study by Mohamed Arafa and colleagues aims to address this gap by reporting their early experience in surgical management of PPF, focusing on indications, functional and radiological outcomes, and complication incidence.

The study was conducted as a prospective case series at a regional Egyptian academic level one trauma center. It included skeletally immature patients with open or closed pelvic fractures who were admitted within 7 days of trauma. The researchers followed a uniform treatment protocol starting with an initial assessment using the ATLS protocol and urgent stabilization with a pelvic binder. Radiographic assessments were performed using various views, and computed tomography was used for pre-operative planning. Fractures were classified based on the modified Tile AO/OTA classification system, guiding the decision for surgical intervention. Surgical approaches varied depending on fracture classification and included percutaneous techniques, Pfannenstiel approach, direct anterior approach, and direct posterior approach. Post-operative follow-up involved regular assessments for functional outcomes using a modified Majeed scoring system and radiological evaluations.

The study achieved acceptable short-term functional and radiological outcomes in surgically treated pediatric patients with PPF. The authors highlight that surgical intervention may be beneficial in preventing long-term complications associated with nonsurgical management. Future studies could focus on determining long-term outcomes and refining surgical guidelines for PPF management. The study also suggests that surgical approaches should be tailored based on patient characteristics, fracture classification, and associated injuries to optimize outcomes. Despite some limitations such as small sample size and short follow-up period, this research contributes valuable insights into the surgical management of pediatric pelvic fractures.

Analysis of Risk Factors Affecting the Prognosis of External Fixation in the Treatment of Unstable Pelvic Fractures in Children: A Retrospective Study of 96 Patients [52]

This is a machine-generated summary of:

Zhang, Hanwen; Zhao, Ronghao; Zhu, Danjiang; Feng, Wei; Song, Baojian; Wang, Qiang Analysis of risk factors affecting the prognosis of external fixation in the treatment of unstable pelvic fractures in children: a retrospective study of 96 patients [52]

Published in: BMC Pediatrics (2025)
Link to original: https://doi.org/10.1186/s12887-025-05485-z
Copyright of the summarized publication:
The Author(s) 2025
License: OpenAccess CC BY-NC-ND 4.0

This article is licensed under a Creative Commons Attribution-NonCommercial-NoDerivatives 4.0 International License, which permits any non-commercial use, sharing, distribution and reproduction in any medium or format, as long as you give appropriate credit to the original author(s) and the source, provide a link to the Creative Commons licence, and indicate if you modified the licensed material. You do not have permission under this licence to share adapted material derived from this article or parts of it. The images or other third party material in this article are included in the article's Creative Commons licence, unless indicated otherwise in a credit line to the material. If material is not included in the article's Creative Commons licence and your intended use is not permitted by statutory regulation or exceeds the permitted use, you will need to obtain permission directly from the copyright holder. To view a copy of this licence, visit http://creativecommons.org/licenses/by-nc-nd/4.0/.

If you want to cite the papers, please refer to the original.

For technical reasons we could not place the page where the original quote is coming from.

Research Highlights

Pelvic fractures, which occur in the ilium, pubis, or ischium, are often linked to high-energy injuries and can result in significant mortality due to the complex anatomy of the pelvis and potential for severe associated injuries. While these fractures are relatively common in adults, they are rare in children, comprising only a small percentage of pediatric fractures. The treatment and prognosis for pediatric pelvic fractures differ significantly from adults due to the unique characteristics of children's skeletal structures. Now, a new study by Hanwen Zhang and colleagues investigates the risk factors affecting the prognosis of external fixation in treating pediatric pelvic fractures by retrospectively analyzing clinical data from pediatric patients with unstable pelvic fractures treated at their center.

The study involved a retrospective analysis of patients with Tile B or C type pelvic fractures who underwent surgical treatment with closed reduction and external fixation. The researchers excluded cases with metabolic bone diseases, pathological fractures, or severe combined lower limb injuries. The surgical procedure involved placing Schanz screws into the iliac bones under C-arm fluoroscopy and using a rectangular frame for fracture reduction. Postoperative management included bed rest, daily disinfection of pin sites, and intravenous antibiotics. Patients were followed up at regular intervals to assess fracture healing and functional outcomes using Cole pelvic fracture functional ratings and WeeFIM scores. Statistical analyses identified independent predictors of prognosis, including age and immediate postoperative displacement values.

The study found that most pediatric patients with unstable pelvic fractures had good outcomes with external fixation; however, children aged 8 years or older with Tile type C fractures and immediate postoperative displacement of 10 mm or more had poorer outcomes. This research highlights the importance of considering age and fracture characteristics when planning treatment for pediatric pelvic fractures. Future study could focus on developing a classification system specifically for pediatric pelvic fractures to guide treatment decisions better. The findings provide valuable insights for pediatric orthopedic surgeons in selecting appropriate treatment plans to improve long-term outcomes for children with unstable pelvic fractures.

Functional Results of Surgically Treated Paediatric Pelvic Fractures Are as Good as Conservatively Treated Ones: Retrospective Evaluation of 64 Patients [53]

This is a machine-generated summary of:

Bozbek, Murat; Aydin, Tahsin; Yavuz, Ibrahim Alper; Ozdemir, Guzelali; Yalcin, Elif; Yildirim, Ahmet Ozgur Functional results of surgically treated paediatric pelvic fractures are as good as conservatively treated ones: retrospective evaluation of 64 patients [53]

Published in: European Journal of Orthopaedic Surgery & Traumatology (2025)
Link to original: https://doi.org/10.1007/s00590-025-04458-3

Copyright of the summarized publication:
The Author(s), under exclusive licence to Springer-Verlag France SAS, part of Springer Nature 2025

Copyright comment: Springer Nature or its licensor (e.g. a society or other partner) holds exclusive rights to this article under a publishing agreement with the author(s) or other rightsholder(s); author self-archiving of the accepted manuscript version of this article is solely governed by the terms of such publishing agreement and applicable law.

All rights reserved.

If you want to cite the papers, please refer to the original.

For technical reasons we could not place the page where the original quote is coming from.

Research Highlights

Paediatric pelvic fractures (PPFs) are uncommon compared to adult cases and typically result from high-energy trauma, often leading to severe complications and mortality. Unlike adults, mortality in children with PPFs is usually due to associated central nervous system or abdominal organ injuries rather than pelvic hemorrhage. Despite the critical nature of these injuries, there is a lack of studies comparing surgical and conservative treatment outcomes in terms of functional parameters. Now, a new study by Murat Bozbek and colleagues addresses this gap by evaluating the functional outcomes of paediatric pelvic fractures using spinopelvic parameters to compare surgical and conservative treatments.

The study was conducted retrospectively at a single trauma center, including patients aged 4–16 years with pelvic ring injuries. Patients were divided into two groups based on their treatment: surgical or conservative. Spinopelvic parameters were measured using video rasterstereography, a radiation-free method that provides quantitative data on spine and pelvis alignment. Surgical treatment was indicated for specific fracture types and performed by an experienced surgeon using standard procedures. The study analyzed various factors such as injury type, additional pathologies, blood transfusion needs, and post-operative spinopelvic parameters to assess functional outcomes.

The findings revealed no significant differences in spinopelvic alignment between surgically and conservatively treated patients at the 12-month follow-up, suggesting that appropriate surgical intervention does not compromise functional pelvic balance. The study also highlighted correlations between pelvic torsion, obliquity measurements, and injury severity scores. Future studies could focus on longer-term follow-up to better understand the evolving functional implications as the paediatric pelvis matures. Additionally, prospective research could further explore the impact of skeletal maturity on fracture patterns and treatment responses to enhance clinical decision-making for paediatric pelvic injuries.

The Application of Lateral-Rectus Approach on Toddlers' Unstable Pelvic Fractures [54]

This is a machine-generated summary of:

Liu, Yuancheng; Zhan, Xiaorui; Huang, Fuming; Wen, Xiangyuan; Chen, Yuhui; Yang, Cheng; Fan, Shicai The application of lateral-rectus approach on toddlers' unstable pelvic fractures [54]

Published in: BMC Musculoskeletal Disorders (2020)

Link to original: https://doi.org/10.1186/s12891-020-3172-1

Copyright of the summarized publication:

The Author(s). 2020

License: OpenAccess CC BY + CC0 4.0

This article is licensed under a Creative Commons Attribution 4.0 International License, which permits use, sharing, adaptation, distribution and reproduction in any medium or format, as long as you give appropriate credit to the original author(s) and the source, provide a link to the Creative Commons licence, and indicate if changes were made. The images or other third party material in this article are included in the article's Creative Commons licence, unless indicated otherwise in a credit line to the material. If material is not included in the article's Creative Commons licence and your intended use is not permitted by statutory regulation or exceeds the permitted use, you will need to obtain permission directly from the copyright holder. To view a copy of this licence, visit http://creativecommons.org/licenses/by/4.0/. The Creative Commons Public Domain Dedication waiver (http://creativecommons.org/publicdomain/zero/1.0/) applies to the data made available in this article, unless otherwise stated in a credit line to the data.

If you want to cite the papers, please refer to the original.

For technical reasons we could not place the page where the original quote is coming from.

Research Highlights

Pelvic fractures in children are uncommon, accounting for a small percentage of all pediatric fractures, yet they often result from severe trauma such as being struck by vehicles. These injuries are frequently accompanied by damage to other systems, leading to significant mortality rates not directly attributable to the fracture itself. Traditionally, conservative treatment has been favored due to the perceived remodeling potential in children; however, recent evidence suggests that this approach may lead to complications affecting quality of life. Now, a new study by Yuancheng Liu and colleagues explores the use of the lateral-rectus approach (LRA) for surgical correction of unstable pelvic fractures in toddlers, providing insights into its effectiveness and safety.

The study involved two female toddlers who sustained unstable pelvic fractures after being hit by cars. Both patients were treated surgically using the LRA by the same trauma orthopedic specialist. Preoperative planning was conducted using advanced imaging techniques and 3D modeling to simulate fracture reduction and screw placement. During surgery, patients were positioned supine, and the LRA incision allowed for clear exposure of the sacroiliac joint. The posterior pelvic ring was fixed with sacroiliac screws, while external fixation was used for the anterior ring. Postoperative care included functional exercises and gradual weight-bearing activities. The study reported successful outcomes with no complications such as screw loosening or infection, and both patients achieved excellent functional recovery.

The application of LRA in this context represents a significant advancement in pediatric orthopedic surgery, offering a viable alternative to traditional approaches with minimal risk of nerve or vascular injury. The study highlights the potential benefits of surgical intervention for unstable pelvic fractures in children, challenging conventional conservative treatment paradigms. Future study could focus on larger sample sizes to validate these findings further and explore long-term outcomes. Additionally, refining surgical techniques and postoperative care protocols may enhance recovery and reduce complications in pediatric patients with similar injuries.

Conclusion

Pediatric pelvic fractures are uncommon compared to adult cases and typically result from high-energy trauma. These fractures often lead to severe complications and death. They are usually managed with external fixation, which generally yields favorable outcomes.

Bibliography

1. Kaye JA, Jick H. Epidemiology of lower limb fractures in general practice in the United Kingdom. Inj Prev. 2004;10:368–74.
2. Lempesis V, et al. Time trends in pediatric fracture incidence in Sweden during the period 1950–2006. Acta Orthop. 2017;88(4):440–5.
3. Joeris A, Lutz N, Wicki B, Slongo T, Audigé L. An epidemiological evaluation of pediatric long bone fractures – a retrospective cohort study of 2716 patients from two Swiss tertiary pediatric hospitals. BMC Pediatr. 2014;20(14):314.

4. Schlickewei W, Keck T. Pelvic and acetabular fractures in childhood. Injury. 2005;36(Suppl 1):A57–63.
5. Signorino PR, Densmore J, Werner M. Pediatric pelvic injury: functional outcome at 6-month follow-up. J Pediatr Surg. 2005;40:107–12; discussion 112–3.
6. Silber JS, Flynn JM. Changing patterns of pediatric pelvic fractures with skeletal maturation: implications for classification and management. J Pediatr Orthop. 2002;22:22–6.
7. Nguyen ATM, Drynan DP, Holland AJA. Paediatric pelvic fractures—an updated literature review. ANZ J Surg. 2022;92:3182–94.
8. Wang X, et al. A brief introduction to the FUTang Updating medical REcords (FUTURE) database. Pediatr Investig. 2021;5(3):247–8.
9. Song F, et al. Epidemiology and the economic burden of pediatric fractures in China: a retrospective study of 14,141 fractures. Bone. 2021;144:115498.
10. Qiu X, Deng H, Zhao Z. Upper limb pediatric fractures in 22 tertiary children's hospitals, China: a multicenter epidemiological investigation and economic factor analysis of 32,832 hospitalized children. J Orthop Surg Res. 2022;17:300.
11. Cullinane DC, Schiller HJ, Zielinski MD, et al. Eastern association for the surgery of trauma practice management guidelines for hemorrhage in pelvic fracture-update and systematic review. J Trauma. 2011;71:1850–68.
12. Falzarano G, Medici A, Carta S, et al. The orthopedic damage control in pelvic ring fractures: when and why-a multicenter experience of 10 years' treatment. J Acute Dis. 2014;3:201–6.
13. American Academy of Orthopaedic Surgeons. Fracture of the pelvis. Medline; 2007.
14. Gross EA, Niedens BA. Validation of a decision instrument to limit pelvic radiography in blunt trauma. J Emerg Med. 2005;28:263–6. https://doi.org/10.1016/j.jemermed.2004.10.013.
15. American College of Surgeons Committee on Trauma. Initial assessment and management. In: Advanced trauma life support for doctors student course manual. Chicago: American College of Surgeons; 2004. p. 11–40.
16. Holden CP, Holman J, Herman MJ. Pediatric pelvic fractures. J Am Acad Orthop Surg. 2007;15(3):172–7. https://doi.org/10.5435/00124635-200703000-00007.
17. Demetriades D, Murray J, Martin M, Velmahos G, Salim A, Alo K, et al. Pedestrians injured by automobiles: relationship of age to injury type and severity. J Am Coll Surg. 2004;199:382–7. https://doi.org/10.1016/j.jamcollsurg.2004.03.027.
18. Gillott A, Rhodes M, Lucke J. Utility of routine pelvic X-ray during blunt trauma resuscitation. J Trauma. 1988;28:1570–4. https://doi.org/10.1097/00005373-198811000-00008.
19. Garvin KL, McCarthy RE, Barnes CL, Dodge BM. Pediatric pelvic ring fractures. J Pediatr Orthop. 1990;10(5):577–82. https://doi.org/10.1097/01241398-199009000-00001.
20. Ismail N, Bellemare JF, Mollitt DL, et al. Death from pelvic fracture: children are different. J Pediatr Surg. 1996;31:82–5.
21. Torode I, Zieg D. Pelvic fractures in children. J Pediatr Orthop. 1985;5(1):76–84. https://doi.org/10.1097/01241398-198501000-00014.
22. Karunakar MA, Goulet JA, Mueller KL, Bedi A, Le TT. Operative treatment of unstable pediatric pelvis and acetabular fractures. J Pediatr Orthop. 2005;25(1):34–8. https://doi.org/10.1097/00004694-200501000-00009.
23. Mulder MB, Maggart MJ, Yang WJ, Perez EA, Namias N, Sola JE, Proctor KG, Thorson CM. Outcomes of pediatric pelvic fractures: a level I trauma center's 20-year experience. J Surg Res. 2019;243:515–23. https://doi.org/10.1016/j.jss.2019.07.011.
24. Hermans E, Cornelisse S, Biert J, Tan E, Edwards M. Paediatric pelvic fractures: how do they differ from adults? J Child Orthop. 2017;11:49–56.
25. Gansslen A, Hildebrand F, Heidari N, Weinberg AM. Pelvic ring injuries in children. Part I: Epidemiology and primary evaluation. A review of the literature. Acta Chir Orthop Traumatol Cechoslov. 2012;79:493–8.
26. Eisa A, Farouk O, Mahran DG, Badran M, Abdelnasser MK, Samir M, Kalampoki V, Hurtado-Chong A, Rometsch E, Mohamedean A, Adam F. Predictors of mortality after pelvic fractures: a retrospective cohort study from a level one trauma centre in Upper Egypt. Int Orthop. 2019;43:2405–13. https://doi.org/10.1007/s00264-018-4230-2.

27. Guillaume JM, Pesenti S, Jouve JL, Launay F. Pelvic fractures in children (pelvic ring and acetabulum). Orthop Traumatol Surg Res. 2020;106:S125–33. https://doi.org/10.1016/j.otsr.2019.05.017.
28. Zwingmann J, Lefering R, Maier D, Hohloch L, Eberbach H, Neumann M, Strohm PC, Sudkamp NP, Hammer T. Pelvic fractures in severely injured children: results from the TraumaRegister DGU. Medicine. 2018;97:e11955. https://doi.org/10.1097/MD.0000000000011955.
29. Sridharan SS, You D, Ponich B, Parsons D, Schneider P. Outcomes following pelvic ring fractures in the paediatric population: a systematic review. J Clin Orthop Trauma. 2020;11:963–9. https://doi.org/10.1016/j.jcot.2020.10.005.
30. Keshishyan RA, Rozinov VM, Malakhov OA, et al. Pelvic polyfractures in children. Radiographic diagnosis and treatment. Clin Orthop Relat Res. 1995;320:28–33. https://pubmed.ncbi.nlm.nih.gov/7586836/
31. Zhu D, Liu D, Song B, Feng W, Zhang X, Wang Q. Therapeutic effect of an external fixator in the treatment of unstable pelvic fractures in children. Orthop Traumatol Surg Res. 2022;108:103150. https://doi.org/10.1016/j.otsr.2021.103150.
32. Blasier RD, McAtee J, White R, Mitchell DT. Disruption of the pelvic ring in pediatric patients. Clin Orthop Relat Res. 2000;376:87–95. https://doi.org/10.1097/00003086-200007000-00013.
33. Calderazzi F, Nosenzo A, Galavotti C, Menozzi M, Pogliacomi F, Ceccarelli F. Apophyseal avulsion fractures of the pelvis. A review. Acta Biomed. 2018;89:470–6. https://doi.org/10.23750/abm.v89i4.7632.
34. Fahmy M, Abdelmoneim MA. Operative intervention of unstable paediatric pelvic fracture: radiological and functional assessment. Eur J Trauma Emerg Surg. 2022;48:187–94. https://doi.org/10.1007/s00068-021-01793-y.
35. Amorosa LF, Kloen P, Helfet DL. High-energy pediatric pelvic and acetabular fractures. Orthop Clin North Am. 2014;4:483–500.
36. Baker JE, Werner NL, Burlew CC. Management of pelvic trauma. Surg Clin North Am. 2024;2:367–84.
37. Igboechi O, Purtell SR, Carry P, Sanders JS. Pediatric pelvic and acetabular fractures: discerning severity by classification and clinical management. J Pediatr Orthop. 2023;7:424–30.
38. Kenawey M. Surgical considerations with the operative fixation of unstable paediatric pelvic ring injuries. Int Orthop. 2017;41:1791–801. https://doi.org/10.1007/s00264-017-3475-5.
39. Pascarella R, Bettuzzi C, Digennaro V. Surgical treatment for pelvic ring fractures in pediatric and adolescence age. Musculoskelet Surg. 2013;3:217–22.
40. Gänsslen A, Heidari N, Weinberg AM. Fractures of the pelvis in children: a review of the literature. Eur J Orthop Surg Traumatol. 2013;23(8):847–61. https://doi.org/10.1007/s00590-012-1102-0.
41. Chotai N, Alazzawi S, Zehra SS, Barry M. Paediatric pelvic fractures: a review of 2 cohorts over 22 years. Injury. 2018;3:613–7.
42. Leonard M, Ibrahim M, McKenna P, Boran S, McCormack D. Paediatric pelvic ring fractures and associated injuries. Injury. 2011;42(10):1027–30. https://doi.org/10.1016/j.injury.2010.08.005.
43. Banerjee S, Barry MJ, Paterson JMH. Paediatric pelvic fractures: 10 years experience in a trauma centre. Injury. 2009;40(4):410–3. https://doi.org/10.1016/j.injury.2008.10.019.
44. Oransky M, Arduini M, Tortora M, Zoppi AR. Surgical treatment of unstable pelvic fracture in children: long term results. Injury. 2010;41:1140–4. https://doi.org/10.1016/j.injury.2010.08.002.
45. Musemeche CA, Fischer RP, Cotler HB, Andrassy RJ. Selective management of pediatric pelvic fractures: a conservative approach. J Pediatr Surg. 1987;22:538–40.
46. Wharton R, Trowbridge S, Simpson A, Sarraf KM, Jabbar Y. Anatomic, diagnostic and management challenges in paediatric pelvic injuries: a review. J Pediatr Orthop B. 2019;5:476–86.
47. Qiu X, Zhu T, Deng H, Chen J, Feng H, Huang Z, Li J, Wang X, Liu S, Wang S, Gu Z, Wu Z, Yang Q, Liu G, Feng G, Sechi LA, Caggiari G, You C, Fu G. Multicenter epidemiological analysis of related factors in 10,808 hospitalized children with lower limb and pelvic fractures in China. Sci Rep. 2024;14:27860. https://doi.org/10.1038/s41598-024-77970-x.

48. Katayama Y, Kitamura T, Hirose T, Kiguchi T, Matsuyama T, Takahashi H, Kiyohara K, Sado J, Adachi S, Noda T, Izawa J, Nakagawa Y, Shimazu T. Pelvic angiography is effective for emergency pediatric patients with pelvic fractures: a propensity-score-matching study with a nationwide trauma registry in Japan. Eur J Trauma Emerg Surg. 2021;47:515–21. https://doi.org/10.1007/s00068-019-01154-w.
49. Nabaweesi R, Arnold MA, Chang DC, Rossberg MI, Ziegfeld S, Sawaya DE, Bathurst MA, Colombani P, Abdullah F. Prehospital predictors of risk for pelvic fractures in pediatric trauma patients. Pediatr Surg Int. 2008;24:1053–6. https://doi.org/10.1007/s00383-008-2195-8.
50. Lu V, Gowrishankar S, Arshad Z, Thahir A, Lenihan J, Mcdonald S, Rawal J, Hull P, Chou D, Carrothers A. The clinical characteristics and management of paediatric pelvic fractures: a changing landscape based on skeletal maturity. Eur J Trauma Emerg Surg. 2023;49:559–70. https://doi.org/10.1007/s00068-022-02108-5.
51. Arafa M, Khalifa AA, Fergany A, Abdelhafez MA, Mohamedean A, Adam FF, Farouk O. Surgical management of paediatric pelvic fractures: a prospective case series and early experience from a level one Egyptian trauma centre. Int Orthop. 2022;46:2315–28. https://doi.org/10.1007/s00264-022-05509-8.
52. Zhang H, Zhao R, Zhu D, Feng W, Song B, Wang Q. Analysis of risk factors affecting the prognosis of external fixation in the treatment of unstable pelvic fractures in children: a retrospective study of 96 patients. BMC Pediatr. 2025;25:360. https://doi.org/10.1186/s12887-025-05485-z.
53. Bozbek M, Aydin T, Yavuz IA, Ozdemir G, Yalcin E, Yildirim AO. Functional results of surgically treated paediatric pelvic fractures are as good as conservatively treated ones: retrospective evaluation of 64 patients. Eur J Orthop Surg Traumatol. 2025;35:347. https://doi.org/10.1007/s00590-025-04458-3.
54. Liu Y, Zhan X, Huang F, Wen X, Chen Y, Yang C, Fan S. The application of lateral-rectus approach on toddlers' unstable pelvic fractures. BMC Musculoskelet Disord. 2020;21:147. https://doi.org/10.1186/s12891-020-3172-1.

21 Compartment Syndrome

Introduction by the Author

Similar to adults, children and adolescents may develop acute compartment syndrome following an injury or surgical procedure. However, the exact incidence of this condition in children remains unclear. The overall incidence of acute compartment syndrome in both children and adults is approximately seven per 100,000 males and one per 100,000 females. In children, as in adults, this condition is most often associated with trauma, particularly tibial shaft fractures, which account for approximately one-third of all cases of acute compartment syndrome.

Acute compartment syndrome predominantly affects young males due to their greater muscle mass and higher likelihood of experiencing high-energy trauma. In children, risk factors include open radius/ulna fractures, humerus fractures concurrent with forearm fractures, open tibia fractures, high-energy trauma, and being male. Conversely, low-energy trauma is linked to a lower risk of acute compartment syndrome. Viper bites can also cause acute compartment syndrome.

Acute compartment syndrome is a time-sensitive condition involving increased pressure within a closed osteofascial compartment, leading to pain and obstructed local circulation. Diagnosing it in children can be challenging due to their limited ability to communicate symptoms effectively, and early fasciotomy is important to prevent severe complications. Despite these difficulties, the key diagnostic sign is pain accompanied by agitation that does not respond to medical treatment.

Prompt diagnosis and intervention, such as fasciotomy, are necessary to prevent severe complications, including tissue necrosis and ischemia. However, compartment pressure measurements are not infallible, and there is

© The Author(s), under exclusive license to Springer Nature Switzerland AG 2026
F. Canavese, *Advances in Pediatric Extremity Fracture Management*,
https://doi.org/10.1007/978-3-032-33306-3_21

no consensus on the diagnostic threshold or the utility of compartment pressure monitoring. Most compartment syndrome diagnoses are based on clinical judgment. While traditional fasciotomy methods involving large incisions are effective, they can result in significant scarring, prolonged hospitalization, and potential complications such as infection. Additionally, about 10% of children require a second operation, such as skin grafting or tissue expansion, to close the wound. To reduce these risks, fasciotomy can be performed through multiple small incisions with similar efficacy in preventing permanent tissue damage.

21.1 Machine Generated Summaries

Disclaimer: The summaries in this chapter were generated from Springer Nature publications using abstractive AI auto-summarization: An abstraction-based summarizer creates new text based on deep learning. New phrases are created to summarize the content. As the constituted sentences are machine selected, they may not fully reflect the body of the work, so we strongly advise that the original content is read and cited. The auto-generated summaries were curated by the author(s) to meet Springer Nature publication standards.

Fasciotomy Through Multiple Small Skin Incisions for the Treatment of Early Acute Osteofascial Compartment Syndrome in Children [17]

This is a machine-generated summary of:

Yuan, Xiaowei; Wu, Jun; Qu, Xiangyang; Li, Ming; Jiang, Linjun; Liu, Xing Fasciotomy through multiple small skin incisions for the treatment of early acute osteofascial compartment syndrome in children [17]
Published in: Journal of Orthopaedic Surgery and Research (2020)
Link to original: https://doi.org/10.1186/s13018-020-01742-2
Copyright of the summarized publication:
The Author(s) 2020
License: OpenAccess CC BY + CC0 4.0

This article is licensed under a Creative Commons Attribution 4.0 International License, which permits use, sharing, adaptation, distribution and reproduction in any medium or format, as long as you give appropriate credit to the original author(s)

and the source, provide a link to the Creative Commons licence, and indicate if changes were made. The images or other third party material in this article are included in the article's Creative Commons licence, unless indicated otherwise in a credit line to the material. If material is not included in the article's Creative Commons licence and your intended use is not permitted by statutory regulation or exceeds the permitted use, you will need to obtain permission directly from the copyright holder. To view a copy of this licence, visit http://creativecommons.org/licenses/by/4.0/. The Creative Commons Public Domain Dedication waiver (http://creativecommons.org/publicdomain/zero/1.0/) applies to the data made available in this article, unless otherwise stated in a credit line to the data.

If you want to cite the papers, please refer to the original.

For technical reasons we could not place the page where the original quote is coming from.

Research Highlights

Osteofascial compartment syndrome (OCS) is a critical emergency condition in pediatric orthopedics, often associated with extremity fractures, vascular injuries, and soft tissue damage. Traditional treatment involves fasciotomy through large incisions, which can lead to complications such as neurovascular injury and infection. Now, a new study by Xiaowei Yuan and colleagues explores the efficacy of fasciotomy through multiple small skin incisions as a treatment for early OCS in children, aiming to reduce complications while effectively decompressing the affected compartments.

The study involved pediatric patients diagnosed with early OCS who were treated at the Children's Hospital of Chongqing Medical University. The researchers employed a method of multiple small skin incisions for decompression after conservative treatments failed to show improvement within 3–6 hours. The procedure involved making small incisions of 0.5–1.0 cm on the affected limb, followed by separation of subcutaneous and deep fascias using a vascular clamp. This approach aimed to relieve pressure without causing significant trauma or requiring secondary surgeries. The study followed up with patients for an average of 2.5 years, assessing outcomes such as wound healing, neuromuscular function, and overall recovery.

The findings suggest that fasciotomy via multiple small skin incisions is a viable alternative to traditional large-incision methods for treating early OCS in children. This technique resulted in fewer complications, such as infections or neurovascular injuries, and facilitated faster recovery with minimal scarring. Future study could focus on refining this method further and exploring its applicability in different clinical settings or more severe cases of OCS. The study highlights the potential for this approach to become a standard practice in managing early OCS in pediatric patients, particularly in resource-limited environments where traditional methods pose greater risks.

Risk Factors for Developing Acute Compartment Syndrome in the Pediatric Population: A Systematic Review and Meta-Analysis [38]

This is a machine-generated summary of:

Mortensen, Sharri J.; Orman, Sebastian; Testa, Edward J.; Mohamadi, Amin; Nazarian, Ara; von Keudell, Arvind G. Risk factors for developing acute compartment syndrome in the pediatric population: a systematic review and meta-analysis [38]

Published in: European Journal of Orthopaedic Surgery & Traumatology (2020)
Link to original: https://doi.org/10.1007/s00590-020-02643-0
Copyright of the summarized publication:
Springer-Verlag France SAS, part of Springer Nature 2020
All rights reserved.

If you want to cite the papers, please refer to the original.

For technical reasons we could not place the page where the original quote is coming from.

Research Highlights

Acute compartment syndrome (ACS) is a critical orthopedic emergency that necessitates prompt diagnosis and intervention to prevent severe complications such as tissue necrosis and ischemia. While ACS is commonly linked to high-energy trauma in both adults and children, the exact incidence in the pediatric population remains unclear, with tibial shaft fractures being a predominant cause. The challenge in diagnosing pediatric ACS is compounded by the varied etiology and symptomatology, as well as children's limited ability to communicate symptoms. Now, a new study by Sharri J. Mortensen and colleagues systematically reviews the literature to identify specific risk factors for pediatric ACS, aiming to aid clinicians in early identification and intervention.

The study conducted a systematic review and meta-analysis following established guidelines, including PRISMA and MOOSE, to consolidate evidence on risk factors for pediatric ACS. Researchers searched multiple databases such as MEDLINE, EMBASE, Web of Science, and Google Scholar for relevant studies. After rigorous screening and quality assessment using the Newcastle–Ottawa Scale, nine retrospective studies were included in the analysis. The study focused on patients aged 18 years or younger with acute traumatic extremity compartment syndrome, excluding cases related to non-traumatic causes or other types of ACS. Statistical analysis was performed using Comprehensive Meta-Analysis software to synthesize effect sizes for risk factors using odds ratios or relative risks.

The study identified several significant risk factors associated with an increased likelihood of developing ACS in children: open radius/ulna fractures, humerus fractures concurrent with forearm fractures, open tibia fractures, high-energy trauma, and male gender. Conversely, low-energy trauma was linked to a lower risk of

ACS. The findings underscore the need for heightened clinical suspicion in patients presenting with these injury patterns. Future study could focus on larger-scale research to further validate these risk factors and explore additional variables such as age or race that may influence ACS development in children. This research contributes valuable insights into pediatric ACS risk factors but highlights the necessity for more high-quality studies in this area.

Mini Approaches Fasciotomy Combined with Vacuum Sealing Drainage for Acute Compartment Syndrome Caused by Fractures in Children [39]

This is a machine-generated summary of:

Hu, Jie; Yan, Jingwen; Su, Yuxi Mini approaches fasciotomy combined with vacuum sealing drainage for acute compartment syndrome caused by fractures in children [39]
Published in: International Orthopaedics (2023)
Link to original: https://doi.org/10.1007/s00264-023-05984-7
Copyright of the summarized publication:
The Author(s) under exclusive licence to SICOT aisbl 2023
Copyright comment: Springer Nature or its licensor (e.g. a society or other partner) holds exclusive rights to this article under a publishing agreement with the author(s) or other rightsholder(s); author self-archiving of the accepted manuscript version of this article is solely governed by the terms of such publishing agreement and applicable law.
All rights reserved.

If you want to cite the papers, please refer to the original.

For technical reasons we could not place the page where the original quote is coming from.

Research Highlights

Acute compartment syndrome (ACS) is a critical condition requiring immediate surgical intervention, typically through fasciotomy, to prevent irreversible muscle and nerve damage. Diagnosing ACS in children poses unique challenges due to communication barriers and the subtlety of symptoms. Traditional fasciotomy methods, while effective, often result in significant scarring, prolonged hospitalization, and potential complications such as infection. Now, a new study by Jie Hu and colleagues explores the efficacy of mini incision fasciotomy combined with vacuum sealing drainage (VSD) in treating ACS in children, aiming to reduce these complications.

In this retrospective cross-sectional study, the researchers reviewed medical records of pediatric patients diagnosed with ACS of the forearms and lower legs at their clinical center. The study included patients who underwent mini incision fasciotomy with or without VSD. The surgical procedure involved making several small incisions to decompress affected compartments while avoiding vital nerves and vessels. Postoperatively, VSD was applied to some patients to enhance healing by improving local microcirculation and reducing edema. The outcomes were assessed using Flynn's evaluation method, focusing on functional recovery, infection rates, and scarring. Statistical analyses were conducted to compare results between groups treated with mini incisions alone versus those combined with VSD.

The study found that mini incision fasciotomy combined with VSD effectively reduced hospitalization time and minimized incision-related infections compared to traditional methods. Patients treated with this approach experienced fewer complications and better aesthetic outcomes due to smaller scars. The findings suggest that this method could be a viable alternative for managing ACS in children, offering a simpler technique that can be easily adopted in various clinical settings. Future studies could focus on larger sample sizes and include other types of ACS to further validate these results and explore broader applications of this technique.

Primary Closure of Fasciotomies Has a Reduced Complication Rate Following Compartment Syndrome in the Paediatric Population [40]

This is a machine-generated summary of:

Walker, Lucy C.; Mullins, Barry M.; Edwards, Caroline; Wadia, Farokh Primary closure of fasciotomies has a reduced complication rate following compartment syndrome in the paediatric population [40]

Published in: International Orthopaedics (2024)
Link to original: https://doi.org/10.1007/s00264-024-06233-1

Copyright of the summarized publication:
The Author(s) under exclusive licence to SICOT aisbl 2024
Copyright comment: Springer Nature or its licensor (e.g. a society or other partner) holds exclusive rights to this article under a publishing agreement with the author(s) or other rightsholder(s); author self-archiving of the accepted manuscript version of this article is solely governed by the terms of such publishing agreement and applicable law.
All rights reserved.

If you want to cite the papers, please refer to the original.

For technical reasons we could not place the page where the original quote is coming from.

Research Highlights

Acute compartment syndrome (ACS) is a serious complication that can occur in pediatric patients with forearm fractures, often resulting from high-energy trauma or crush injuries. While extensive guidelines exist for managing ACS in adults, there is a lack of comparable diagnostic criteria and management protocols for the pediatric population. This gap in knowledge is compounded by the limited evidence on long-term outcomes and the appropriate timing for surgical intervention in children. Now, a new study by Lucy C. Walker and colleagues addresses these issues by examining the presentation, intra-compartmental pressures, and management factors influencing outcomes in pediatric ACS cases.

The study conducted a retrospective cohort analysis of pediatric patients diagnosed with ACS at a tertiary referral center for pediatric orthopedic surgery. The researchers reviewed electronic medical records to gather data on patient demographics, injury mechanisms, and treatment details. They focused on the timing of surgical interventions, specifically fasciotomies, and their impact on long-term outcomes. Statistical analyses were performed to compare variables such as complication rates and the number of operations required between different patient groups. The study found that direct closure of fasciotomy wounds was associated with significantly fewer complications and shorter recovery times compared to other wound closure methods.

The findings suggest that direct wound closure after fasciotomy may lead to better outcomes in pediatric ACS patients, potentially due to less severe initial injuries or more favorable physiological conditions. This study highlights the need for further research into the specific factors that allow for direct closure and how they might predict recovery trajectories. Future studies could explore these aspects in larger cohorts or multi-center settings to validate these findings and refine treatment protocols for pediatric ACS, ultimately improving patient care and long-term outcomes.

Pathophysiology of an Adolescent with Compartment Syndrome: A Case Report and Review of the Literature [41]

This is a machine-generated summary of:

Alamoudi, Naela B.; AlJoaid, Rinad; Alaithan, Tajah M.; Alqithmi, Mohammed
Pathophysiology of an adolescent with compartment syndrome: a case report and review of the literature [41]
Published in: Journal of Medical Case Reports (2025)
Link to original: https://doi.org/10.1186/s13256-025-05189-z
Copyright of the summarized publication:
The Author(s) 2025
License: OpenAccess CC BY-NC-ND 4.0

This article is licensed under a Creative Commons Attribution-NonCommercial-NoDerivatives 4.0 International License, which permits any non-commercial use, sharing, distribution and reproduction in any medium or format, as long as you give appropriate credit to the original author(s) and the source, provide a link to the Creative Commons licence, and indicate if you modified the licensed material. You do not have permission under this licence to share adapted material derived from this article or parts of it. The images or other third party material in this article are included in the article's Creative Commons licence, unless indicated otherwise in a credit line to the material. If material is not included in the article's Creative Commons licence and your intended use is not permitted by statutory regulation or exceeds the permitted use, you will need to obtain permission directly from the copyright holder. To view a copy of this licence, visit http://creativecommons.org/licenses/by-nc-nd/4.0/.

If you want to cite the papers, please refer to the original.

For technical reasons we could not place the page where the original quote is coming from.

Research Highlights

Acute compartment syndrome (ACS) is a critical emergency in orthopedics, characterized by increased intracompartmental pressure within a closed osteofascial compartment, leading to pain and obstructed local circulation. The condition is most commonly associated with trauma, particularly tibial shaft fractures, and predominantly affects young males due to their higher muscle mass and likelihood of high-energy trauma. Now, a new study by Naela B. Alamoudi and colleagues presents an exceptional case of atraumatic acute myonecrosis leading to ACS in a patient without sickle cell disease (SCD), highlighting a rare presentation of non-traumatic isolated compartment syndrome.

The study details the case of a 21-year-old Saudi male with juvenile myoclonic epilepsy who presented with severe anterior leg pain and swelling after climbing stairs. Despite no history of trauma or SCD, the patient developed rhabdomyolysis and ACS in the anterior compartment of the left leg. Initial treatment included intravenous fluids and analgesia, but due to increasing pain, an orthopedic consultation led to the diagnosis of compartment syndrome. A fasciotomy was performed under general anesthesia, revealing necrotic muscle tissue in the anterior compartment. Post-surgery, the patient showed improvement with physical therapy and was able to bear weight on the leg.

This case underscores the complexity of diagnosing ACS when it presents atypically without trauma or common risk factors like SCD. The study highlights the importance of maintaining a high index of suspicion for ACS in patients with disproportionate pain and swelling, even in the absence of typical triggers. Future study could focus on understanding the pathophysiology of myonecrosis in such cases to improve diagnostic accuracy and treatment strategies. The authors emphasize interdisciplinary collaboration for timely intervention and optimal outcomes in managing atypical presentations of ACS.

Acute Compartment Syndrome and Fasciotomy After a Viper Bite in Italy: A Case Report [42]

This is a machine-generated summary of:

Sassoè-Pognetto, Marco; Cavalcante, Riccardo; Paonessa, Matteo Acute compartment syndrome and fasciotomy after a viper bite in Italy: a case report [42]

Published in: Italian Journal of Pediatrics (2024)
Link to original: https://doi.org/10.1186/s13052-024-01638-5
Copyright of the summarized publication:
The Author(s) 2024
License: OpenAccess CC BY + CC0 4.0

This article is licensed under a Creative Commons Attribution 4.0 International License, which permits use, sharing, adaptation, distribution and reproduction in any medium or format, as long as you give appropriate credit to the original author(s) and the source, provide a link to the Creative Commons licence, and indicate if changes were made. The images or other third party material in this article are included in the article's Creative Commons licence, unless indicated otherwise in a credit line to the material. If material is not included in the article's Creative Commons licence and your intended use is not permitted by statutory regulation or exceeds the permitted use, you will need to obtain permission directly from the copyright holder. To view a copy of this licence, visit http://creativecommons.org/licenses/by/4.0/. The Creative Commons Public Domain Dedication waiver (http://creativecommons.org/publicdomain/zero/1.0/) applies to the data made available in this article, unless otherwise stated in a credit line to the data.

If you want to cite the papers, please refer to the original.

For technical reasons we could not place the page where the original quote is coming from.

Research Highlights

Vipers are the only medically significant snakes in Europe, and while envenomation by these snakes is rare, it can lead to symptoms of varying severity that may necessitate antivenom treatment and extended hospitalization. The clinical manifestations of viper bites depend on several factors, including the bite location, venom characteristics, and the victim's overall health. Although children are often considered at higher risk due to their smaller body size, some studies have not found significant differences in envenomation severity between adults and children. Now, a new study by Marco Sassoè-Pognetto and colleagues reports a case of a young girl who developed severe compartment syndrome following a viper bite, requiring surgical intervention.

The study details the case of a girl bitten on her right leg while hiking near Bielmonte, Italy. Despite not seeing the snake, photographic evidence suggested a viper bite due to the presence of fang marks and edema. The girl was quickly transported to a hospital where initial treatments included paracetamol and rehydration therapy. However, her condition worsened with increased edema and drowsiness. Blood tests revealed neutrophilic leukocytosis and elevated D-dimer levels. Although antivenom was recommended by the Pavia Poison Center, it was not administered immediately. As her condition deteriorated further, she was transferred to a pediatric intensive care unit where she received antivenom and underwent fasciotomy to relieve compartment syndrome. Post-surgery, her recovery was monitored closely with regular dressing changes until discharge.

This case highlights the importance of timely assessment and treatment in viper envenomation cases to prevent severe complications like compartment syndrome. The study underscores that fasciotomy should be considered when compartment syndrome persists despite antivenom therapy. Future study could focus on refining guidelines for surgical intervention timing in snakebite cases to improve patient outcomes. Additionally, examining fang punctures for multiple bite marks can provide valuable information about venom quantity and potential clinical severity, aiding in more effective treatment planning.

Conclusion

Acute compartment syndrome is a critical condition requiring immediate surgical intervention, such as fasciotomy, to prevent irreversible damage to muscles and nerves. Open fractures, high-energy trauma, concurrent humerus and forearm fractures, and being male significantly increase the risk of developing acute compartment syndrome in children. While invasive intracompartmental pressure measurement can aid in diagnosis, clinical judgment remains essential.

Bibliography

1. Lin JS, Balch Samora J. Pediatric acute compartment syndrome: a systematic review and meta-analysis. J Pediatr Orthop B. 2019;29:90–6. https://doi.org/10.1097/BPB.0000000000000593.
2. Garner MR, Taylor SA, Gausden E, Lyden JP. Compartment syndrome: diagnosis, management, and unique concerns in the twenty-first century. HSS J. 2014;10(2):143–52. https://doi.org/10.1007/s11420-014-9386-8.
3. Grottkau BE, Epps HR, Di Scala C. Compartment syndrome in children and adolescents. J Pediatr Surg. 2005;40(4):678–82. https://doi.org/10.1016/j.jpedsurg.2004.12.007.
4. Dickersin K, Berlin JA. Meta-analysis: state-of-the-science. Epidemiol Rev. 1992;14:154–76. https://doi.org/10.1093/oxfordjournals.epirev.a036084.
5. Mohamadi A, Chan JJ, Lian J, Wright CL, Marin AM, Rodriguez EK, von Keudell A, Nazarian A. Risk factors and pooled rate of prolonged opioid use following trauma or surgery: a systematic review and meta-(regression) analysis. J Bone Joint Surg Am. 2018;100(15):1332–40. https://doi.org/10.2106/JBJS.17.01239.
6. Xu W, Tan L, Wang HF, Jiang T, Tan MS, Tan L, Zhao QF, Li JQ, Wang J, Yu JT. Meta-analysis of modifiable risk factors for Alzheimer's disease. J Neurol Neurosurg Psychiatry. 2015;86(12):1299–306. https://doi.org/10.1136/jnnp-2015-310548.
7. Blackman AJ, Wall LB, Keeler KA, Schoenecker PL, Luhmann SJ, O'Donnell JC, Gordon JE. Acute compartment syndrome after intramedullary nailing of isolated radius and ulna fractures in children. J Pediatr Orthop. 2014;34(1):50–4. https://doi.org/10.1097/BPO.0b013e31829527de.
8. Blakemore LC, Cooperman DR, Thompson GH, Wathey C, Ballock RT. Compartment syndrome in ipsilateral humerus and forearm fractures in children. Clin Orthop Relat Res. 2000;376:32–8.
9. Ferlic PW, Singer G, Kraus T, et al. The acute compartment syndrome following fractures of the lower leg in children. Injury. 2012;43(10):1743–6.

10. Harris LR, Arkader A, Broom A, Flynn J, Yellin J, Whitlock P, Miller A, Sawyer J, Roaten J, Skaggs DL, Choi PD. Pulseless supracondylar humerus fracture with anterior interosseous nerve or median nerve injury-an absolute indication for open reduction? J Pediatr Orthop. 2019;39(1):E1–7. https://doi.org/10.1097/bpo.0000000000001238.
11. Robertson AK, Snow E, Browne TS, Brownell S, Inneh I, Hill JF. Who gets compartment syndrome?: a retrospective analysis of the national and local incidence of compartment syndrome in patients with supracondylar humerus fractures. J Pediatr Orthop. 2018;38(5):e252–6. https://doi.org/10.1097/bpo.0000000000001144.
12. Sees JA, Cutler GJ, Ortega HW. Risk factors for compartment syndrome in pediatric trauma patients. Pediatr Emerg Care. 2020;36:e115–9. https://doi.org/10.1097/pec.0000000000001636.
13. Shore BJ, Glotzbecker MP, Zurakowski D, Gelbard E, Hedequist DJ, Matheney TH. Acute compartment syndrome in children and teenagers with tibial shaft fractures: incidence and multivariable risk factors. J Orthop Trauma. 2013;27(11):616–21. https://doi.org/10.1097/BOT.0b013e31828f949c.
14. Villarreal ED, Wrenn JO, Sheffer BW, Sawyer JR, Spence DD, Kelly DM. Do patient-specific or fracture-specific factors predict the development of acute compartment syndrome after pediatric tibial shaft fractures? J Pediatr Orthop. 2020;40:e193–7. https://doi.org/10.1097/BPO.0000000000001410.
15. Wind TC, Saunders SM, Barfield WR, Mooney JF 3rd, Hartsock LA. Compartment syndrome after low-energy tibia fractures sustained during athletic competition. J Orthop Trauma. 2012;26(1):33–6. https://doi.org/10.1097/BOT.0b013e3182163367.
16. McQueen MM, Gaston P, Court-Brown CM. Acute compartment syndrome. Who is at risk? J Bone Joint Surg Br. 2000;82(2):200–3. https://doi.org/10.1302/0301-620x.82b2.9799.
17. Yuan X, Wu J, Qu X, Li M, Jiang L, Liu X. Fasciotomy through multiple small skin incisions for the treatment of early acute osteofascial compartment syndrome in children. J Orthop Surg Res. 2020;15:269. https://doi.org/10.1186/s13018-020-01742-2.
18. Mars M, Hadley GP. Raised compartmental pressure in children: a basis for management. Injury. 1998;29(3):183–5.
19. Tharakan SJ, Subotic U, Kalisch M, Staubli G, Weber DM. Compartment pressures in children with normal and fractured forearms: a preliminary report. J Pediatr Orthop. 2016;36(4):410–5.
20. Torlincasi A, Lopez R, Waseem M. Acute compartment syndrome. In: StatPearls [Internet]. Treasure Island: StatPearls Publishing; 2023. https://www.ncbi.nlm.nih.gov/books/NBK448124/#:~:text=The%20anterior%20compartment%20of%20the,nerve%2C%20and%20the%20tibial%20artery.
21. Al Moosawi M, Ezzat H. A rare case of compartment syndrome and myonecrosis in a patient with hemoglobin SC disease. Clin Case Rep. 2021;9:3899. https://doi.org/10.1002/ccr3.3899.
22. Biedert R. Compartment syndromes of thigh and lower leg. In: Doral MN, Karlsson J, editors. Sports injuries. Berlin, Heidelberg: Springer; 2015.
23. Griffith M, Hattaway J, Griffith R, O'Brien F, Huh J. Acute exertional compartment syndrome: a case series and review of the literature. Foot Ankle Surg Tech Rep Cases. 2021;1(3):100040.
24. Chippaux JP. Epidemiology of snakebites in Europe: a systematic review of the literature. Toxicon. 2012;59:86–99.
25. de Haro L, Glaizal M, Tichadou L, Blanc-Brisset I, Hayek-Lanthois M. *Vipera aspis* envenomation: experience of the Marseille Poison Center from 1996 to 2008. Toxins. 2009;1:100–12.
26. Di Nicola MR, Pontara A, Kass GEN, Kramer NI, Avella I, Pampena R, Mercuri SR, Dorne JLCM, Paolino G. Vipers of major clinical relevance in Europe: taxonomy, venom composition, toxicology and clinical management of human bites. Toxicology. 2021;453:152724.
27. Fuchs J, Gessner T, Kupferschmidt H, Weiler S. Indigenous venomous snakebites in Switzerland: analysis of reports to the National Poisons Information Centre over 22 years. Swiss Med Wkly. 2021;151:w30085.
28. Lonati D, Giampreti A, Rossetto O, Petrolini V, Vecchio S, Buscaglia E, Mazzoleni M, Chiara F, Aloise M, Gentilli A, Montecucco C, Coccini T, Locatelli CA. Neurotoxicity of

European viperids in Italy: Pavia Poison Control Center case series 2001–2011. Clin Toxicol. 2014;52:269–76.
29. Paolino G, Di Nicola MR, Pontara A, Didona D, Moliterni E, Mercuri SR, Grano M, Borgianni N, Kumar R, Pampena R. Vipera snakebite in Europe: a systematic review of a neglected disease. J Eur Acad Dermatol Venereol. 2020;34:2247–60.
30. Barani C, Mortamet G, Forli A. Upper limb compartment syndrome after a viper bite in a child: a case report. Hand Surg Rehabil. 2021;40:97–100.
31. Cawrse NH, Palmer JH, Hayes C, Inglefield CJ. A snake in the clinical grass: late compartment syndrome in a child bitten by an adder. Br J Plast Surg. 2002;55(5):434–5.
32. Evers LH, Bartscher T, Lange T, et al. Adder bite: an uncommon cause of compartment syndrome in northern hemisphere. Scand J Trauma Resusc Emerg Med. 2010;18(1):1–5.
33. Frangides CY, Koulouras V, Kouni SN, Tzortzatos GV, Nikolaou A, Pneumaticos J, Pierrakeas C, Niarchos C, Kounis NG, Koutsojannis CM. Snake venom poisoning in Greece. Experiences with 147 cases. Eur J Intern Med. 2006;17:24–7.
34. Pietrangiolillo Z, Frassoldati R, Leonelli V, Freschi R, Russomando A, Lucaccioni L, Lughetti L. Compartment syndrome after viper-bite in toddler: case report and review of literature. Acta Biomed. 2012;83:44–50.
35. Tucker SC, Josty I. Compartment syndrome in the hand following an adder bite. J Hand Surg Eur. 2005;30:434–5.
36. Vigasio A, Battiston B, De Filippo G, Brunelli G, Calabrese S. Compartmental syndrome due to viper bite. Arch Orthop Trauma Surg. 1991;110:175–7.
37. Avila-Agüero ML, Valverde K, Gutiérrez J, París MM, Faingezicht I. Venomous snakebites in children and adolescents: a 12-year retrospective review. J Venom Anim Toxins. 2001;7:69–84.
38. Mortensen SJ, Orman S, Testa EJ, Mohamadi A, Nazarian A, von Keudell AG. Risk factors for developing acute compartment syndrome in the pediatric population: a systematic review and meta-analysis. Eur J Orthop Surg Traumatol. 2020;30:839–44. https://doi.org/10.1007/s00590-020-02643-0.
39. Hu J, Yan J, Su Y. Mini approaches fasciotomy combined with vacuum sealing drainage for acute compartment syndrome caused by fractures in children. Int Orthop. 2024;48:1481–7. https://doi.org/10.1007/s00264-023-05984-7.
40. Walker LC, Mullins BM, Edwards C, Wadia F. Primary closure of fasciotomies has a reduced complication rate following compartment syndrome in the paediatric population. Int Orthop. 2024;48:2475–81. https://doi.org/10.1007/s00264-024-06233-1.
41. Alamoudi NB, AlJoaid R, Alaithan TM, Alqithmi M. Pathophysiology of an adolescent with compartment syndrome: a case report and review of the literature. J Med Case Rep. 2025;19:144. https://doi.org/10.1186/s13256-025-05189-z.
42. Sassoè-Pognetto M, Cavalcante R, Paonessa M. Acute compartment syndrome and fasciotomy after a viper bite in Italy: a case report. Ital J Pediatr. 2024;50:70. https://doi.org/10.1186/s13052-024-01638-5.

Conclusion

This volume synthesizes contemporary evidence and clinical insight on upper- and lower limb fractures in skeletally immature patients, emphasizing when conservative care is appropriate, when surgery is indicated, and which surgical techniques are most commonly used.

When dealing with pediatric fractures, surgeons must remember three important points: remodeling potential supports treatment; age and displacement determine surgery; and minimally invasive fixation is favored.

Younger children frequently tolerate greater residual angulation or translation because of significant remodeling potential, so nonoperative care remains the default for many pediatric fractures. On the other hand, older children with limited remodeling capacity, significant displacement, intra-articular involvement, neurovascular compromise, or instability more often require surgical fixation. When surgery is indicated, minimally invasive procedures should be favored. In particular, elastic stable intramedullary nailing is a preferred, less invasive option for many long bone fractures because it balances stability with early mobilization and low complication rates. Kirschner wires and percutaneous pinning remain, however, important alternatives for many pediatric fractures.

The book is organized by anatomical location, allowing key information to be summarized according to the anatomy, from proximal to distal with respect to the appendicular skeleton.

The standard treatment for clavicle fractures is conservative care. Surgery is only considered for older patients who experience significant shortening or functional impairment. However, the superiority of surgery over nonoperative care remains unclear. Supracondylar fractures require careful neurovascular assessment, and closed reduction and pinning are indicated for displaced fractures. Lateral condyle and medial epicondyle injuries often require fixation to stabilize the elbow joint and prevent nonunion or entrapment. An MRI can help detect hidden injuries. Redisplacement after reduction of distal radius fractures is common, so pinning or elastic stable intramedullary nailing is recommended when remodeling potential is limited. Elastic stable intramedullary nailing is the preferred surgical option for two-bone forearm fractures. Femoral neck fractures are rare but carry a high risk of

© The Editor(s) (if applicable) and The Author(s), under exclusive license to Springer Nature Switzerland AG 2026
F. Canavese, *Advances in Pediatric Extremity Fracture Management*,
https://doi.org/10.1007/978-3-032-33306-3

avascular necrosis and are usually managed surgically. For diaphyseal fractures of the femur or tibia in older children, elastic stable intramedullary nailing, more rigid nails, or external fixation may be used, depending on the child's weight and the complexity of the fracture. Pediatric pelvic fractures are uncommon and are often associated with high-energy trauma. They require multidisciplinary care.

Orthopedic surgeons must be aware of the possibility of complications when dealing with pediatric fractures. Physeal fractures of the distal femur and the proximal and distal tibia can lead to growth arrest, resulting in subsequent shortening and/or angular deformity. Anatomic reduction and CT guidance are necessary when displacement exceeds 2–3 mm. While this does not prevent growth arrest, it reduces the risk of early osteoarthritis.

Missed injuries, such as chronic Monteggia lesions, require corrective osteotomy and careful planning. Early diagnosis of acute injuries is essential to avoid complications. Acute compartment syndrome is a time-critical emergency in children. Prompt diagnosis and fasciotomy are essential to avoid irreversible damage.

Following a thorough literature review, this book recommends a personalized approach based on the patient's age and fracture type. This approach involves conservative management when remodeling potential is high, fixation when displacement, joint involvement, or skeletal maturation indicates poor remodeling or a high risk of secondary displacement, and minimally invasive fixation when surgery is necessary. Advances in imaging technology, such as ultrasound, magnetic resonance imaging, and computed tomography, as well as the proper use of modern implants, improve diagnosis and management, resulting in better outcomes. However, many controversies remain, particularly concerning surgical thresholds and the best fixation methods for specific fractures.

Since pediatric orthopedic traumatology is an evolving field, this book should not be considered definitive. Rather, it should be considered a tool that provides patients and their families with up-to-date knowledge and expertise. It should also encourage orthopedic professionals to address existing gaps in order to optimize care for children with fractures.

GPSR Compliance

The European Union's (EU) General Product Safety Regulation (GPSR) is a set of rules that requires consumer products to be safe and our obligations to ensure this.

If you have any concerns about our products, you can contact us on ProductSafety@springernature.com

In case Publisher is established outside the EU, the EU authorized representative is:

Springer Nature Customer Service Center GmbH
Europaplatz 3
69115 Heidelberg, Germany

Batch number: 10732031

Printed by Printforce, the Netherlands